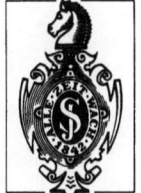

H. M. Emrich   M. Wiegand (Eds.)

Integrative Biological Psychiatry

With 64 Figures

Springer-Verlag

Berlin Heidelberg New York
London Paris Tokyo
Hong Kong Barcelona
Budapest

Prof.Dr.med.habil. HINDERK M. EMRICH
Max-Planck-Institut für Psychiatrie
Kraepelinstraße 10
W-8000 München 40, FRG

Dr.med.Dipl.-Psych. MICHAEL WIEGAND
Psychiatrische Klinik der Technischen Universität
Ismaninger Straße 22
W-8000 München 80, FRG

ISBN-13:978-3-642-77170-5   e-ISBN-13:978-3-642-77168-2
DOI: 10.1007/978-3-642-77168-2

Typesetting: Camera-ready by authors
25/3130–543210 – Printed on acid-free paper

Foreword

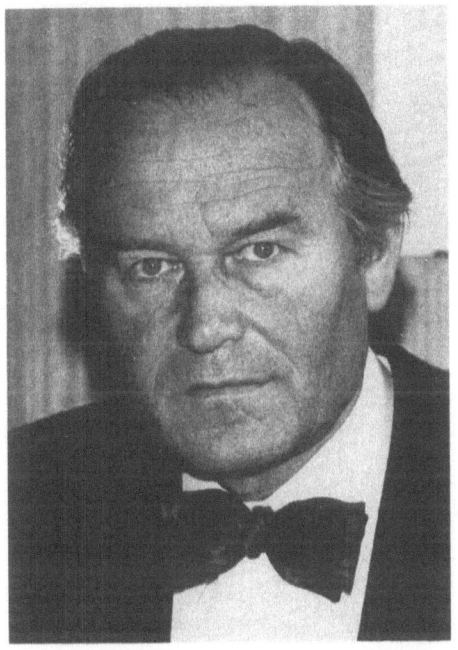

Professor Detlev Ploog

On March 19-21, 1989, a symposium entitled "Integrative Biological Psychiatry" was held at the Ringberg Castle (Bavaria) to honor the scientific work of Detlev Ploog, who retired at that time from his position as the Director of the Max Planck Institute of Psychiatry in Munich. The lectures represent an overview of the scientific work conducted at the Max Planck Institute within the recent past and thus also reflect the scientific intentions and research strategies of Detlev Ploog, who brought together extremely divergent tendencies within basic and clinical research and integrated the findings to elucidate new perspectives for fundamental psychiatric problems. His ability to combine topics such as brain and behavior with neuropsychological, neuroethological, psychopharmacological, and behavioral aspects generated a scientific climate in which psychiatric research flourished. The chapters in the present volume represent a documentation of this integrative view on psychiatry, and we, who worked together with Detlev Ploog as his university colleagues at the Ludwig Maximilians University (H.H.), the Technical University of Munich (H.L.) and as his successor at the Max Planck Institute (F.H.) wish him, also after his retirement, continued scientific success, with many additional contributions to modern psychiatry.

Hanns Hippius
Florian Holsboer
Hans Lauter

Preface

One of the main purposes of science is to elaborate models of natural processes that should be as realistic as possible. From this point of view two divergent tendencies in research strategies can be derived: on the one hand, scientific work has to be as reductionist as possible, since without reductionism, in principle, it is impossible to attain any understanding at all — even the simplest orientation within "the world" is only made possible by simplified internal "models" of it. On the other hand, research has — in the beginning — to be as nonreductionist as possible, since complex phenomena, such as psychiatric disorders, would otherwise be overlooked. An initially overly reductionist view would lead psychiatry to bypass its object. This paradoxical situation is reflected by the title of this book, *Integrative Biological Psychiatry*, a conception that aims at combining both of these divergent research strategies, the reductionist and the holistic or integrative view.

The present volume provides an overview of research topics pursued at the Max Planck Institute of Psychiatry in Munich in the recent past, including relevant findings in the fields of ethology, systems theory of psychosis, psychopharmacology, chronobiology, sleep research, and therapy. It constitutes a festschrift in honour of the former director of the Institute, Professor Detlev Ploog.

We wish to thank the authors for their good cooperation, and we are very grateful to Vera Rosburg and Ruth Wiegand for their valuable secretarial assistance. Finally, we would like to express our appreciation to Professor Detlev Ploog and wish him the best for the future.

Hinderk M. Emrich
Michael Wiegand

Contents

Part III: Psychiatric Aspects of Chronobiology and Sleep

Part IV: Diagnostic and Therapeutic Aspects

Contents

List of Contributors

At the Max Planck Institute of Psychiatry, Kraepelinstraße 2-10, W-8000 München 40 (Germany):

Bronisch, T.	241	Pirke, K.M.	129
Deisz, R.A.	93	Ploog, D.	3
Dirlich, G.	181	Schreiber, W.	207
Dodt, H.U.	93	Schweiger, U.	129
Emrich, H.M.	81,123,181	Strian, F.	269
Feuerlein, W.	251	Wever, R.A.	159
Hansert, E.	283	(Chronobiology Workgroup,	
Krieg, J.-C.	135	W-8138 Andechs, Germany)	
Lauer, C.	207	Zaudig, M.	229
Mombour, W.	221	Zerbin-Rüdin, E.	71
Papoušek, H.	45	von Zerssen, D.	181
Papoušek, M.	45	Zieglgänsberger, W.	93
Pawelzik, H.	93		

Other affiliations:

Amorosa, H.   61
  Heckscher Klinik Solln, Wolfratshauser Str. 350, W-8000 München 71, Germany[*]

Aschoff, J.   145
  Max Planck Institute of Behavioral Physiology, W-8138 Andechs, Germany

Berger, M.   207
  Psychiatric University Clinic, Hauptstraße 5, W-7800 Freiburg, Germany[*]

---

[*] Formerly: Max Planck Institute of Psychiatry, Munich

Broocks, A.   129
National Institute of Mental Health, Bethesda, Maryland, USA*

Dose, M.   123
District Hospital, Feuchtwangerstraße 38, W-8800 Ansbach, Germany*

Hartung, H.-D.   105
Psychiatric Clinic of the University of Munich, Nußbaumstraße 7,
W-8000 München 2, Germany

Hellweg, R.   105
Department of Psychiatry of the Free University of Berlin, Eschenallee 3,
W-1000 Berlin 19, Germany*

Hock, C.   105
Psychiatric Clinic of the University of Munich, Nußbaumstraße 7,
W-8000 München 2, Germany

Jürgens, U.   37
German Primate Center, Kellnerweg 4, W-3400 Göttingen, Germany*

Küfner, H.   251
Instititute for Therapy Research, Parzivalstraße 25, W-8000 München 40,
Germany*

Noterdaeme, M.   61
Heckscher Klinik Solln, Wolfratshauser Straße 350, W-8000 München 71,
Germany*

Riemann, D.   207
Central Institute of Mental Health, POB 5970, W-6800 Mannheim,
Germany*

Wiegand,M.   207
Psychiatric Clinic of Technical University, Ismaninger Straße 22,
W-8000 München 80, Germany*

---

* Formerly: Max Planck Institute of Psychiatry, Munich

Part I: Perspectives of Ethology, Development, and Systems Biology

1 Ethological Foundations of Biological Psychiatry

D. Ploog

> Men ought to know that from the brain and from the brain only arise our pleasures, joys, laughter, and jests as well as our sorrows, pains, griefs and tears....It is the same thing which makes us mad or delirious, inspires us with dread and fear, whether by night or by day, brings sleeplessness, inopportune mistakes, aimless anxieties, absent mindedness and acts that are contrary to habit...
>
> Hippocrates (c. 310-250 B.C.), *The Sacred Disease*

Introduction

In the above quotation the emotional states and behaviors inherent in the species of man are described. By studying the underlying brain mechanisms we strive to explain these conditions and, where relevant, cure them. My hypothesis in this contribution is that only an approach based on evolutionary biology and a comparison of species, i.e. on an ethological approach, can lead to a neurobiological explanation of the normal and pathological states mentioned by Hippocrates.

Both biologists and physicians are generally quite familiar with the approach used in the fields of comparative anatomy and physiology; they have no difficulty recognizing that, say, the spinal column of fish and man have a common structural organization, the *Bauplan* that is laid down in the genome. It is much more difficult, however, to make evolutionary comparisons relating to behavior or emotions and affects or even cognition, although it is clear that evolution has also occurred at these levels and that it is very closely connected to morphological, and in particular cerebral, evolution. As the behavior of the vertebrates has become increasingly complex there have been corresponding evolutionary changes in the brain.

In any attempt to understand the functioning of the brain it should always be kept in mind that the pressure of natural selection leading to further development of old structures and to the establishment of new structures is on the behavior of the organism. Adaptive behavior modifies or changes old structures and thus brings about new ones. This statement cannot be reversed, however. The investigation of cerebral structures and functions can lead to a valid explanation of brain mechanisms only if we can determine which behavior is related to the structure or function being investigated. It is exactly this question which the ethologist and neuroethologist addresses. Neuroethology then is the study of causal relationships between species-specific types of behavior and their neural substrates. As psychopathologists and psychiatrists we too begin with behavior, including the patient's verbal behavior. We make our diagnosis on the basis of behavioral signs and symptoms. We then attribute a certain etiology to the disease or disturbance, an etiology that is still usually hypothetical, for instance the "dopamine hypothesis of schizophrenia" (Carlsson 1987). And because many psychopathological disorders have multiple causes, etiology will probably always be hypothetical in certain areas of psychiatry, where the analysis of behavior will remain the method of choice. Whereas we have neuroanatomy as the foundation of neuropathology and physiology as the foundation of pathophysiology, behavior cannot yet serve as the foundation of the pathology of behavior, i.e., of psychiatry, because we do not have enough knowledge about the causal mechanisms involved. (Here the causal mechanisms are to be understood in the sense of Karl Jaspers' causal connections.) The science of ethology and neuroethology serves this purpose for psychiatry at least as far as systems analysis and evolutionary perspectives of behavior are concerned.

Concept of Innate Behavior

To illustrate the concept of innateness I have chosen an example from the evolution of the vertebrates. It has to do with the prey-catching toad (Ewert 1989). The behavior has four components which are integrated into one achievement, the catching of prey.

If a hungry toad is put under a glass cylinder and a rectangular object with certain dimensions is moved around the cylinder in a horizontal position, this dummy prey, the "worm," elicits the whole instinctive action (Lorenz 1937/1950) of prey-catching:

The sign stimulus typical for this species elicits an orienting movement (taxis) and snapping (fixed action pattern). The taxis component is adapted to the stimulus situation, e.g., the speed at which the prey is moving, whereas the fixed action pattern consists of more or less stereotyped movements: If the prey is removed during binocular fixation the toad is unable to correct the course of the instinctive action and snaps at the air. The fixed (or modal) action pattern consists of opening the mouth, flicking out the tongue, grasping the prey, closing the mouth, and gulping. The toad's motivation to eat is evident in its appetitive behavior, i.e., in the number of turning movements per minute. It decreases with the degree of satiation, the sign stimulus becoming less and less effective. Charles Whitman (1899) already realized that instinctive actions are not always consistent in intensity and duration, even under the same stimulus conditions. The conclusion was later drawn that any given behavior is dependent not only on external stimuli but also on internal processes which underlie the changes in behavior. To explain the selective responsiveness of a fixed action pattern to a sign stimulus an Innate Releasing Mechanism (IRM) is assumed which, like a stimulus filter, releases the species-specific movements (Tinbergen 1951). This mechanism is equivalent to Lorenz's (1935) Innate Releasing Schema.

Each of these four components of the prey-catching action — appetitive behavior, sign stimulus, taxis and snapping — has been investigated as to its CNS correlate with adequate neurobiological methods. This has made it possible to identify the anatomical pathways and neuronal network from the muscle periphery to the midbrain level, to classify neurons with recognition and localization properties, and to search for putative tectal command neurons acting toward the sensory (visual) side and the motor side, providing a link between the two systems.

Now what does the prey-catching of toads have to do with psychiatry? First, this is a way of showing in a nutshell what a complex innate behavior is like. It consists of several parts and culminates in a multistage action. The behavior develops during maturation of the organism. It does not require learning, but may be improved upon by experience. The neural apparatus for this behavior is used throughout the vertebrates and, with increasing complexity, up to the mammals (nipple searching, orienting movements, nipple grasping, sucking, gulping). It is employed in orienting behavior and visual pursuit; it may be activated in REM sleep and dreaming. It is a mechanism which serves the survival of the individual as well as of the species. How far it is also involved in abnormal human behavior is unclear, but the phylogenetically old machinery is certainly at work in human eating disorders as I discuss later on.

At this point I should state that in principle very little gets lost in phylogeny, neither structures nor functions nor behavior, no matter how subordinate they may become. Yawning and scratching, seen in all terrestrial vertebrates, are perhaps good examples. However, old structures, functions, and behaviors may be used for newly emerging adaptive behavior. And this is true not only for motor behavior but also for the evolution of emotion and cognition.

Concept of Social Behavior and Communication

Social behavior plays a prominent role in the evolution of the vertebrates. Life in some sort of a social grouping appears to be of advantage to both the individual and the species. Because every species has its characteristic social behavior and all species in a genus, a family, or even an order show similarities in their social behavior, as for example iguanas or the primates, the assumption can be made that there is also a close relationship between cerebral structures and cerebral functions that produces species-typical social behavior.

There are at least four classes of social behavior: first, the interactions of the male and female for the purpose of reproduction; second, the actions and interactions of female and male for the care of the young and the interactions of the young with parents and siblings; third, all forms of cohesive interactions and bonding; and fourth, all kinds of agonistic interactions among members of the same species, such as displaying, attacking, defending, threatening, and avoiding. All four classes play a fundamental role in human social behavior, and severe disturbances and deviations can occur in all of them. Thus the study of simpler systems of social behavior may help to explain the biological roots of such psychopathologies.

The key to understanding the social behavior of a species lies in the question of how the animals communicate with each other.

From an evolutionary perspective we might speculate that in the beginning the simplest modes of social behavior were nothing but approach and avoidance among members of the same species. The outcome of such encounters was unpredictable. Because communication between partners was advantageous, social signals evolved to permit more flexibility in encounters and a greater degree of information about the outcome. There seems to be a basic rule in the evolution of social signals: If it is of advantage to a sender for a recipient to perceive the disposition or state of the sender through a specific behavior, that behavior pattern is likely to be modified until it becomes conspicuous. This transformation of a behavior into a social signal is called ritualization. It constitutes an adaptive channeling of expressive behavior, produced by natural selection. It has a built-in genetic basis, although learning may play a part. Ritualized behavior patterns can be characterized as displays. They are based on motivated intention movements (Huxley 1966).

This can be explained by an example. The green iguana belongs to the large family of Iguanidae. It is a gregarious animal whose life is hierarchically organized. The top animal is a male easily recognizable by its whitish head, which is distinctly brighter than the heads of the other group members. If a top male loses a fight and thereby the top rank, it loses its bright color; within minutes head and body assume a brownish-green color. With the loss of status the animal's social behavior is subject to drastic changes. The color of its head is an indicator of its internal state and the involvement of the autonomic nervous system and hormones. Among the small number of social signals in the family of Iguanidae, head nodding is the most conspicuous (Distel and Veazey, 1982). It consists of a sequence of up-and-down movements of the head, highly stereotyped in amplitude, frequency, and time course — a typical fixed action pattern (see Fig. 1). Head nodding is accompanied by an extension of the dewlap that makes this signal even more conspicuous. It is used in a number of competitive social encounters but can also be observed in isolated males in situations lacking a detectable releasing stimulus. Lorenz (1937/1950) termed this the vacuum activity of fixed action patterns. A defeated or low-ranking animal will never show this display.

In systematic electrical brain stimulation studies of the Iguana in our laboratory (see Fig. 2) it was possible to elicit various behavior patterns that are used as

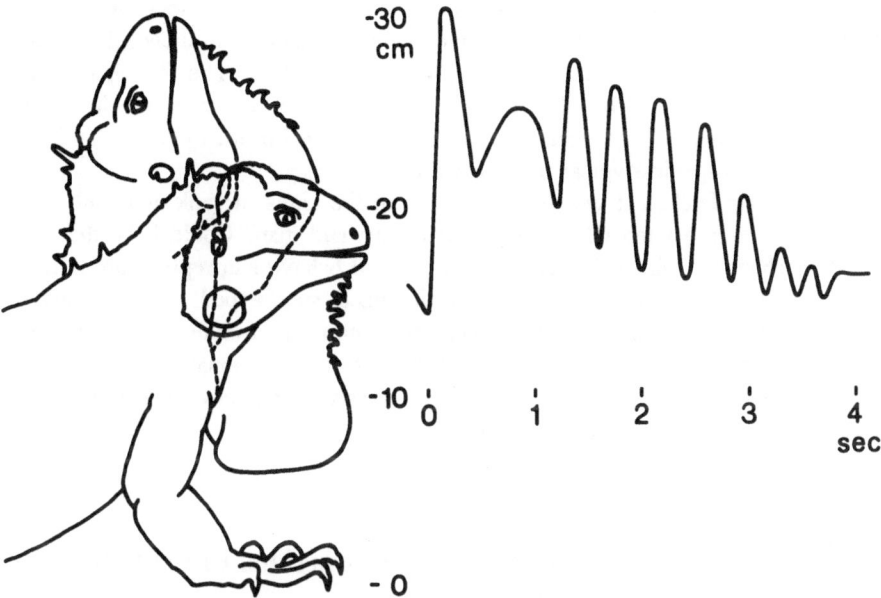

Fig. 1. The head-nodding display of *Iguana iguana*, a South American lizard. Onset and termination of the conspicuous social signal. Amplitude, frequency, and time course of the nodding shown by the line. (From Distel and Veazey 1982)

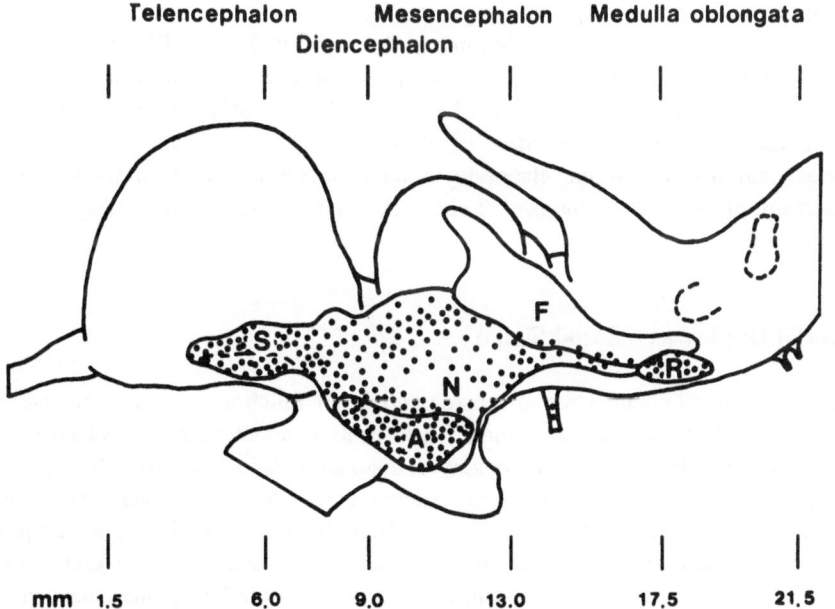

Fig. 2. The brain of Iguana in a sagittal diagram, delineating areas of electrical brain stimulation with behavioral consequences. *A*, aggressive defense (hypothalamus); *F*, violent flight (tectum); *N*, axial turning movements and head raising (ventral thalamus); *S*, septum; *R*, raphe; *dotted areas*, strong arousal. (After Distel 1978)

social signals, including head nodding and head brightening. The loci for eliciting these stereotyped but nevertheless complex behavior patterns in diencephalic and mesencephalic structures have been mapped (Distel 1978). The fact that social signals can be elicited by electrical stimulation of certain areas of the brain indicates that this class of behavior is somehow encoded in the brain mechanisms which mediate species-typical social behavior.

Is it too far-fetched if we see similarities in the signs of rank and rank loss including the associated CNS changes in Iguana and man? Could it be that the brain mechanisms which mediate ritualized social behavior in reptiles are homologous to the mechanisms which mediate ritualized, stereotyped, and compulsive behavior in man (MacLean 1990)? There are a number of studies in nonhuman primates which show significant correlations between hormonal state and rank. There are also reports on psychosurgery for obsessive-compulsive neuroses which relieved the patients from their severe suffering.

Communication Processes and Brain Functions in Primates

The increasing refinement and differentiation of social behavior and communication, and of the brain functions involved, has been studied in the squirrel monkey (*Saimiri sciureus*) over the years.

When we began our studies in Munich in the early 1960s, very little was known about the brain mechanisms of social behavior and communication processes in primates. Because of the experience I had gained previously working with Paul MacLean at the National Institute of Mental Health in Bethesda, Md, United States, and because of the elaborate social behavior and rich communication repertoire of the squirrel monkey, I chose this small New World monkey as our model animal.

Genital Display as a Social Signal

The study of communication processes and brain functions gained momentum through a rather exciting observation. To learn more about the social behavior of the squirrel monkey I observed a colony of these animals in MacLean's laboratory and found, among other social signals, one that is best described as genital display (Ploog and MacLean 1963; Ploog et al. 1963). This signal is used in various types of agonistic, dominance, and courtship behaviors. It consists of several components: penile erection, lateral positioning of the leg with the hip and knee bent, and marked supination of the foot and abduction of the big toe. In displaying females, enlargement of the clitoris replaces erection (Maurus et al. 1965). The display is frequently accompanied by a specific vocalization and sometimes, in young animals, by a few spurts of urine. Figure 3 shows four variations of genital

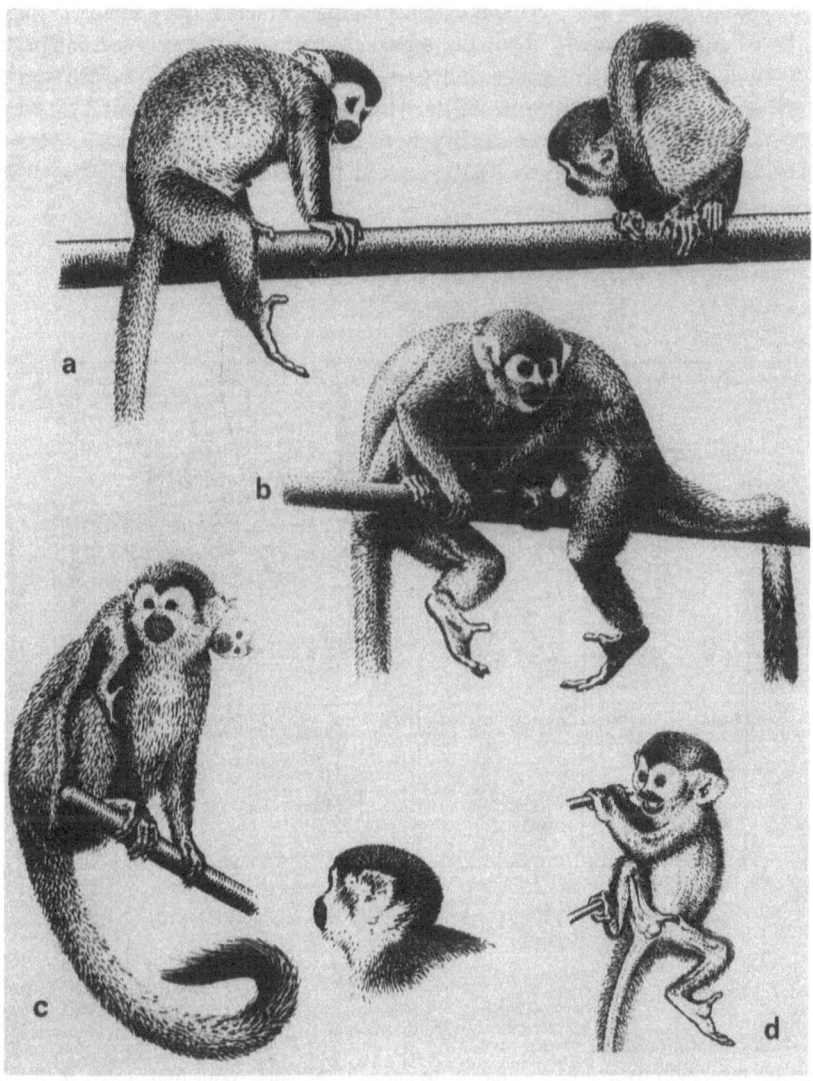

Fig. 3. Genital display, a social signal of the squirrel monkey. *a*, display at a distance; *b*, counterdisplay in proximity; *c*, displaying at a conspecific from the back of mother on the 2nd day of life; *d*, 49-day-old male displaying at his mirror image and vocalizing. (From Ploog 1974)

display. In the open position the displaying dominant animal looks at the partner to be subdued from a distance. In the closed position, sometimes seen as counterdisplay in rivaling males, partners touch each other but do not look at each other. The signal may be exhibited as early as the 1st or 2nd day of life, directed to a cage-mate; it is also seen in monkeys displaying to their mirror image (Ploog et al. 1963; MacLean 1964). Thus the signal is used in different types of partner interactions with slightly varying functions whose core appears to be the function of self-assertion. From sociometric data I have concluded that genital display is a social signal that contributes decisively to the formation of group structure and to regulatory processes which I have termed "social homeostasis" (Ploog 1967; Ploog and Melnechuk 1972) (see Fig. 4).

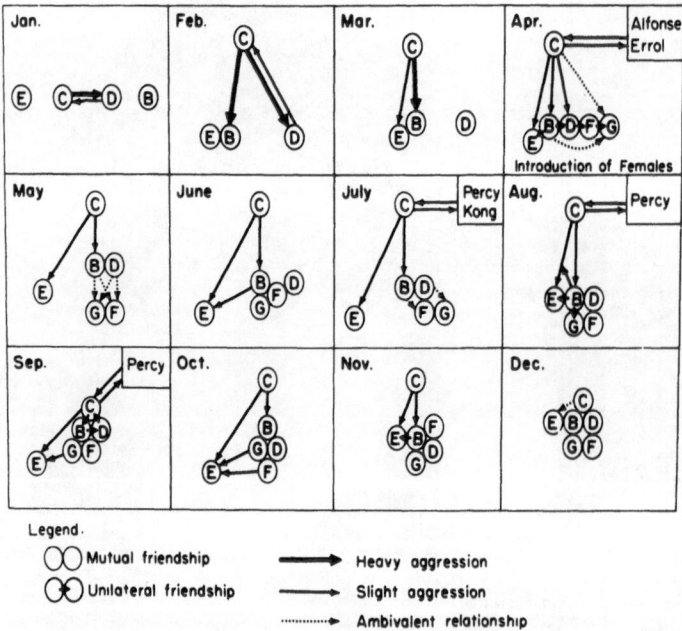

Fig. 4. Social homeostasis: group formation in a colony of squirrel monkeys. The dynamics of group formation over 1 year is based on sociometric data. With four males *(E,B,C,D)* and two females *(F,G)*, the group has an abnormal gender composition. *C* establishes himself as alpha male, *B* is second and attains the mediating role; *D* is a male in puberty opposing *C* from the beginning by genital display and other "undue" signals. *F* and *G* are mature females, close to *B* and *D* but never to *C*; and *E* is the omega animal and often the scapegoat of the group but sometimes protected by *B* (see August section). *C* defends the group against strange males. He exhibits genital display often to all males and rarely to females. He never courts the females but masturbates often. (In a later group composition of two males and four females he becomes the alpha animal again, displays to all members, courts and copulates with one female, and does not masturbate.) After 3 months no more severe aggressive acts *(heavy arrows)* occur. Genital display is included in the "slight aggression" *(light)* arrows. *Broken arrows* indicate indifferent interactions. "Friendship" means all cohesive interactions (Ploog 1963; Ploog et al. 1963)

Here, as in the case of head nodding, we have a process of ritualization. When functioning as part of copulatory behavior, genital organs serve to maintain the species. When used in genital display, these same organs function as a ritualized social signal that provides the individual with a means of intraspecific communication. As in head nodding, the complex motor program for the social signal is innate — exhibited even by neonates and by monkeys socially isolated at birth — but the rules under which it may be used or suppressed change with maturation and develop with social experience (Ploog et al. 1967; Ploog 1969; Hopf 1970). From the contexts in which the signal occurs and the sometimes concurrent vocal expression it is obvious that genital display is a signal and, at the same time, an expression of a distinct emotion or, considering the slightly varying functions, a spectrum of distinct emotions.

Cerebral Representation of Penile Erection

At the time of the first observations on genital display a brain stimulation study was conducted which aimed at the localization of genital function in the brain. The most conspicuous component of genital display, the penile erection, can be elicited by electrical stimulation of three subdivisions of the limbic system (MacLean and Ploog, 1962).

The following structures are involved:

1. The distribution of hippocampal projections to part of the septum, anterior and midline thalamic nuclei, and hypothalamus.
2. Structures comprising the mamillary bodies, mamillothalamic tract, anterior thalamus, and cingulate gyrus.
3. Loci in the gyrus rectus, the medial part of the medial dorsal nucleus of the thalamus, and regions of their known connections; the inferior thalamic peduncle, which contains projections from the medial dorsal nucleus that subsequently proceed caudally in association with the medial forebrain bundle.

The results suggest that excitatory influences descend medially in the periventricular fiber system and laterally by way of the medial forebrain bundle. Figure 5 depicts most of the structures. For the detailed mapping of loci for penile erection the reader is referred to the original publication.

These results were rather surprising because of the large extent of the system from which penile erection was elicitable. Until then sexual functioning was thought to be located mainly in the hypothalamus. In the light of the observations on genital display, however, it became obvious that we were dealing here with a brain system which mediates not merely sexual functions but also social behavior with its manifold implications.

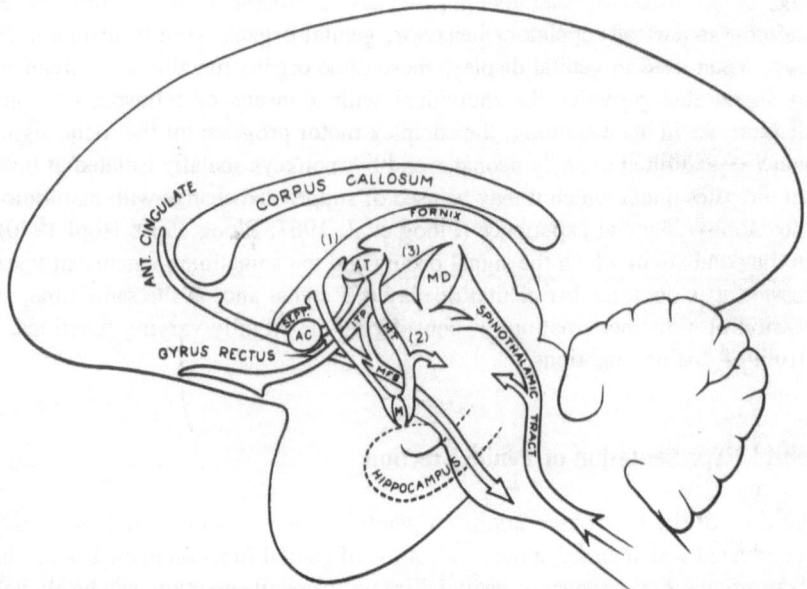

Fig. 5. Cerebral representation of penile erection found in parts of three cortico-subcortical subdivisions of the limbic system schematically depicted and labeled (*1*), (*2*), and (*3*). See text for definitions. The septum (*SEPT*) and medial parts of the medial dorsal nucleus (*MD*) are nodal points with respect to erection. The medial forebrain bundle (*MFB*) and inferior thalamic peduncle (*ITP*) are important descending pathways. Other abbreviations: *AC*, anterior commissure; *AT*, anterior thalamus; *M*, mamillary bodies (from MacLean 1962)

Homologies of Genital Display in Man

Observations and numerous cultural documents show that man too uses genital signals for communication — in earlier times more frequently than today (MacLean 1962; Ploog 1966b; Wickler 1966) (see Fig. 6). In this communication signals by males showing the penis directly or indirectly are most common, but "genital mocking" by young girls who lift their loincloth in a teasing manner is also known (Eibl-Eibesfeldt 1984). As in the monkey, the function and meaning of the male signals are complex and multiply determined. One component is the demonstration of power. Rulers and gods are shown with big phalli. In a different context genital display has a defensive component, as for example in the "guardians" who display in front of the houses and at the edges of the fields they are guarding. In some places, such as in Borneo and on the island of Nias, such figures are still in use as house guardians. In New Guinea penis sheaths of different shapes and sizes are still worn. They serve for display — as decoration and as insignia of rank. In Europe too signs of virility were used for centuries as ornaments on suits of armor, military uniforms, and other warriors' garments. One relic of this custom is the ornamented flap on Bavarian lederhosen (Koenig 1970).

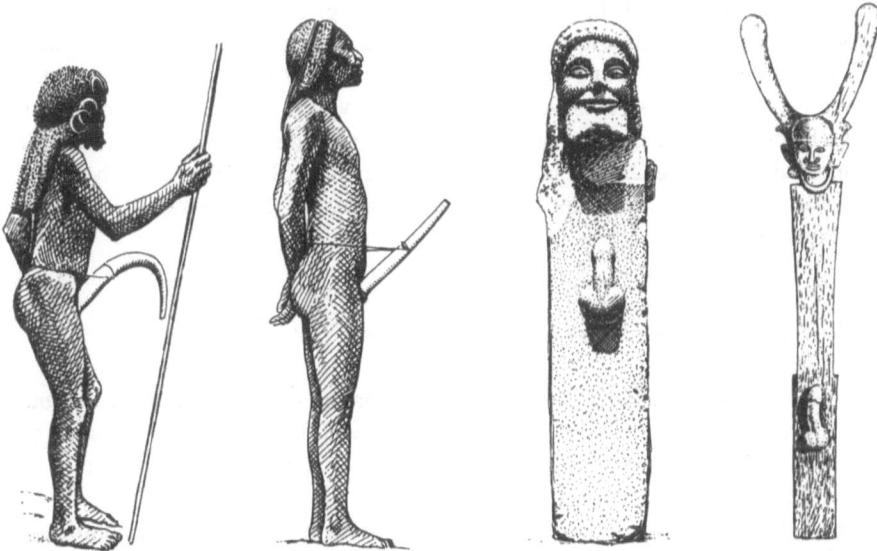

Fig. 6. Genital display in man. *Left,* two Papuans of Cogume on the River Conca. *Next to them,* herm of Sifnos (490 B.C.), National Museum, Athens. *Right,* house guardian ("Siraha") of the natives of the island of Nias. Such figures as tall as a man are still in use. (From Eibl-Eibesfeldt 1984)

In discussions of genital display the question arises of whether any insights can be gained about the exhibitionist, his motivation, and his behavior. This comparison almost suggests itself when one reads of folkways in which girls are shocked by boys who show them penis dummies (Ujváry 1966). Without going into the psychopathology of exhibitionism, which is by no means uniform, it should be emphasized that through exhibiting a sociogenital signal is secondarily transformed back into a sexual action. What genital displaying and exhibiting have in common is the ambivalence of advance and retreat that is typical of genital display. Both occur in an agonistic social context and should be seen as acts of self-assertion. In both cases distance from the partner plays an important role. The exhibitionist tries to keep his distance and to avoid proximity, unless he is in a safe place while exhibiting, e.g., on a river bank, with girls passing by in boats (Ploog 1980).

Genital display lends itself very well to a discussion of Freud's widely known and still mostly accepted doctrine that social (and cultural) life of the human kind has its roots in sexuality and is driven by it. From our studies we have learned that genital display is a built-in pattern of social, not sexual, behavior which is used by the individual as a social signal for the purpose of intraspecific communication long before sexual behavior emerges. In addition, all developmental primate behavior studies show that adverse conditions of social life during ontogeny lead to severe deficiencies and aberrations in social *and* sexual behavior. Since especially during the early developmental phases humans share a lot of primate-specific social behavior, such as mothering, bonding, and cohesive and agonistic behavior, with the nonhuman primates, it may be time to turn Freud's doctrine around: The sexual behavior of primates rests on social behavior, and social behavior has its roots in a set of species-typical behavior patterns which serve as the basis for the formation and the organization of social structures and communal life that secure the survival of the individual. To make sexual behavior dependent upon social behavior has consequences for the treatment of the majority of sexual neuroses.

Audiovocal Communication in Primates

The voice is an outstanding means of social signaling in nonhuman primates and man. Interest in the evolution and biological foundations of human language and speech inspired our experimental studies on the audiovocal communication of squirrel monkeys.

The voice has a long evolutionary history ranging from fish, amphibians, reptiles, and birds to mammals and primates. Together with the complexity of the sound-producing apparatus, the variety of vocal expression and the complexity of the cerebral mechanisms controlling the peripheral apparatus have increased, reaching their apex in man. The vocalizations at the "base" of the phylogenetic vocal tree are stereotypic in form and limited in number, whereas at the "top" of the tree there is the extensive, vocally modulated repertoire of primates (Ploog 1970). Inasmuch as most forms of vocalizations serve two purposes, namely as expressions of emotion and, at the same time, as communicative signals, primates have the most highly refined means of expressing emotions and of communicating (Ploog, in press). How these two faculties are linked — in behavior and brain function — is exemplified by the vocal repertoire of the squirrel monkey.

In a first approach to the classification of vocal signals we assumed that calls with a similar acoustic structure have a similar function. Therefore, the sonagrams of all calls recorded were grouped according to structural similarities. Five classes (plus one "mixed bag"), each containing several call types, emerged and were assigned to a general function that was based on carefully recorded observation of the monkey's behavior while he was calling or receiving a call from a conspecific (see Fig. 7). For several calls more specific functions could be designated and experimentally confirmed. For instance, the isolation peep is emitted if an animal gets separated from the group; furthermore, there are two types of alarm calls, one for aerial predators and one for terrestrial predators, both of which can be elicited by presenting an appropriate visual stimulus (Winter et al. 1966; Schott 1975;

Fig. 7. Vocal repertoire of the squirrel monkey, schematic representation with sound spectrograms. *Abbreviations: aggress.*, aggression; *alarm p.*, alarm peep; *l. grunt*, labor grunt. For division into six groups and for further explanation, see text. (From Winter et al. 1966)

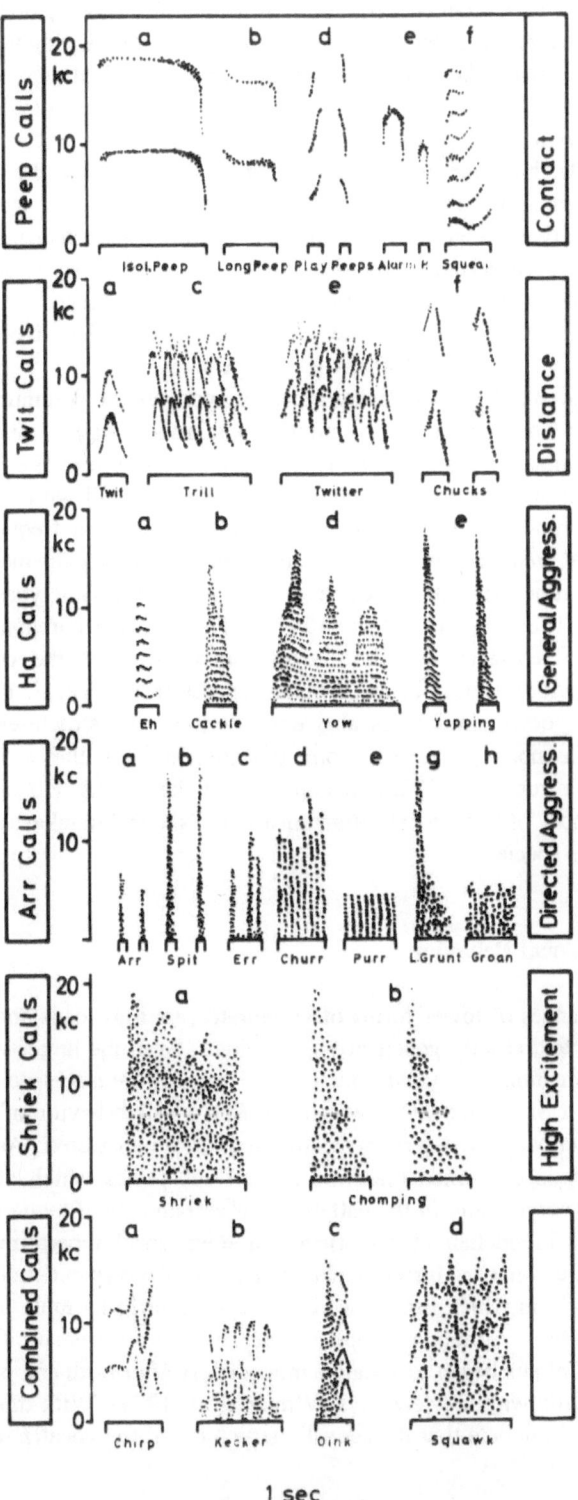

1 sec

Herzog and Hopf 1986). Other methods were also used to investigate the meaning (or function) of calls, e.g., playbacks of tape recordings for eliciting vocal or other motor responses from the listeners; or varying the motivational state of the animals, e.g., by food deprivation or the introduction of a strange male, and recording the event-related vocal behavior in a group.

These methods, however, yielded results which could explain the functions of signals only in bits and pieces and not in a systematic manner. Hence, a new approach had to be worked out that is not based on observer decision but solely on the monkey's vocal responses to vocal input from conspecifics — spontaneously or in dialogues (Maurus et al. 1985). This can be achieved technically by telemetering the calls on a tape, whereby the monkeys under investigation are distinguishable by their individual carrier frequencies.

Supposing the monkeys use categorical components in communication, as humans do; then one might expect accumulations in the statistical distribution of the physical parameters of such components (Maurus and Ploog 1984; Maurus et al. 1988). The search for such accumulations was successful with regard to the communicative function of amplitude modulation, changes in frequency power distribution, and frequency modulation and with regard to other more complex communicative functions, all of which operate across the call types of Fig. 7 (Maurus et al. 1986; Barclay et al. 1987). The acoustic components in the monkey's vocal repertoire found to significantly influence the conspecific's succeeding behavior are also present in human speech (Maurus et al. 1989). There is evidence that other similarities also exist between the structures of human speech and of the monkey's acoustic communication and how they are used in the two species (Maurus et al. 1988). It appears that the results will contribute to "cracking the code" of audiovocal communication in squirrel monkeys and perhaps in other primate species.

Innateness of Vocal Behavior

The vocal utterances of lower forms of vertebrates, such as toads and frogs, are species-specific and strictly genetically determined. Even the larger vocal repertoires of some mammals, e.g., various Felidae species, are also species-specific. But the question of the extent to which the rich vocal behavior of nonhuman primates is genetically predetermined still needs to be answered. As far as the squirrel monkey is concerned there are several subspecies which differ in appearance, in karyotype, and in the patterning of certain calls (Ploog et al. 1975). Hybrids exhibit Mendelian characteristics in their vocal repertoire (Newman 1985). To find out what a squirrel monkey must learn from an external model, we performed a study in which infants were raised from birth by mute mothers and in acoustic isolation. Although completely deprived of species-specific auditory experience, the infants began to vocalize immediately after birth and produced all types of adult calls within a few days (Winter et al. 1973). With this and other evidence we can conclude that the acoustic structures of the vocalizations of this primate species are genetically preprogrammed fixed action patterns similar to the monkey's genital display and to the head nodding of the iguana. Hence species-specific calls are social signals par excellence.

The monkey's vocal behavior can be compared with that of the human infant during his first 3 months of vocal development. Both monkey and infant vocalize regardless of exteroceptive input or deafness. Like the monkey, the human infant vocalizes in a species-typical manner, independent of the language spoken in his presence. Nevertheless there are profound differences. While the monkey's vocal repertoire remains more or less invariant, the human infant's vocal production undergoes preprogrammed changes that are universal in all languages. The fascinating aspect, however, is that both monkey and preverbal infant use their vocal behavior to express emotions *and* to communicate.

Cerebral Organization of Vocal Behavior

How is vocal behavior represented and organized in the brain? Answers to this question contribute in two ways to basic issues in biological psychiatry. Firstly, we gain direct access to the brain system which is responsible for the expression of emotions and thereby indirect information on the system which generates and controls emotions. Secondly, we gain access to a nonverbal communication system which we largely share with the nonhuman primates. This system operates not only in our nonverbal communication with our conspecifics but also through prosodic features in our language — in conversation, in songs without words, in complaining and cursing . The introductory quotation from Hippocrates includes not only some pronounced emotional states, often vocally expressed, but also emotional states which are subject to treatment in psychiatry.

The squirrel monkey has been studied more thoroughly than any other primate with regard to vocal repertoire and the brain structures involved (Jürgens 1979; Jürgens and Ploog 1981; Ploog 1981a; Jürgens 1988). For our purpose the results of electrical brain stimulation are sufficient for an outline of the system involved in vocal behavior. Surprisingly, only species-specific, i.e., natural, calls can be elicited by electrical stimulation of the brain sites above a certain level in the pons. The four diagrams of Fig. 8 show the extent of the structures (in black) yielding calls, and spectrographic samples of the call types elicited. The responsive structures reach from orbito-frontal and temporal subcortical structures, through thalamic and hypothalamic structures, into the midbrain and pons and their intimate connections with the limbic system. Note that not a single vocally responsive site was detected in the neocortex (Jürgens and Ploog 1970).

The great extent of the vocalization-yielding structures, the fact that elicited calls are often accompanied by other motor and autonomic reactions, and the results of latency measurements between stimulus onset and the beginning of vocalization suggest that not all of the structures are directly involved in the production of calls. Rather, stimulation of these structures causes a motivational change in the animal that is then expressed by the call. This hypothesis was tested in self-

18   D.Ploog

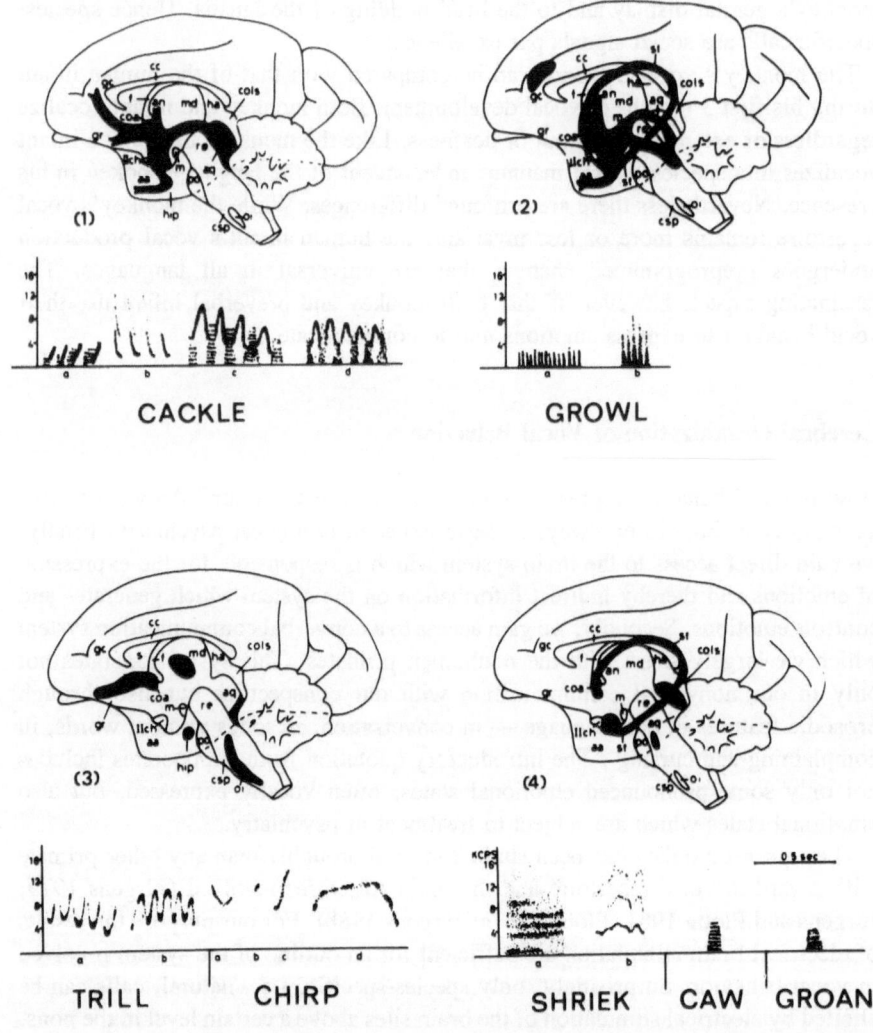

Fig. 8. Vocalization elicited by electrical stimulation of the squirrel monkey's brain. General view of the cerebral system (*in black*) yielding: (*1*) cackling calls, (*2*) growling calls, (*3*) chirping calls, and (*4*) shrieking calls. The calls are represented as frequency-time diagrams. *Abbreviations: aa*, area anterior amygdalae; *an*, nucleus anterior; *aq*, substantia grisea centralis; *cc*, corpus callosum; *coa*, commissura anterior; *cols*, colliculus superior; *csp*, tractus corticospinalis; *f*, fornix; *gc*, gyrus cinguli; *gr*, gyrus rectus; *ha*, nucleus habenularis; *hip*, hippocampus; *m*, corpus mamillare; *md*, nucleus medialis thalami; *oi*, nucleus olivaris inferior; *po*, griseum pontis; *re*, formatio reticularis tegmenti; *st*, stria terminalis; *Ilch*, chiasma opticum (Jürgens 1979b; Ploog 1981a)

stimulation experiments in which the animal could switch the electrical stimulation on and off. In this way it could be determined whether stimulation of a specific vocalization area was aversive, neutral or pleasant. The experiments revealed that there are two subsystems of vocalization-producing brain structures, one system in which the electrically elicited vocalization is independent of the accompanying reinforcement effect, if any, and a second system in which vocalization and reinforcement are strictly correlated. The first system consists of the anterior limbic cortex and the ventromedial capsula interna, on the one hand, and the caudalmost periaqueductal gray and adjacent parabrachial region, on the other. The second system includes the rest of the vocalization-eliciting areas. The first system represents primary vocalization areas where the stimulus directly triggers the activity of a vocalization center. The areas of the second system mediate secondary reactions due to stimulus-induced motivational changes (Jürgens 1976a).

Figure 9 summarizes the results on the cerebral representation of vocal behavior and demonstrates the hierarchical organization. In a diagram of the simian brain those areas are depicted which are functionally important for phonation in monkeys and man. The lowest level (I) is represented by the nucleus ambiguus, whose neurons supply the larynx with the innervation required for the execution of vocal movements, by respiratory motoneurons, and by the lateral pontine and medullary reticular formation, which have coordinating functions.

The central gray in the lower midbrain and upper pons (II) is the phylogenetically oldest structure for the generation of species-specific calls. It receives input from motivation-controlling brain structures (III). Electrical stimulation yields species-specific vocalizations in amphibians, reptiles, mammals, and man. Its destruction — experimentally or traumatically — causes mutism. In the primate, this area receives direct input from and is controlled by the anterior cingulate gyrus (IV). This structure is involved in the initiation and voluntary control of the voice, although to a different degree in monkeys and man. Monkeys can control their vocal behavior to a rather limited extent in regard to the frequency and amplitude of a species-specific vocalization, but not in regard to the acoustic structure of the utterance. In an experiment, monkeys were required to produce a "coo" of a certain duration and intensity contingent upon conditional stimuli and reward. After bilateral ablation of the cingulate area, this instrumental response was abolished, although the monkeys were still able to vocalize spontaneously and adequately in the communal situation as well as vocally respond to external fearful stimuli (Sutton et al. 1974; Kirzinger and Jürgens 1982). On the other hand, clinical work has shown that patients with bilateral lesions of the cingulate area may lose spontaneous speech completely. After a state of akinetic mutism is overcome and the initiation of speech is possible again, the voice sounds monotonous, the speech is aprosodic, and the patient continues to have difficulties in initiating verbal communication (Jürgens and von Cramon 1982).

Although I am not dealing directly with language and speech in this contribution, the obvious question about the role of the primary motor cortex in phonation should be briefly answered. It is well known that this cortex is crucial for the voluntary control of movements. Destruction of the face area in the speech

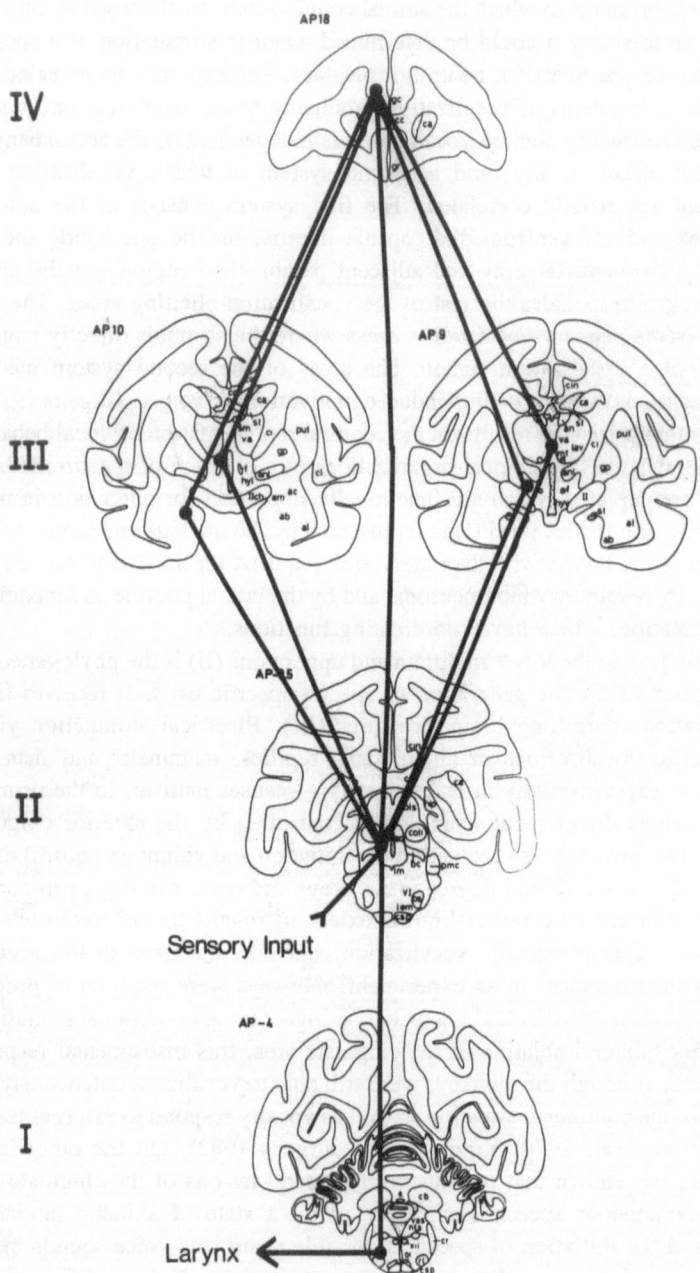

Fig. 9. Diagram of hierarchical control of vocalization. All brain areas indicated by a dot yield vocalization when electrically stimulated. All lines interconnecting the dots represent anatomically verified direct projections (leading in a rostrocaudal direction). The dots indicate in (*IV*) the anterior cingulate gyrus; in (*III*) the basal amygdaloid nucleus, dor-

somedial and lateral hypothalamus, and midline thalamus; in (*II*) the periaqueductal gray and laterally bordering tegmentum; and in (*I*) the nucleus ambiguus and surrounding reticular formation (the nucleus ambiguus itself yields only isolated movements of the vocal folds; phonation can be obtained, however, from its immediate vicinity). For a further explanation, see the text. (Jürgens and Ploog 1981)

hemisphere in man will result in severe anarthria and aphonia. A bilateral lesion of this area in the monkey will, however, leave its vocalization completely unimpaired (Jürgens et al. 1982). This profound functional difference is based on different anatomical projections. While in man there is a direct connection between the primary motor cortex and the laryngeal motoneurons, obviously an outgrowth of the pyramidal tract in both directions, such a connection is lacking in the monkey (Jürgens 1976b). Thus man can exert a direct voluntary control over his vocal cords, but apes and monkeys cannot. This new pathway is clearly a prerequisite for the emergence of social communication in the speaking mode since the acquisition of learned vocal gestures is required. This difference explains why nonhuman primates can learn neither to speak nor to sing (Ploog 1988 a,b).

When human evolution and the unprecedented increase in neocortex are discussed, however, concomitant changes in subcortical structures are usually neglected. The limbic system is one of these structures. Since this system is heavily involved in vocal behavior, as just outlined, it is important to know that morphometric analyses of limbic structures revealed more neurons in the human anterior thalamic limbic nuclei than expected in an anthropoid with a brain the size of ours. The increased number of neurons produces an increased limbic input into the human neocortex, especially into the supplementary motor area and the premotor and orbitofrontal cortex. The enlargement of the thalamic limbic pool of neurons may represent an increased differentiation of the limbic message being sent to the cortex. And vice versa, through reciprocal connections the enlarged thalamic limbic pool may represent an increased ability to activate and control limbic structures via neocortical input (Armstrong 1986).

This anatomical excursion makes it quite clear that the subcortical vocal communication system, basic for the emergence of speech, is intimately and reciprocally connected with those neocortical areas which, on the one hand, have this system under control and, on the other, are informed about the processes going on there. The fact that great emotional excitement makes our voice tremble or can even make us speechless can be explained by these connections. This system may also represent the window which permits self-awareness and verbal reports on our emotions and feelings (Ploog 1989a,b).

Disconnection of Emotions from the Expressions of Emotion

The electrical elicitation of vocal expressions confirms the old contention that the limbic system is instrumental in the elaboration of emotions (Kleist 1934; MacLean 1949, 1955; Papez 1937). Over and above this, the finely graded vocal actions indicate in detail what kind of emotion is being elaborated and what structures within the limbic system are involved at any time. Furthermore, according to the hierarchical organization of the system those parts of the system where the emotions (the motivational states) are worked out (level III in Fig. 9) can be separated from the part which releases the appropriate vocal signal (emotional expression), which is on level II. As I have outlined elsewhere (Ploog 1989a), the facial expressions of emotion are organized in a similar fashion, and hence the two main social signaling systems in primates, including man, are rather intertwined and follow the same functional rules.

Since there are a number of mental diseases, foremost the affective and schizophrenic psychoses, where emotions are out of kilter (revealed by verbal reports from the patient) and the expression of emotions is disturbed (revealed by the observations of the psychiatrist), one would like to know more about the brain structures and functions that are involved in the malfunction.

There is clinical evidence that vocal, as well as facial, expressions of emotions can be separated from emotions as subjective feelings. This evidence can be provided only by man since only he is able to report in words on emotional experience.

One of the most common diseases of the extrapyramidal system is Parkinson's disease, affecting the neurotransmitter system of the basal ganglia. Patients with this disease commonly display a mimetic facial paresis, a condition in which they retain the ability to move the facial muscles to verbal command (voluntary control), but gradually lose spontaneous emotional facial expressions. Likewise, they can employ their voice at will, but their speech gradually loses the prosodic features and sounds flat in affect. In spite of this expressive motor deficiency, the subjective feelings of these patients are not impaired, as becomes evident from listening to their subtle descriptions of their emotions.

In contrast to the loss of emotional expression with intact subjective feelings, patients suffering from pathological laughing and crying involuntarily display extremely pronounced forms of these emotional expressions, but they report no corresponding emotional experience during these bouts. The emotional expressions occur against their will and cannot be inhibited voluntarily. The automatic expressions are probably caused by "the interruption of a control system, presumably lying at the base of the brain stem" (Poeck 1969). These clinical and neuropathological findings are corroborated by observations of infants with anencephalic malformations, who exhibit expressions of crying and smiling if the midbrain is intact (Gamper 1926; Steiner 1974). Be reminded of Fig. 9, level II!

Yet another dichotomy of function is seen in facial apraxia: The patient is unable to execute facial movements, including facial expressions of emotions, on command but can do so spontaneously. Similarly, there is the akinetic mutism in which the patient is unable to use his or her voice on command but can produce emotional utterances, for example, groans indicating pain. Our patient had a bilateral infarction in the anterior cingulate gyrus (Jürgens and von Cramon 1982). See Fig. 9, level IV. The problem here is that voluntary control over the peripheral apparatus, which serves emotional expression, has been lost at a high CNS level, while the appropriate emotional expression is still intact (Ploog 1986).

Considering the disconnection (Geschwind 1965) of emotions and the expressions of emotion on the one hand and the hierarchical organization of expressive behavior (vocal as well as facial) on the other, it is now easier to understand why a voluntarily produced social signal, whether vocal or facial, evokes the specific central state to which the produced signal belongs (Ekman, Levenson and Friesen 1983). It can be maintained that the emotional *experience* is as specific as the evoked central nervous state and the (uninhibited) emotional *expression* (Ploog 1989a).

Integration and Disintegration of Communication and Social Behavior

So far it has been my aim to present examples of animal communication with the respective brain mechanisms involved to characterize the important building blocks of social communication processes of a respectable phylogenetic age. The components typical for each species are the releasing stimuli (social or environmental), the elicited neural programs for the expressions of emotion (e.g., vocal or facial), which at the same time function as social signals, and the receiver's context-dependent responses of a similar kind.

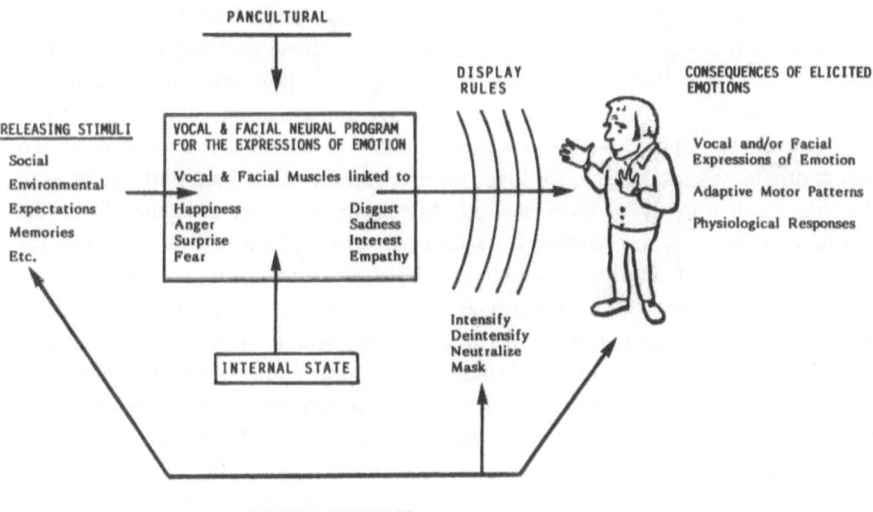

Fig. 10. Determinants of the expressions of emotion and nonverbal communication processes. See text for further explanation. (After Ekman 1971, modified)

Figure 10 illustrates these basic components still present in man but now developed into a system of the highest complexity. In fact, the basic component system is involved not only in all nonverbal but also in all verbal human communication and in everyday direct partner interaction, but it is dominated by or even hidden in human language, which has become the basis for cultural evolution. The new linguistic faculty functions within a structural framework of older functions whose biology has been adapted to the new situation. This has been discussed in the section on the cerebral organization of vocal behavior.

The contribution of ethology and neuroethology to psychiatry rests on investigations of the structural framework of those basic components that form species-typical nonverbal communication and social behavior. If one takes the bird's eye view on the psychopathology of mental disorders, it is social behavior and communication which is disintegrated in various ways in a great many of them. It is as if this species-typical system of *Homo sapiens* is the most vulnerable one and is easily involved in mental disorders of different categories as we see them today. One may speculate whether awareness of this human-specific vulnerability provides us with a lead in the quest for causal mechanisms in mental disorders.

Eating Disorders

I have chosen anorexia nervosa and bulimia as an example of the disintegration of social behavior and communication because of the integrated research and combined effort within our Clinical Institute to explain this psychosocial and psychosomatic disorder. There are several contributions on this topic in this volume. I therefore restrict myself to the ethological aspects of this disease (Ploog 1981b). Some quotations of what anorexic girls have said about their motivation to starve themselves clearly reveal the social motives that drive them to act as they do. "To me," a patient said, "to be slim meant to be powerful. It made me the center of attraction. I was finally given the love and attention I had longed for." Or: "Whenever I gained weight, I felt as if I had lost what I loved most of all. To me, anorexia was a substitute for love, for everything." Or: "I am nothing without the disease, a nobody, a bore, a void. My anorexia is my existence." As the disorder progresses, the striving for social recognition (and self-realization), for feeling strong and special, gradually declines and turns into social isolation, loneliness, and despair. This emotional state was portrayed by a bulimic girl: "I slowly turned into a primitive animal, all I did was search for food." And another bulimic, even more desperately: "I had lost my self-respect. I had failed completely, had never really lived; had I taken heroin during that time, it could not have done more damage to my body and my personality" (Gerlinghoff 1985).

The consequences of starvation and malnutrition influence the CNS regulation of the hunger drive. Normally, the releasing effect of food stimuli varies with hunger and satiation, i.e., with the internal state of the organism as outlined in the example of the prey-catching toad. In mammals, including humans, the basic behavioral patterns and neural control mechanisms for obtaining food, feeding, food rejection, and even food aversion are present at birth. This means that the most important primary drive system, which yields pleasure (positive reinforcement) by feeding and pain (negative reinforcement) by hunger, is subject to change in anorexia nervosa and bulimia. The change into the fully developed syndrome of this disease results in a perversion of the hunger drive: Although the feeling of hunger may still cause discomfort, the consequence of hunger, the weight loss, causes pleasure and significant reward, whereas food stimuli take on an ambivalent value, they are something to be avoided and yet at the same time something that completely occupies the mind. This extremely ambivalent state of approach (mentally) and avoidance (physically) can be overridden by attacks of bulimia, wherein food stimuli indiscriminately elicit voracious eating. In extreme cases where even spoiled, bad-smelling food is eaten, one is reminded of the Klüver-Bucy syndrome, and thus the question arises as to whether the sudden central disinhibition of feeding behavior includes a temporary dysfunction of the amygdala, which are involved in food recognition. In the full-blown syndrome nothing but thoughts about food and about how to obtain food is on the minds of the girls, and daily life is reduced to the level of the four-stage prey-catching which I discussed in the beginning.

If one compares the signs and symptoms of anorexics with the large body of literature on what is known about lateral and medial hypothalamic as well as amygdalar functions and feeding behavior in mammals, including monkeys, one can draw parallels that may help to explain the brain and behavior mechanisms of this drive-dependent perverted behavior, in which the subjects seem to develop starvation dependence (Szmukler and Tantam 1984; Ploog 1985).

I postulate that the hunger drive and its regulating cerebral machinery are disintegrated. The craving for food and the stubborn determination not to eat it lead to a continuous neural irritation of the hypothalamus and other parts of the feeding system similar to certain self-stimulation effects in animals. The gastrointestinal peptides could be involved in this process (Ploog 1981b; 1990). The behavior of anorexics follows a vicious circle which is similar to addictive behavior, and so is the course and often the outcome of the disease. Chronic anorexics, like addicts, show loss of zest, appear to be anhedonic, are without partners and are unfit for social relations (Ploog and Pirke 1987).

Social Behavior and Goal Attainment

Social species in general and primates in particular develop and maintain social support networks by means of communicative behavior. Each member of the group fulfills a certain role which depends on strength, age, sex, kinship, and special bonds and alliances among group members. Each member knows each other member and learns to predict the behavior of his conspecifics, at least to a certain degree. The social network rests on fluent communication as exemplified in Fig. 4. The study of the means of communication — e.g. gestural, audiovocal, visuofacial — has shown that specific behaviors carry distinct functions which have mutual consequences. The human social network has similar traits. It secures mutual assistance, resource sharing, emotional support, information sharing, and participation in child care and upbringing. In sociobiological terms, these are the benefits. The costs for this highly developed system are considerable and require time and effort. Individuals may suffer resource depletion from unreciprocated giving, they must be able to tolerate having emotional debts, and they may be vulnerable to the acts of others (McGuire 1979).

This is not the place to outline sociobiological concepts and achievements, despite their importance for evolutionary psychiatry (Hamilton 1964; Wilson 1975; Dawkins 1976; Voland and Voland 1989). It can be said, however, that each individual living in a social system is equipped with species-typical behavior patterns which enable biologically relevant goals to be pursued by means of ordered sets of adaptive behavior referred to as strategies, essential for survival and reproduction. A behavior is adaptive if it enhances an individual's everyday actions contributing to the pursuit of the biological goals.

Clinical psychiatrists know that many psychiatric illnesses are marked by severe deficits in social behavior, social competence, and social skills. Psychiatric illnesses reduce one's capacity for goal attainment. There are increased disruptions of kinship and friendship bonds, disrupted pair bonds with a decreased probability of offspring, difficulties in establishing efficient time-energy budgets; there is imprecise communication, a lack of behavioral and learning flexibility, a higher chance of offspring suffering from medical and psychiatric disorders; and financial resources tend to be unpredictable (McGuire and Essock-Vitale 1981). Most clinicians and psychiatric patients would agree that the functional disability associated with mental illness is an impairment in the capacity to carry out activities necessary for daily living.

McGuire and Essock-Vitale (1982) tested the hypothesis that experienced clinicians associate a decreased ability to generate adaptive behavior with both the exacerbation and remission states of psychiatric illnesses. To investigate this hypothesis they established a functional classification of adaptive behavior (Tab. 1), which consists of 7 behavior categories with 48 adaptive behaviors. It is applicable to both nonpsychiatric and psychiatric populations. Note that the classification does not deal with signs and symptoms but rather with functions of behavior and can therefore be used to assess the consequences of illness. Fifteen psychiatrists used the behavior classification system for their ratings. Seven diagnostic categories were to be rated. The clinicians' ratings clearly indicate that they associate reduced behavioral capacities with psychiatric disorders. Although the score in the category of normal subjects was always the highest and the score in the simple schizophrenic category was always the lowest for each behavior category, the relative depression of adaptive behavior ratings varied across the diagnostic categories (Fig. 11). That is to say, each diagnostic category had a characteristic profile of adaptive behavior deficiency.

Table 1. The 7 behavior categories and the 48 adaptive behaviors which compose them

---

Information processing (the reception and manipulation of information)
         Memory
         Thinking
         Operation of senses
         Observational learning
         Active learning

Social understanding (an awareness of the norms of interaction among members of a group)
         Understanding group norms among strangers
         Understanding norms, familiar group
         Understanding group goals and goal-oriented behaviors
         Understanding others' motives, behaviors, feelings
         Anticipating needs of others
         Understanding one's effects on others
         Understanding social support systems
         Understanding one's social options
         Monitoring others' behavior

Social maintenance (the preservation and continuation of behaviors which are useful in ordinary social interactions)
  o   Verbal behavior
         Nonverbal behavior
         Behaving according to group norms among strangers
         Behaving according to norms, familiar group
         Behaving according to group goals and goal-oriented behaviors
  o   Communicating one's motives, thoughts
         Tolerating conflict with individuals

Social manipulation (influencing the outcomes of interactions with others to one's own advantage)
         Using one's social options
         Altering others' behavior through their emotions
  o   Promising rewards
  o   Extracting promises
         Signaling, defending territory
         Disguising cheating

Social exchanges (giving or receiving any commodity)
         Meeting needs of others
         Using social support systems
         Engaging in altruistic behavior
         Receiving altruistic behavior

Self-understanding (an awareness of one's own being and needs)
         Feeling
         Anticipating own needs
         Identifying essential material resources
         Understanding material environment
         Anticipating material needs
  o   Monitoring own physical and mental health
  o   Understanding own motives regarding feelings

Self-maintenance (providing for the preservation and continuation of one's own well-being)
         Meeting own needs
  o   Acquiring essential material resources
         Altering priorities
         Tolerating conflict in material environment
         Enjoying own affects and behaviors
         Tolerating reciprocity imbalance
  o   Tolerating physical fatigue, pain
         Altering material environment
         Being physically adroit
  o   Maintaining physical attractiveness

      Circles indicate adaptive behaviors seen in humans only

28   D.Ploog

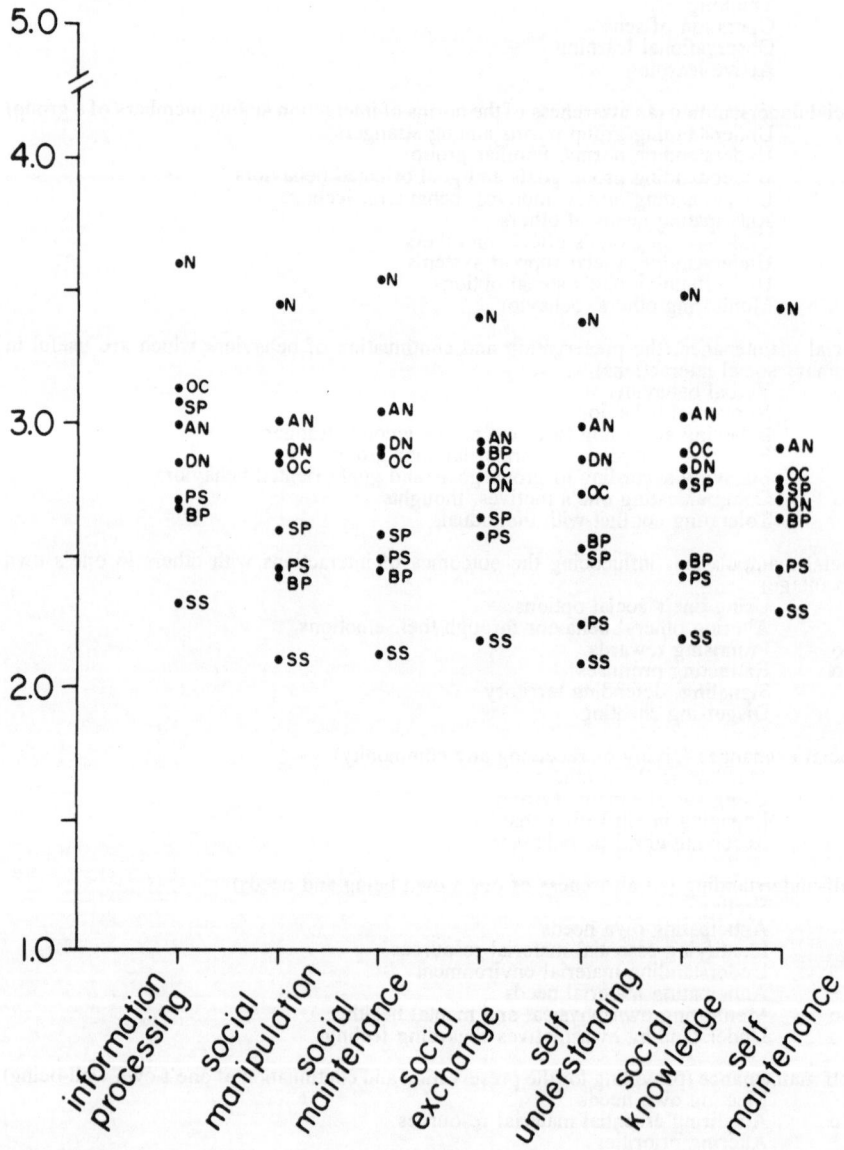

Fig. 11. Mean adaptive behavior ratings for each disorder for each behavior category. *PS*, paranoid schizophrenia; *SS*, simple schizophrenia; *BP*, bipolar illness (manic type); *AN*, anxiety neurosis; *DN*, depressive neurosis; *OC*, obsessive-compulsive personality; *SP*, schizoid personality; *N*, normal. See text for further explanation. (From McGuire and Essock-Vitale 1982)

Examination of the 7 behavioral categories with their respective adaptive behavior shows that 4 of the 7 concern social behavior, and only 4 of the 26 adaptive behaviors within these categories are specific for man and not for other primates, including apes.

These 4 are language-dependent. Two further behavior categories concern the self. Even there, only 5 or 6 out of 17 behaviors are exclusively reserved for the human, and 3 of the 6 require introspection the content of which can only become known to others by language. Finally, the first behavior category, which is functionally involved in the other six, applies in total to simians and apes provided that "thinking" is meant to be correspondent to problem solving.

What does this mean? It certainly does not mean that the behavior of monkeys and man does not differ. But it does mean that monkeys and man share an astonishing number of ethologically adaptive social behaviors which are similar in kind, though not the same in refinement and diversification. In my opinion it is justified to consider these adaptive behaviors as homologues to human social functioning. And it is social functioning that is the target system for mental illness. This system is based on and mediated by the cerebral mechanisms which have been addressed in the previous sections.

Synopsis

Highly preprogrammed animals, such as toads, can make only a limited number of behavioral choices in a given motivational state and to a given stimulus. This is also the case in infants with anencephalic malformations and in severely demented patients. In Jacksonian terms, such a dissolution of behavior indicates that phyletically old brain structures and functions are preserved in the human brain. Preprogrammed social behavior, for example in the green iguana, plays a prominent role in the evolution of the vertebrates. The key to understanding the social behavior of a species lies in the question of how the animals communicate with each other. Most communication is based on motivated intention movements which have become ritualized and are used as social signals. A perfect example of such a transformation into a social signal is the genital display of the squirrel monkey. The fact that social signals can be elicited by electrical stimulation of certain subcortical neuronal systems in the brain indicates that this class of complex behavior is somehow encoded in the brain mechanisms which mediate species-typical social behavior. The social communication system has a long evolutionary line of descent. Body gestures, facial expressions, and vocal gestures have become most refined in nonhuman primates. In man, the communication system has reached a new dimension, by acquisition of language and speech, but remains intimately tied up with the nonverbal communication system, which resides in structures of the limbic system, the striatal complex (MacLean 1990), and of the midbrain and pons.

In regard to basic issues in psychopathology and psychiatry, a continuous and special effort has been made to identify and delineate the cerebral organization of vocal behavior in a nonhuman primate. This communicative behavior yields direct access to the brain system responsible for the refined expression of emotions and thereby to information on the system which generates and controls emotions. We also gain access to a nonverbal communication system which man largely shares with the nonhuman primate; it constitutes the biological foundation of the only recently evolved form of communication in the speaking mode.

As with other systems in the brain, the vocal system is hierarchically organized and consists of various structural and functional levels and subsystems which serve differential functions, ranging from a voluntary induction of vocal signals at the top of the system (anterior cingulate gyrus) to an automatic but integrated vocal signal production at the lower midbrain level down to a level where partial vocal functions only, but not integrated signal patterns, can be generated.

With the hierarchical organization of this signaling system in mind, the concept of the disconnection of emotions (subjective feelings) from the expressions of emotions was applied to Parkinson's disease with loss of spontaneous facial and vocal emotional expressions on the one hand and pathological laughing and crying with loss of control over emotional expressions on the other. There are further clinical examples of functional disintegration of emotional expressions, e.g., in facial apraxia and akinetic mutism.

After component analysis of communication processes at various levels of complexity, the concept of the disintegration of social behavior is taken a step further, with application to the most complex levels of mental disorders.

As an example of a drive-dependent disorder anorexia nervosa and bulimia nervosa is discussed. Social stimuli and motives elicit starvation the consequences of which upset the CNS regulation of the hunger drive. The daily life of the afflicted persons regresses to thinking of and craving food. The hypothesis is advanced that the subjects develop starvation dependence, which is similar to addictive behavior. Their social behavior is severely impaired and they become unfit for social relations.

Many mental illnesses are marked by severe deficits in social behavior. Normally the social communication system is the backbone of the social support networks which nonhuman and human primates develop and maintain. The functions of this system regulate communal life. In mental illness, especially in the major psychoses, the social communication system disintegrates. This can lead to either blocking of the expression of emotions, as in severe depressive states or in catatonia, or to disinhibition of the expression of emotions, dependent on the internal state. The response choices to social and other external signals in a given situation become limited or even distorted, and reasoning no longer assists in making decisions.

Whether it is in the acute episode or in remission, experienced psychiatrists can detect the deficits in their patients' social behavior. It is very likely that they get the clues for these deficits via the communication system, which appears to be the target system for mental illness.

References

Armstrong E (1986) Enlarged limbic structures in the human brain: the anterior thalamus and medial mamillary body. Brain Res 362:394-397

Barclay D, Streit K-M, Maurus M, Steinleitner M, Haeglsperger R (1987) Linguistic strategies to detect frequency modulation patterns relevant to primate vocal communication. Lang Comm 7:255-265

Carlsson A (1987) The dopamine hypothesis of schizophrenia 20 years later. In: Häfner H, Gattaz WF, Janzarik W (eds) Search for the causes of schizophrenia. Springer, Berlin Heidelberg New York, pp 223-235

Dawkins R (1976) The selfish gene. Oxford University Press, New York

Distel H (1978) Behavior and electrical brain stimulation in the green iguana, *Iguana iguana* L. II. Stimulation effects. Exp Brain Res 31:353-367

Distel H, Veazey J (1982) The behavioral inventory of the green iguana, *Iguana iguana*. In: Burghardt GM, Rand AS (eds) Iguanas of the world. Their behavior, ecology, and conversation. Noyes, Park Ridge

Eibl-Eibesfeldt I (1979) Ritual and ritualization from a biological perspective. In: Cranach M v, Foppa K, Lepenies W, Ploog D (eds) Human ethology. Cambridge University Press, Cambridge, pp 3-55

Eibl-Eibesfeldt I (1984) Die Biologie des menschlichen Verhaltens. Grundriß der Humanethologie. Piper, München

Eibl-Eibesfeldt I (1984) Grundriß der vergleichenden Verhaltensforschung, 7. edn. Piper, München

Ekman P (1972) Universals and cultural differences in facial expressions of emotion. Nebraska symposium on motivation. University of Nebraska Press, Lincoln, pp 207-283

Ekman P, Levenson RW, Friesen WV (1983) Autonomic nervous system activity distinguishes among emotions. Science 221:1208-1210

Ellgring H (1989) Nonverbal communication in depression. Cambridge University Press, Cambridge

Ewert J-P (1989) The release of visual behavior in toads: stages of parallel/hierarchical information processing. In: Ewert J-P, Arbib MA (eds) Visuomotor coordination. Amphibians, comparisons, models, and robots. Plenum, New York, pp 39-120

Gamper E (1926) Bau und Leistungen eines menschlichen Mittelhirnwesens. Neurologie 102:154-235

Gerlinghoff M (1985) Magersüchtig. Piper, München

Geschwind N (1965) Disconnexion syndromes in animals and man. Brain 88:237-294, 585-644

Hamilton WD (1964) The genetical evolution of social behavior. J Theor Biol 7:1-16

Herzog M, Hopf S (1986) Recognition of visual pattern components in squirrel monkeys. Eur Arch Psychiatr Neurol Sci 236:10-16

Hopf S (1970) Report on a hand-reared squirrel monkey (*Saimiri sciureus*). Z Tierpsychol 27:610-621

Huxley J (1966) Introduction. In: Huxley J (ed) A discussion on the ritualization of behavior in animals and man. Philosophical transactions, vol 251, B 772. Royal Society, London, pp 247-524

Jaspers K (1923) Allgemeine Psychopathologie, 3. edn. Springer, Berlin

Jürgens U (1976a) Reinforcing concomitants of electrically elicited vocalizations. Exp Brain Res 26:203-214

Jürgens U (1976b) Projections from the cortical larynx area in the squirrel monkey. Exp Brain Res 25:401-411

Jürgens U (1979) Neural control of vocalization in nonhuman primates. In: Steklis HD, Raleigh MJ (eds) Neurobiology of social communication in primates. Academic, New York, pp 11-44

Jürgens U (1988) Central control of monkey calls. In: Todt D, Goedeking P, Symmes D (eds) Primate vocal communication. Springer, Berlin, pp 162-167

Jürgens U, Cramon D v (1982) On the role of the anterior cingulate cortex in phonation: a case report. Brain Lang 15:234-248

Jürgens U, Kirzinger A, Cramon D v (1982) The effects of deep-reaching lesions in the cortical face area on phonation. A combined case report and experimental monkey study. Cortex 18:125-140

Jürgens U, Ploog D (1970) Cerebral representation of vocalization in the squirrel monkey. Exp Brain Res 10:532-554

Jürgens U, Ploog D (1981) On the neural control of mammalian vocalization. Trends Neurosci, 4: 135-137

Kirzinger A, Jürgens U (1982) Cortical lesion effects and vocalization in the squirrel monkey. Brain Res 233:299-315

Kleist K (1934) Gehirnpathologie. Barth, Leipzig

Koenig O (1970) Kultur und Verhaltensforschung. Einführung in die Kulturethologie. dtv, München

Lorenz K (1935) Der Kumpan in der Umwelt des Vogels. J Ornithol 83:137-213, 289-413

Lorenz K (1937) Über die Bildung des Instinktbegriffes. Naturwissenschaften 25:289-300, 307-318, 324-331

Lorenz K (1950) The comparative method in studying innate behavior patterns. Symp Soc Exp Biol 4:221-268

Lorenz K (1965) Evolution and modification of behavior. Chicago University Press, Chicago

MacLean PD (1949) Psychosomatic disease and the "visceral brain." Psychosom Med 11:338-353

MacLean PD (1955) The limbic system ("visceral brain") and emotional behavior. Am Med Assoc Neurol Psychiatry 73:130-134

MacLean PD (1962) New findings relevant to the evolution of psychosexual functions of the brain. J Nerv Ment Dis 135:289-301

MacLean PD (1964) Mirror display in the squirrel monkey, *Saimiri sciureus*. Science 146:950-952

MacLean PD (1990) The triune brain in evolution. Plenum, New York

Maurus M, Barclay D, Kühlmorgen B, Wiesner E, Llorach-Forner V (1989) Synonymy in squirrel monkey calls? Lang Comm 9:69-76

Maurus M, Barclay D, Streit K-M (1988) Acoustic patterns common to human communication and communication between monkeys. Lang Comm 2:87-94

Maurus M, Kühlmorgen B, Wiesner E, Barclay D, Streit K-M (1985) "Dialogues" between squirrel monkeys. Lang Comm 5(3): 185-191

Maurus M, Mitra J, Ploog D (1965) Cerebral representation of the clitoris in ovariectomized squirrel monkeys. Exp Neurol 13:283-288

Maurus M, Ploog D (1984) Categorization of social signals as derived from quantitative analyses of communication processes. In: Harré R, Reynolds V (eds) The meaning of primate signals. Cambridge University Press, Cambridge, pp 226-241

Maurus M, Streit K-M, Barclay D, Wiesner E, Kuehlmorgen B (1988) A new approach to finding components essential for intraspecific communication. In: Todt D, Goedeking P, Symmes D (eds) Primate vocal communication. Springer, Berlin, pp 69-87

Maurus M, Streit K-M, Barclay D, Wiesner E, Kühlmorgen B (1986) Interrelations between structure and function in the vocal repertoire of Saimiri. Eur Arch Psychiatr Neurol Sci 236:35-39

McGuire MT (1979) Sociobiology: its potential contribution to psychiatry. Perspect Biol Med 23:50-69

McGuire MT, Essock-Vitale SM (1981) Psychiatric disorders in the context of evolutionary biology. A functional classification of behavior. J Nerv Ment Dis 169:672-686

McGuire MT, Essock-Vitale SM (1982) Psychiatric disorders in the context of evolutionary biology. The impairment of adaptive behavior during exacerbation and remission of psychiatric illnesses. J Nerv Ment Dis 170:19-20

Newman JD (1985) Squirrel monkey communication. In: Rosenblum LA, Coe CL (eds) Handbook of squirrel monkey research. Plenum, New York, pp 99-126

Newman JD, Symmes D (1982) Inheritance and experience in the acquisition of primate acoustic behavior. In: Snowdon CT, Brown CH, Petersen MR (eds) Primate communication. Cambridge University Press, Cambridge, pp 259-278

Papez JW (1937) A proposed mechanism of emotion. Arch Neurol Psychiatry 38:725-743

Ploog D (1958) Endogene Psychosen und Instinktverhalten. Fortschr Neurol 26:83-98

Ploog D (1963) Vergleichend quantitative Verhaltensstudien an zwei Totenkopfaffen-Kolonien. Z Morphol Anthropol 53:92-108

Ploog D (1966) Biological bases for instinct and behavior: studies on the development of social behavior in squirrel monkeys. In: Wortis J (ed) Recent advances in biological psychiatry, vol VIII. Plenum, New York, pp 199-223

Ploog D (1967) The behavior of squirrel monkeys (*Saimiri sciureus*) as revealed by sociometry, bioacoustics, and brain stimulation. In: Altmann SA (ed) Social communication among primates. University of Chicago Press, Chicago, pp 149-184

Ploog D (1969) Early communication processes in squirrel monkeys. In: Robinson RJ (ed) Brain and early behavior. Development in the fetus and infant. Academic, London, pp 269-298

Ploog D (1970) Social communication among animals. In: Schmitt FO (ed) The neurosciences. Rockefeller University Press, New York, pp 349-361

Ploog D (1974) Die Sprache der Affen und ihre Bedeutung für die Verständigungsweisen des Menschen. Kindler, München (Kindler Taschenbücher 2133)

Ploog D (1980) Soziobiologie der Primaten. In: Kisker KP, Meyer J-E, Müller C, Strömgren E (eds) Psychiatrie der Gegenwart, 2. edn, vol I/2. Springer, Berlin Heidelberg New York, pp 379-544

Ploog D (1981a) Neurobiology of primate audio-vocal behavior. Brain Res Rev 3:35-61

Ploog D (1981b) Neuroethological aspects of anorexia nervosa. In: Perris C, Struwe G, Jansson B (eds) Biological psychiatry 1981. Biomedical, Amsterdam, pp 1027-1034

Ploog D (1985) Anorexia nervosa — an addiction. In: Pichot P, Berner P, Wolf R, Thau K (eds) Psychiatry, vol 2. Plenum, New York, pp 717-720

Ploog D (1988a) An outline of human neuroethology. Human Neurobiol 6:227-238

Ploog D (1988b) Neurobiology and pathology of subhuman vocal communication and human speech. In: Todt D, Goedeking P, Symmes D (eds) Primate vocal communication. Springer, Berlin, pp 195-212

Ploog D (1989a) Psychopathology of emotions in view of neuroethology. In: Davison K, Kerr A (eds) Contemporary themes in psychiatry. Royal College of Psychiatrists, London, pp 441-458

Ploog D (1989b) Zur Evolution des Bewuβtseins. In: Pöppel E (ed) Gehirn und Bewuβtsein. VCH, Weinheim, pp 1-15

Ploog D (1990) Neuronale Substrate der Lust und Unlust. In: Heimann H (ed) Anhedonie. Verlust der Lebensfreude. Fischer, Stuttgart, pp 31-57

Ploog D (to be published) Evolution of vocal communication. In: Papousek H, Jürgens U, Papousek M (eds) Non-verbal vocal communication: comparative and developmental approaches. Cambridge University Press, Cambridge

Ploog D, Blitz J, Ploog F (1963) Studies on social and sexual behavior of the squirrel monkey (Saimiri sciureus). Folia Primatol (Basel) 1:29-66

Ploog D, Hopf S, Winter P (1967) Ontogenese des Verhaltens von Totenkopf-Affen (Saimiri sciureus). Psychol Forsch 31:1-41

Ploog D, Hupfer K, Jürgens U, Newman JD (1975) Neuroethologic studies of vocalization in squirrel monkeys with special reference to genetic differences of calling in two subspecies. In: Brazier MAB (ed) Growth and development of the brain. Raven, New York, pp 231-254

Ploog D, MacLean PD (1963) Display of penile erection in squirrel monkey (Saimiri sciureus). Anim Behav 11:32-39

Ploog D, Melnechuk T (1970) Primate communication. In: Schmitt FO, Melnechuk T, Quarton GC, Adelman G (eds) Neuroscience research symposium summaries, vol 4. The M.I.T.Press, Cambridge MA, pp 103-190

Ploog D, Melnechuk T (1972) Are apes capable of language? In: Schmitt FO, Adelman G, Melnechuk T, Worden FG (eds) Neuroscience research symposium summaries, vol. 6. The M.I.T.Press, Cambridge MA, pp 599-700

Ploog D, Pirke KM (1987) Psychobiology of anorexia nervosa. Psychol Med 17:843-859

Poeck K (1969) Pathophysiology of emotional disorders associated with brain damage. In: Vinken PJ, Bruyn GW (eds) Handbook of clinical neurology, vol 3. North Holland, Amsterdam, pp 343-367

Schott D (1975) Quantitative analysis of the vocal repertoire of squirrel monkeys (Saimiri sciureus). Z Tierpsychol 38:225-250

Steiner JE (1974) Innate, discriminative human facial expressions to taste and smell stimulation. Ann N Y Acad Sci 237:229-233

Sutton D, Larson C, Lindemann RC (1974) Neocortical and limbic lesion effects on primate phonation. Brain Res 71:61-75

Szmukler GI, Tantam D (1984) Anorexia nervosa: starvation dependence. Br J Med Psychol 57:303-310

Tinbergen N (1951) The study of instinct. Clarendon, Oxford

Ujváry Z (1966) Das Begräbnis parodierende Spiele in der ungarischen Volksüberlieferung. Österr Z Volkskd 69:267-275

Voland E, Voland R (1989) Evolutionary biology in psychiatry: the case of anorexia nervosa. Ethol Sociobiol 10:223-240

Whitman CO (1899) Animal behavior. In: Biol Lect Mar Biol Lab, Woods Hole. Ginn, Boston, pp 285-338

Wickler W (1966) Ursprung und biologische Bedeutung des Genitalpräsentierens männlicher Primaten. Z Tierpsychol 23:422-437

Wilson EO (1975) Sociobiology: The new synthesis. Harvard University Press, Cambridge

Winter P, Handley P, Ploog D, Schott D (1973) Ontogeny of squirrel monkey calls under normal conditions and under acoustic isolation. Behavior 47:230-239

Winter P, Ploog D, Latta J (1966) Vocal repertoire of the squirrel monkey (*Saimiri sciureus*), its analysis and significance. Exp Brain Res 1:359-384

Wolff PH (1987) The development of behavioral states and the expression of emotions in early infancy. University of Chicago Press, Chicago

2 Monkey Calls as a Model for the Neurobiological Investigation of Emotional Vocal Expression in Man

U. Jürgens

Monkeys possess a rich repertoire of vocal utterances expressing a variety of emotional states. In the squirrel monkey, for instance, there are calls that are uttered when an animal has lost contact with its group mates, thus expressing, in anthropomorphic terms, loneliness. There are other calls uttered during the sudden occurrence of unexpected, nondangerous events attracting the attention of the vocalizer, thus corresponding to the human surprise. There are numerous agonistic call types expressing all shades from self-confident threat through defensive threat and protest to frustration, submission, and panic — to mention only a few (Winter et al. 1966). Monkey calls thus represent highly differentiated emotional indicators.

Monkey calls differ from human speech in that they do not have to be learnt. More specifically, squirrel monkey infants that are raised by surgically muted mothers under acoustic isolation nevertheless produce all call types of the species-specific repertoire — despite the fact that they never had an opportunity to hear another monkey's calls (Winter et al. 1973). Monkey calls, furthermore, differ from verbal utterances by the fact that articulation, i.e., movements of the supra-laryngeal tract, does not play an essential role in the production of the calls: while human words are specified predominantly by different tongue, lip, jaw, and velum movements, the different monkey vocal patterns are determined almost exclusively by different laryngeal maneuvers.

Not all human vocal activity is verbal, however. There is a wealth of nonverbal emotional vocal utterances, such as laughing, crying, whimpering, moaning, and jubilating. Furthermore, the verbal component of speech is often superimposed by an emotional intonation component that adds to the verbal content an item of information about the emotional state of the speaker. Such emotional vocal expressions have in common with monkey calls that they are, to a large extent, genetically determined in their acoustic structure. This is suggested firstly by the fact that several nonverbal emotional utterances also occur in deaf-and-blind born, i.e., in persons who do not have the opportunity to learn these patterns from others, and must thus rely on genetically preprogrammed vocal patterns (Eibl-Eibesfeldt 1973). Secondly, transcultural comparisons of the emotional intonations used during anger, sadness, happiness, or disgust reveal common features for specific emotions across different languages and thus also suggest a genetic basis for this type of vocal behavior (Beier and Zautra 1972; Kramer 1964).

Human emotional vocal expression, furthermore, has in common with monkey calls that differences in emotional state are expressed by different laryngeal activity rather than different articulatory gestures. That is, vocal differentiation is

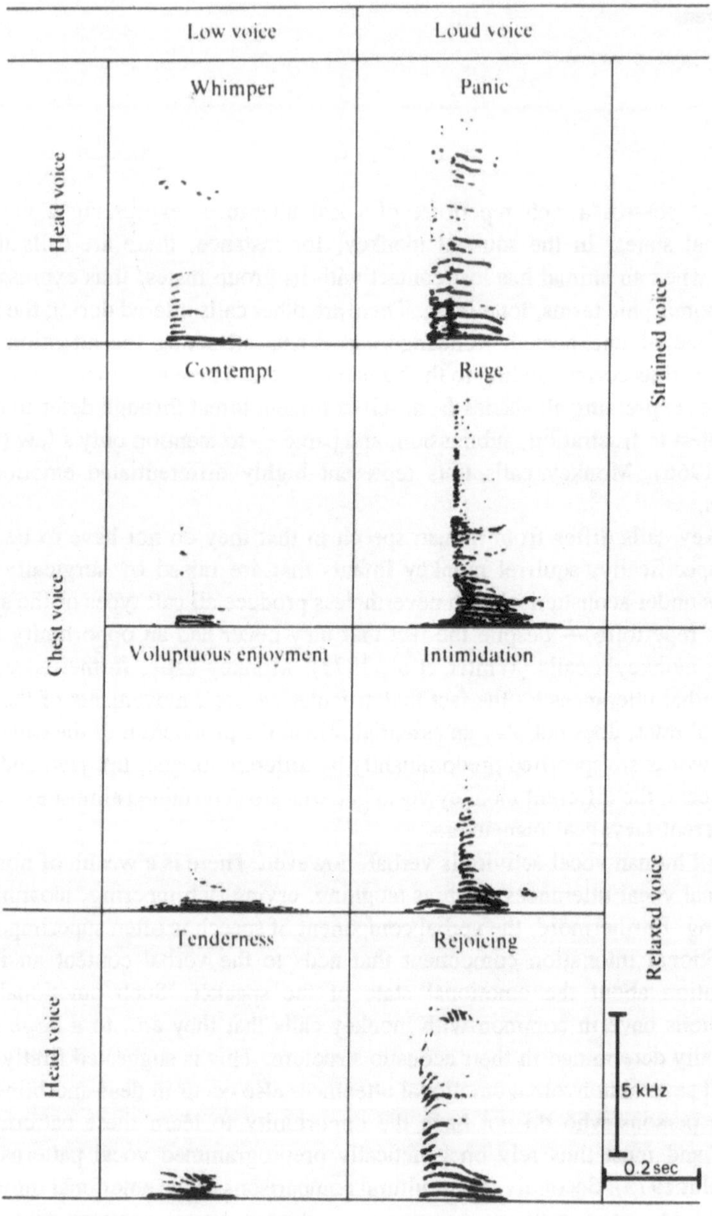

Fig. 1. Spectrographic representation of the German word *Du* in eight different intonations

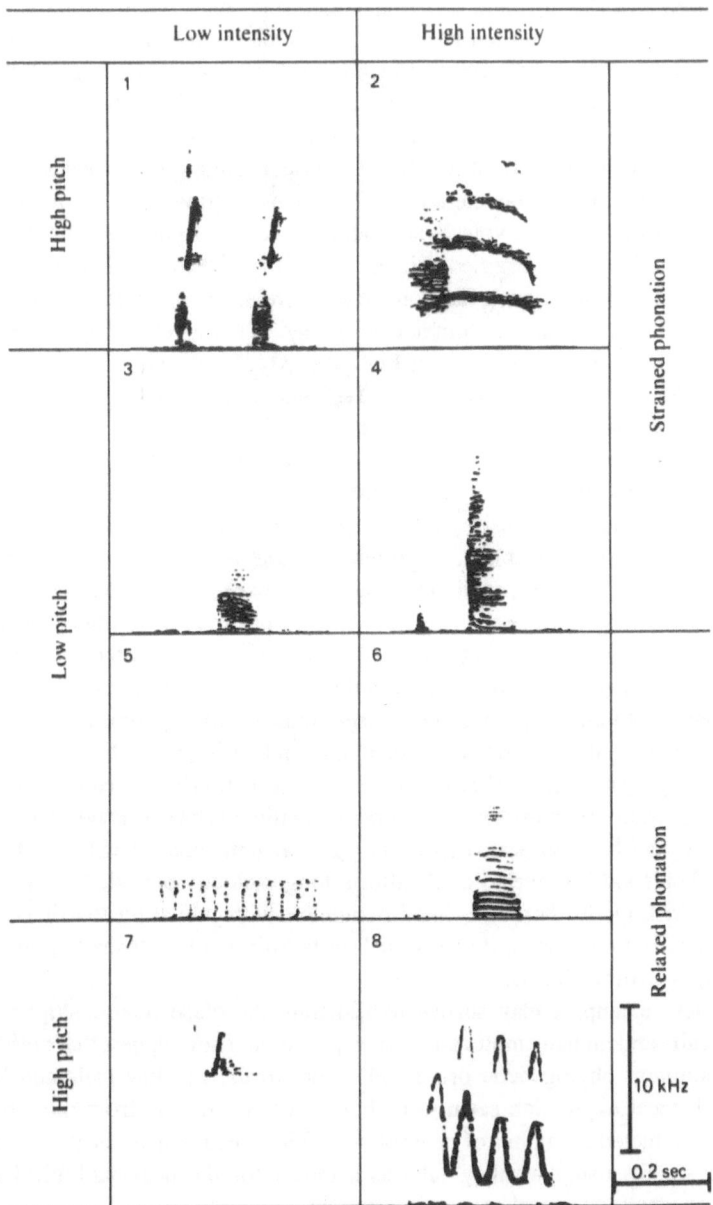

Fig. 2. Spectrographic representation of eight different vocalizations of the squirrel monkey (*Saimiri sciureus*). Call 1 is uttered by infants trying to regain their mother's back. Calls 2 and 3 express extreme distress and slight uneasiness, respectively. Call 4 is used during mobbing of potential predators. Call 5 is uttered by infants during suckling, and by adults during huddling and between copulatory activity. Call 6 represents a threatening call. Call 7 is a contact call and serves to draw other group members' attention to the vocalizer. Call 8 announces pleasurable external events (see text)

based on changes in fundamental frequency, frequency modulation, amplitude modulation, and ratio between harmonic and nonharmonic energy rather than on formants and formant transitions. Finally, preliminary results suggest that the acoustic features characterizing specific emotional states are similar in monkey and man. This follows from a classification scheme for human emotional intonations proposed by Trojan (1975). According to Trojan, emotional intonations can be characterized by three parameters (Fig. 1): intensity (low voice — loud voice), pitch (head voice — chest voice), and ratio between harmonic and nonharmonic energy (relaxed voice — strained voice). For example, tenderness is expressed by a relatively high proportion of harmonic energy (relaxed voice), low intensity, and high pitch. Jubilating has in common with tenderness a relaxed voice and high pitch; it differs from tenderness in its high intensity. If intensity and pitch are kept high, but phonation changes from a relaxed to a strained mode, a panic-stricken voice, expressing terror or intensive pain, emerges.

The same three parameters underlying the classification of intonations can be used also to classify monkey calls. In other words, monkey calls can be distinguished according to intensity, pitch, and proportion of nonharmonic energy (strain). In the squirrel monkey, a call which combines low intensity, high pitch, and lack of strain — a combination typical for the expression of tenderness in man — is the so-called "short peep" (Fig. 2, call 7). Short peeps are uttered whenever an animal wants to draw the attention of group mates near to the vocalizer in a nonagonistic situation. Their function is thus very similar to the human acoustic counterpart: both aim at getting into closer contact with a partner.

The squirrel monkey's acoustic pendant to the jubilating intonation — i.e., high intensity, high pitch, lack of strain — is the trill call (Fig. 2, call 8). Trilling, similar to jubilating, expresses a pleasurable emotional state: it is uttered when an animal that had been separated from its group regains contact with it; it is also uttered when food is detected or if, after a longer cloudy period, the sun breaks through. Trilling, furthermore, has in common with jubilating that it is a contagious vocalization; that is, if one animal starts trilling, others usually join it, thus producing a trilling chorus.

These few examples may suffice to illustrate the close relationship between monkey calls and human emotional vocal expression. They suggest that both forms have a common phylogenetic origin; in other words, monkey calls and human emotional vocal expression seem to be homologous. Starting from this premise, we have conducted a number of neurophysiological, neuroanatomical, and neurochemical studies using monkey calls as a model for the neurobiological investigation of emotional vocal expression in man.

In our first study, the squirrel monkey's brain was explored systematically for areas yielding vocalization when electrically stimulated (Jürgens and Ploog 1970). Figure 3 summarizes the results of this study. It can be seen that there are in fact a number of structures the activation of which produces species-specific calls. The majority of these structures belong to the limbic system, i.e., a group of phylogenetically old forebrain structures known to play a crucial role in the control of emotional behavior. Such limbic vocalization-eliciting structures are, e.g., the anterior cingulate cortex, amygdala, bed nucleus of the stria terminalis, septum, hypothalamus, and midline thalamus. Figure 3, furthermore, shows that not all of these structures produce the same call type. The midline thalamus, for instance, produces only a whistle-type warning call; the posterior periventricular hypothalamus yields exclusively cackling-like mobbing calls; the stria terminalis produces purring, a call normally uttered during huddling of group mates or suckling of infants. Some areas produce more than one call type, but these call types are usually functionally related.

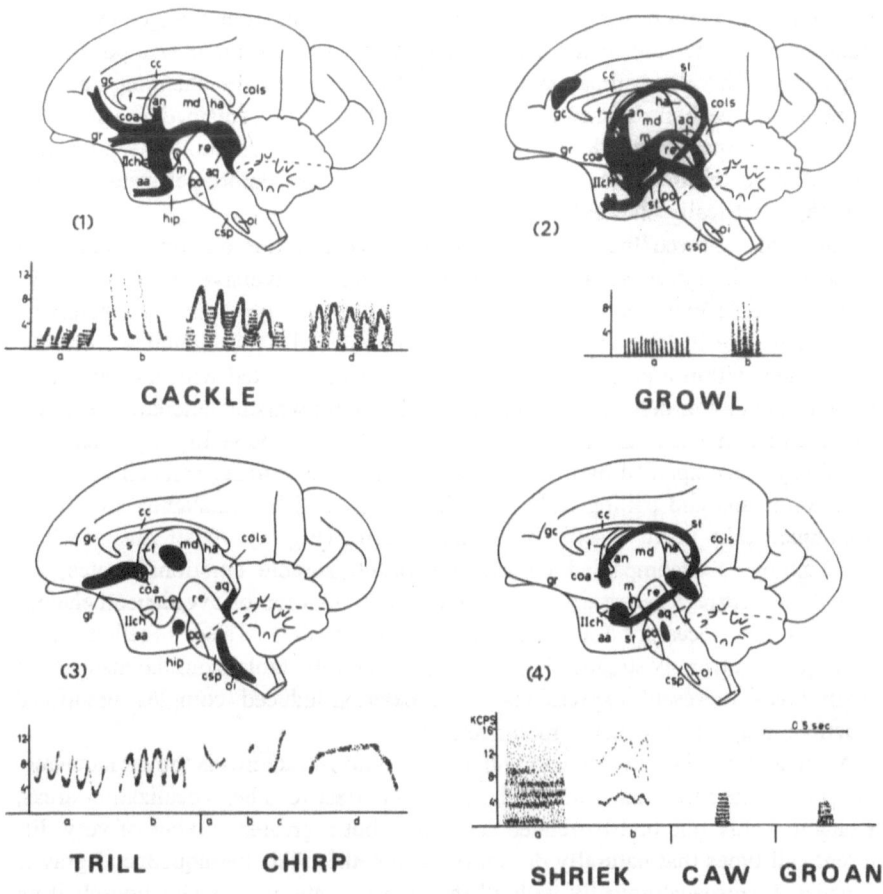

Fig. 3. Vocalization control areas in the squirrel monkey. The *black areas* represent brain structures the electrical stimulation of which yields vocalization. Below the brain diagrams, there are spectrographic representations of the call types elicitable. *Abbreviations:* aa, area anterior amygdalae; *an,* nucleus anterior thalami; *aq,* periaqueductal gray, *cc,* corpus callosum; *coa,* commissura anterior; *cols,* colliculus superior; *csp,* corticospinal tract; *f,* fornix; *gc,* gyrus cinguli; *gr,* gyrus rectus; *ha,* habenula; *hip,* hippocampus; *m,* corpus mamillare; *md,* nucleus medialis dorsalis thalami; *oi,* oliva inferior; *po,* griseum pontis; *re,* formatio reticularis mesencephali; *s,* septum; *st,* stria terminalis; *llch,* chiasma opticum.

From this the question arises of how the electrically elicited vocalizations must be interpreted: do they represent pure motor responses or are they expressions of electrically induced emotional states. In order to answer this question, we have carried out a self-stimulation study (Jürgens 1976). The study was carried out in such a way that squirrel monkeys were implanted with vocalization-eliciting electrodes and then placed into a cage consisting of two compartments. Presence in one compartment led automatically to stimulation of a vocalization-eliciting brain site; presence in the other compartment was devoid of stimulation. As the animal was free to move from one compartment to the other, it could switch on and off the vocalization-eliciting brain stimulation at will. The compartment in which the stimulation was given was not always the same, but changed every few minutes from one side of the cage to the other. In this way, it was possible to register whether the animal avoided stimulation by always changing into the stimulation-free compartment, followed stimulation, or remained in one compartment irrespective of the presence or absence of stimulation. The procedure thus allowed the detection of aversive and pleasurable emotional states accompanying electrically elicited vocalizations.

The study showed that in all, except two, vocalization-eliciting brain areas vocalization is indeed accompanied by pleasurable or aversive states. There is, furthermore, a close correlation between elicited call type and accompanying emotional state in the sense that one and the same call type elicitable from different sites within a particular structure is always associated with the same type of self-stimulation behavior. For instance, the alarm whistles elicitable from the midline thalamus and the shrieking calls elicitable from the ventral hypothalamus are always accompanied by avoidance behavior, while purring calls all along the stria terminalis and trilling calls from the dorsolateral hypothalamus are always accompanied by positive self-stimulation behavior (Fig. 4). At all sites at which vocalization is accompanied by aversive or pleasurable emotional states, the stimulation current necessary for positive self-stimulation or avoidance behavior is below that necessary for making the animal vocalize. Taken together, these observations strongly suggest that the vocalizations elicitable from the majority of brain areas represent expressions of stimulation-induced complex emotional reactions rather than isolated motor responses.

An area of special interest among the vocalization structures is the periaqueductal gray of the midbrain. Its stimulation, in contrast to other vocalization areas, yields not only one or two related call types, but a greater number of very different call types that naturally do not occur together. The periaqueductal gray is connected neuroanatomically with all the above-mentioned vocalization-eliciting areas, on the one hand, and the oro-laryngorespiratory motor coordination center in the reticular formation of the lower brain stem, on the other hand (Jürgens and Pratt 1979). After destruction of the periaqueductal gray, vocalizations can no longer be elicited from other brain structures; spontaneous vocalizations are also abolished. These observations suggest that the periaqueductal gray represents a central relay station of the vocalization system interconnecting the diverse motivation-controlling limbic structures with the phonatory motor-coordination apparatus.

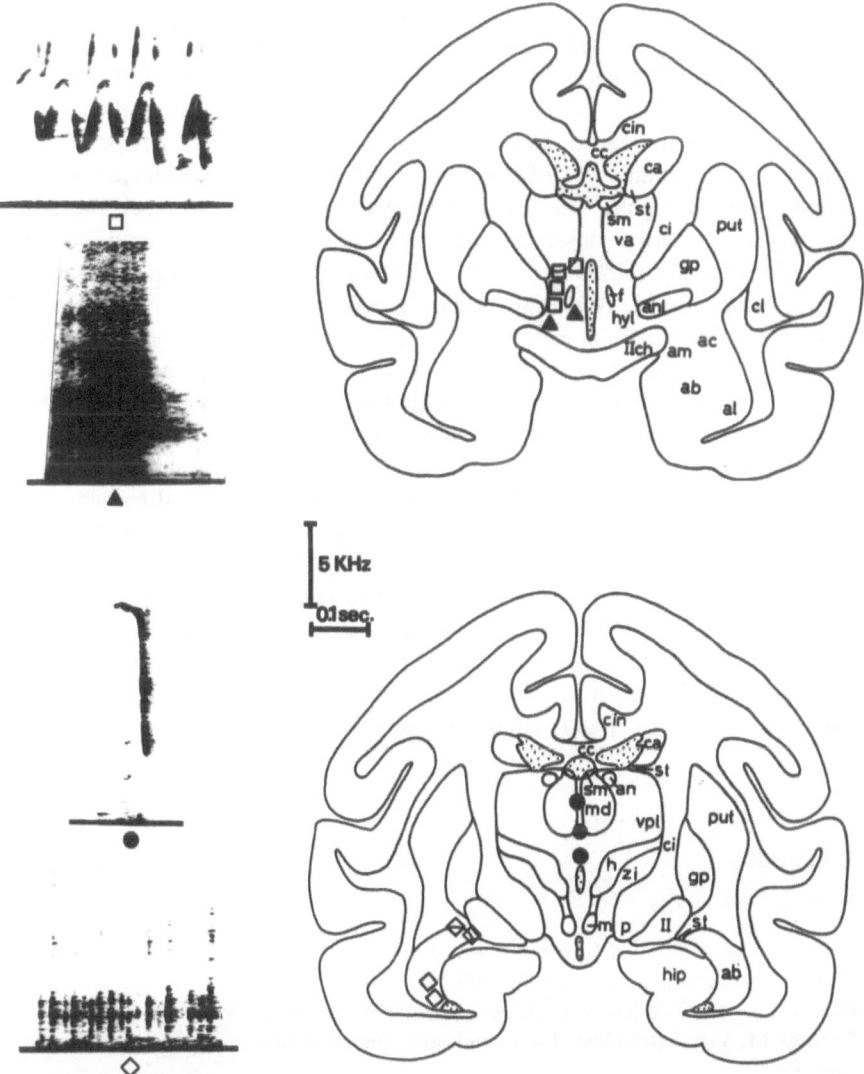

Fig. 4. Frontal sections of the squirrel monkey's brain with sites yielding trilling (*square*), shrieking (*triangle*), alarm whistles (*circle*), and purring (*rhomb*). The calls are represented in spectrographic form *on the left side*. All vocalization-eliciting sites yielding self-stimulation behavior are indicated by *white symbols*; those yielding escape/avoidance behavior are indicated *in black*. *Abbreviations: ab*, nucleus basalis amygdalae; *ac*, nucleus centralis amygdalae; *al*, nucleus lateralis amygdalae; *am*, nucleus medialis amygdalae; *an*, nucleus anterior thalami; *anl*, ansa lenticularis; *ca*, nucleus caudatus; *cc*, corpus callosum; *ci*, capsula interna; *cin*, cingulum; *cl*, claustrum; *f*, fornix; *gp*, globus pallidus; *h*, field H (Forel); *hip*, hippocampus; *hyl*, lateral hypothalamus; *m*, corpus mamillare; *md*, nucleus medialis dorsalis thalami; *p*, pedunculus cerebri; *put*, putamen; *sm*, stria medullaris; *st*, stria terminalis; *va*, nucleus ventralis anterior thalami; *vpl*, nucleus ventralis posterior lateralis; *zi*, zona incerta; *II*, nervus opticus; *IIch*, chiasma opticum.

In order to find out which neurotransmitters are involved in the information transfer in the periaqueductal vocalization center, we recently started a neuropharmacological study (Jürgens and Lu, to be published), in which we injected neurotransmitter antagonists into the periaqueductal gray and then tested the elicitability of vocalization from the forebrain. Until now we have tested antagonists of glutamate, acetylcholine, GABA, glycine, dopamine, norepinephrine, serotonin, histamine, and endorphin. The only antagonists that were able to block vocalization completely were the nonselective glutamate antagonists kynurenic acid and the *N*-methyl-D-aspartate (NMDA) receptor-specific glutamate antagonist 2-amino-5-phosphonovaleric acid. A partial inhibition, i.e., an increase in threshold, is obtained with glutamylaminomethyl-sulfonic acid, a glutamate antagonist that binds to quisqualate and kainate receptors, while no effect is obtained with glutamic acid diethyl ester that antagonizes specifically the quisqualate receptor. Blockade of a more recently proposed fourth type of glutamate receptor that binds to 2-amino-4-phosphonobutyric acid is also without effect. These findings suggest that glutamate or a related excitatory amino acid plays a crucial role in the neural transmission processes underlying the periaqueductal gray's control of emotional vocal expression. The responsible receptors seem to be of the NMDA and kainate subtype. It should be added that the antagonists of GABA, glycine and endorphin, when injected into the periaqueductal gray, in some cases lower the threshold for the elicitation of vocalization, i.e., have a facilitatory effect. This means that the periaqueductal glutamatergic vocalization control mechanism is modulated by GABAergic, glycinergic, and endorphinergic neurons.

References

Beier EG, Zautra AJ (1972) Identification of vocal communication of emotions across cultures. J Consult Clin Psychol 39: 166

Eibl-Eibesfeldt I (1973) The expressive behaviour of the deaf- and-blind-born. In: Von Cranach M, Vine J (eds) Social communication and movement. Academic, London, pp 163-194

Jürgens U (1976) Reinforcing concomitants of electrically elicited vocalizations. Exp Brain Res 26: 203-214

Jürgens U, Ploog D (1970) Cerebral representation of vocalization in the squirrel monkey. Exp Brain Res 10:532-554

Jürgens U, Pratt R (1979) Role of the periaqueductal gray in vocal expression of emotion. Brain Res 167: 367-378

Kramer E (1964) Elimination of verbal cues in judgment of emotion from voice. J Abnorm Psychol 68: 390-396

Trojan F (1975) Biophonetik. Wissenschaftsverlag, Mannheim

Winter P, Ploog D, Latta J (1966) Vocal repertoire of the squirrel monkey, its analysis and significance. Exp Brain Res 1: 359-384

Winter P, Handley P, Ploog D, Schott D (1973) Ontogeny of squirrel monkey calls under normal conditions and under acoustic isolation. Behaviour 47:230-239

3 Early Integrative and Communicative Development: Pointers to Humanity

H. Papoušek, M. Papoušek

Introduction

Complex interrelationships between the human brain and behavioral correlates have obliged research psychiatrists to seek interdisciplinary cooperation in attempts to define mental health and detect pathways of mental disorders. Comparative and developmental approaches have proven particularly profitable for several good reasons:

1. Progress in research on a neuronal base remains fruitless unless its involvement in behavioral regulation can be manifested.

2. The use of experimental animals and the search for animal models of human behavior have necessitated a thorough knowledge of similarities and dissimilarities between human and animal organisms.

3. Speculations on the critical significance of infantile experience for later mental health have been contrasted by a lack of detailed understanding of the needs and supportive interventions that might specifically operate on infant mental development.

4. Social interactions between infants and caretakers have long been disregarded in both etiopathogenetic and therapeutic concepts in psychiatry and have only vaguely been conceptualized as matters of mere emotional bonding.

Cooperation with other disciplines has not been a one-way avenue; psychiatrists have not only profited from but also contributed to research in related areas while, for instance, drawing attention to clinical entities which represent nature's experiments. Chronobiological aspects of endogenous manic-depressive disorders, differential involvement of Korsakoff's syndrome in procedural and declarative amnesias, or interrelations between consciousness and hemispheric division of brain functions may serve as examples of beneficial interchanges between psychiatry and neurosciences or other disciplines.

Biological approaches in psychiatry have drawn attention to the evolutionary past of mankind, and behavioral evolution in particular. Although paleontologists cannot interpret the evolution of behavioral patterns as clearly as the morphological evolution, behavioral evolution appeals to psychiatrists for good reasons. Evolutionary approaches have proven useful in elucidating the adaptive significance of behavioral patterns as well as the proportion of genetic determination in those patterns. For ethical reasons, innateness of behavioral patterns can seldom be directly evidenced in experimental designs. Human researchers have, therefore, looked for indirect indices and have considered comparative and developmental sources of evidence.

For instance, the following parameters in behavioral patterns have been suggested as indirect criteria of innateness by Papoušek and Papoušek (1987, to be published): involvement in species-specific means of evolutionary adaptation; universality across sex, age, culture, or species; early emergence during ontogeny; coevolution of behavioral counterparts in conspecifics; minimal conscious awareness and rational control; conceptual congruity in interpretation with respect to functionally interrelated behavioral patterns. From this viewpoint, developmental, comparative, or cross-cultural studies serve to test the borders of universality and help differentiate the relative contributions of biological and cultural determinants in human behavior.

Perhaps more important — and certainly much more difficult — is man's desire to understand the heritage and destiny of mankind and to differentiate adaptive from maladaptive tendencies in human behavior. The goal is — perhaps a fruit, perhaps an *agent movens* of human cultures — to define the borders between achievements and failures or mental health and mental disease. In terms of theory systems, the question is where the border lies between order and chaos; where do the dynamics become unpredictable and may lead to catastrophies. Here the interests of psychiatrists coincide with those of many other scientists, philosophers, educators, and artists. If this area of interest is not to be given up due to despair or superstitions, it is necessary — among other things — to extend the knowledge on long-term trends beyond the span of a mere few generations, be it with the help of paleontology, on the one hand, or cybernetic simulators on the other. This need is closely related to a better understanding of similarities and dissimilarities between man and other animals.

The Human Heritage

An increasing amount of paleontological and anthropological evidence has indicated that the pivotal role in the evolution of bipedality and of a large neocortex cannot be narrowed down to the use of tools, which was originally stressed in Darwin's interpretations (Darwin 1871). The earliest recognized tools are about 2 million years old whereas the marked expansion of the hominid cerebral cortex took place during the past 2 or 3 million years, and a complete morphological adaptation to bipedality during the period of *Australopithecus afarensis*, 3 or 4 million years ago.

Alternative interpretations indicate the influence of demographic factors upon the differentiation of hominids. For instance, Lovejoy (1981) believes that bipedality may have resulted from a mere variation in genetic reproduction. It represented a disadvantageous nonsaltatory form of walking; however, it might have been adopted due to advantages related to the demographic propagation, according to Lovejoy. Free hands facilitate caring for two or more dependent offsprings simultaneously, an advantage of particular importance in the case that offspring are produced at relatively short intervals and an infant is born before the preceding one has become independent. Birth spacing is shorter in man (2 - 4 years) than in other primates (for instance, 5 - 7 years in chimpanzees) and the difference becomes even more significant in relation to longevity. Thus it is possible that hominid ancestors of human parents had to cope with the presence of more than one dependent offspring. Disadvantages of bipedality in slower locomotion may have forced the selection of strong social bonds with advanced forms of communication in order to successfully protect one's self against predators.

Lovejoy's arguments require further verification and may be modified by future findings in paleontology; however, they have brought about a new view of the role of parent-infant interactions during human evolution. This view can no longer be disregarded in theories on behavioral development. The new concepts on human evolution focus much more attention on altruistic forms of social interactions than preceding theories which stressed aggressive behavior under the influence of animal research. The relatively long period of infant dependency is no longer viewed as a mere disadvantage in locomotion, but foremost as an advantageous prolongation of intense parenting with an early chance to support the progeny's integrative and communicative competence (Papoušek and Papoušek 1982).

While discussing the demographic propagation in hominids, Lovejoy also considers differences in reproductive behaviors as potential factors of divergence in hominids from pongids. For example, the continuous sexual receptiveness of hominid females, the absence of an externally recognizable estrous cycle, the shift from external signs of an estrous cycle to more variable epigamic features and to sexual uniqueness, together with the changing environmental conditions during Miocene, might have led to an equally stable male approach, to stable pair bonding, to the direct involvement of males in the survival of the offspring, and to a bifocal distribution of parenting. Monogamy, as Lovejoy points out, can be found only among those primates in which the male distinctly engages in the parenting process.

The continuous sexual receptiveness and the absence of synchronization between copulation and the estrous cycle have to be counterbalanced with some regulation of birth spacing if they are not to interfere with nursing as long as the youngest infant depends on maternal milk. A cross-cultural study of birth-spacing factors in the !Kung San hunters-gatherers in the Kalahari desert (Konner and Worthman 1980; Konner 1982) helped elucidate the problem of birth spacing and at the same time detected another aspect of mother-infant bonding, which — in addition to the protection against predators — may have influenced human evolution.

The span between births is around 44 months in the !Kung San families, although sexual activity continues and no contraception is used during those months; mild seasonal forms of undernutrition alone cannot explain the delay in further pregnancies. Unlike Western mothers, however, the !Kung San mothers

nurse children for up to 2 or 3 years in frequent intervals, which are shorter than
15 min on the average. The stimulation of the breast nipple elicits the hormone
prolactin which may effectively suppress gonadal functions and thus prevent the
next contraception but only if nursing intervals are shorter than the half-time of
prolactin in plasma, namely, 30 min. Consequently, mother-infant bonding may
have been selected as an effective control of birth spacing in addition to other
adaptive functions.

On the whole, unlike former concepts on attachment, the present scenario of
human evolution offers a much broader psychobiological view of early interactions
between human infants and caretaking environments. Moreover, two additional
aspects require attention in studies on early social interactions. First, the display
of emotional feelings and their processing by social counterparts may be more
complex in man than in other primates. Second, the selection of parent-infant
bonding may have been related to the selection of capacities necessary for social
communication and learning. The gaps in paleontological evidence on such
interrelationships call for more attention to processes detectable in early ontogeny.

Although parental care for infants' mental development may seem to be
determined culturally, we can hardly imagine that human culture may have
emerged independently of biological selection pressures or could neglect biological
determinants without dangerous consequences. Both human speech and human
culture have precursors in the animal world, for instance, in the capacity of
abstract symbolization in the honeybee *Apis mellifera* (von Frisch 1965), in the use
of categorical vocal signals in vervet monkeys (Seyfarth et al. 1980), in the
capacity of learning sign language in chimpanzees (Gardner and Gardner 1969),
or in the culture of "cleanliness" in the Japanese macaque monkeys (Kawai 1963).
Humans seem to be unique only in that they possess all prerequisites of speech
simultaneously: both a vocal tract which allows fast streams of finely differentiated
vocal sounds, and an intellectual competence which allows a many-sided application of verbal symbols in cultural communication have developed during
human evolution (Lieberman 1984).

The capability of using abstract verbal symbols enabled man to create a symbolic
world in which exploration and problem-solving could go beyond the physical
limits of the real world and of the individual's organism. In the symbolic world,
man found means of communication crossing the borders separating continents,
cultures, and strange species. Such a capacity allows man to accumulate and
process enormous amounts of knowledge and develop immensely powerful
technologies. In the same vein, however, the capacity helps man to overcome
biological constraints, to increase demographic propagation, and to improve
biological resistance. Thus, speech and culture have not only emerged from
biological roots but have also brought about biological consequences. Communication has doubtlessly been selected as a very effective means of human
adaptation. As such, communication can share the properties of biologically
relevant forms of adaptation: universality across sex, age, and culture; early
emergence during ontogeny; coevolution of behavioral counterparts in conspeci-

fics; and minimal conscious awareness and control (Papoušek and Papoušek 1987; to be published).

The Beginning of Integrative and Communicative Abilities

Let us now consider the potential effects of early parenting on infants' mental development. Two assumptions seem to be crucial for a successful interindividual sharing of experience between parents and infants. The infant should, at least, be capable of perceiving and processing parental information with the help of fundamental learning and cognitive operations. In Latin, *infans* means "incapable of speech" and clearly indicates the initial handicap in communication which is caused by immaturity of both the vocal tract and the intellectual competence. Conversely, the parent should be able to meet the infant's constraints, to adjust mode, amount, and timing of information to the infant's actual state of integrative capacities, and thus to facilitate didactically infant processing of information.

From the perspective of systems theory, the parent-infant dyad is a prototype of a didactic system with polar differences between the two partners in the amount of integrated life experience and in the level of communicative competence. Unfortunately, both the common means of communication within the dyad, and the mechanisms of intrinsic motivation — for acquisition of knowledge in the infant, and for sharing knowledge in the parent — have only recently met adequate degrees of interest in research. Theoretically significant aspects of early teaching and learning still wait for further experimental verification.

The paucity of studies on the earliest forms of educational processes may be caused by the lack of adequate models in animal behavior. The present literature concerns only simple forms of learning in the young of some species, and only anecdotal evidence on parental teaching. For instance, chimpanzees — in whom sufficient prerequisites may be available — show minimal inventiveness in teaching activities, although the cognitive development in the young is comparable with that in human infants (Chevalier-Skolnikoff 1982). Jane Lawick-Goodall (1967) observed situations in which young chimpanzees were obviously learning skills displayed by parents, however, parents showed no tendency didactically to utilize and control such opportunities as if they were not motivated for teaching interventions at all.

Human infants are predisposed very early not only for simple forms of learning but also for elementary forms of more complex cognitive operations. Habituation and basic forms of conditioning have been demonstrated in newborns (for a detailed survey see Rovee-Collier and Lipsitt 1982; Rovee-Collier 1987), including premature newborns (Solkoff and Cotton 1975). Similarly, imitation (Meltzoff and Moore 1983) and intentionality (Papoušek 1967), at least within the range of sufficiently coordinated motor patterns, function in newborns as well. During the rest of preverbal age, more complex capacities of discriminatory learning, detection and acquisition of rules, and concept formation including simple numerical concepts appear and have been studied in numerous projects (for surveys see Harris 1983; Papoušek 1977).

Long-term analyses of the developmental process in integrative capacities are rare; however, they evidence important circumstances. First, the early capacities are slow and unstable; for instance, they significantly fluctuate with changes in the infant's behavioral and emotional states. Second, the early capacities allow the infant to cope adaptively only with simple and frequently repeated environmental events. Third, the course of coping is accompanied with distinct affective expressions in the infant's facial and vocal behavior (Papoušek 1967, 1977). Therefore, the experimenter has to carefully design teaching situations along principles which do not substantially differ from didactic principles in teachers' activities. Stimulations have to be easily perceivable; their structure, amount, and timing have to be adjusted to the pupil's level of integrative competence.

For less dependent coping with highly variable environments and particularly for speech acquisition, the early integrative capacities necessarily have to be carried out faster and more economically. From this point of view, it is very important to realize that such acceleration and economization depends not only on maturation but also on training as demonstrated by Papoušek (1967, 1977). In his studies, the rate of infant learning depended significantly not only on age but also on experience from similar learning situations or on the arrangement of experiments which confronted infants first with easy and only then with more complex learning situations. These findings indicated that infants might profit from educational interventions and raised the question of whether there are natural learning situations in the infant's everyday life which could fulfill the assumptions of successful learning.

The search for natural learning situations has led to surprising results. Firstly, the most frequent learning situations have been found in infant interactions with social environment. Secondly — and more surprisingly — unpretended teaching capacities have been detected in unintentional, consciously uncontrolled patterns of parental behavior (Papoušek and Papoušek 1978, 1984, 1987). The non-conscious character of such teaching interventions explains why they had escaped observers' attention or traditional attempts to analyze parental behavior with the help of questionnaires. Moreover, it indicates a biological origin in behavioral tendencies to give the infant's mental development not only a nonspecific emotional but also a specific empirical support. Since the support — as we are going to show in more detail — corresponds to the principles of scholarly didactics and yet may be a product of evolutionary selection, it seems to represent a primary biological model of didactics (Papoušek and Papoušek 1987).

Microanalyses of parent-infant interactions which have helped detect natural teaching capacities in parents also evidence further important aspects. Due to typically short periods of latency in unintentional, intuitive responses, parents can easily cope with the fast flow of interactional episodes without being worn out by a multitude of rational decisions. On the contrary, they can enjoy the interaction, enrich it with emotional engagement and playful modifications, and thus increase its effect upon infants.

Similarly to schoolteachers, parents of infants are also confronted with the necessity to establish adequate conditions for infant learning such as an optimal level of infant attention, application of simple and repetitive messages, gradual ordering of skills to be trained, and adjustments to feedback signals indicating limits of infant tolerance. Unlike teachers, however, parents are neither aware of these conditions, nor academically prepared to fulfill them, nor can they rely upon verbal communication with infants. Yet, parents are preadapted for teaching infants, according to the Papoušeks (1987).

A few examples should illustrate parental preadaptedness. Since facial behavior plays a particularly important role both in nonvocal communication and in demonstrations of how to produce vocal sounds, parents tend strongly to attract the newborn's visual attention to parental face, position themselves *en face* in the newborn's visual field, and shorten the eye-to-eye distance to approximately 22.5 cm in order to facilitate visual perception. They reinforce the achievement of visual contact with a "greeting response" (retroflection of head, half-opened mouth, and raised eyebrows). Interestingly, such facilitation is fully independent of the parental belief that newborns may be unable to see anything during the first weeks of life (Schoetzau and Papoušek 1977; Papoušek and Papoušek 1987).

Correct estimates of the infant's behavioral state and responsiveness are crucial to teaching interventions but are difficult to read from young infants. Micro-analyses reveal that parents frequently test muscle tone either in the perioral area or in hands whenever they are to decide whether to entertain, feed, sooth, or lullaby the infant. Their attempts elicit distinguishable types of infant responses which help select the most suitable intervention (Papoušek and Papoušek 1982). Again, parents may respond to visible hand movements and believe that they respond to facial expression, according to experimental verification (Kestermann 1982). The rate and adequacy of parental behaviors are independent of parental sex but depend significantly on the amount of experience in infant care, according to Kestermann's study.

Parental preadaptedness is particularly evident in relation to vocal communication. There is a strong tendency for both parents and strangers to speak to newborns (Rheingold and Adams 1980). More important, they use a specific modification of speech — the so-called babytalk or motherese — when addressing newborns or preverbal infants, independent of the belief whether newborns can hear at all or whether infants should always hear only a correct form of adult speech. The characteristics of babytalk are very interesting. For instance, its average fundamental frequency is higher than that of narrative speech, its structure is simple and repetitive, vowels and intersegmental pauses are prolonged, and the melody of prosodic contours is strikingly enhanced and follows rules other than in adult narrative speech. Parents switch instantly from narrative speech to babytalk and vice versa if speaking alternatively to infants and adults.

If we consider the newborn's state of vocal competence and attempt to conceptualize suitable directions for environmental support and guidance, we find that characteristic babytalk corresponds to resulting directives in astonishing ways. The difference in average fundamental frequency may function as a signal that messages are directed toward the infant. Prolonged vowels may represent models for training the necessary control of respiration since newborns are not yet able to prolong expirium for the sake of quiet noncry vocalizations. Moreover, the initial vowel-like fundamental vocalization in very young infants allows the first modulations only in one feature — the melody — before the first consonants can be produced. Therefore, it is adaptive for the parent to display prolonged vowels in strikingly melodic forms and reward infant imitations (Papoušek and Papoušek 1981).

Melodic modulations are not as variable in parental babytalk as they could be. On the contrary, parents use only a small set of melodic contours but repeat them many times. They also free the contours from dependence on semantic rules of the narrative adult speech where contours — in far less conspicuous forms — give the sentence characters of statement, question, commands, etc. In babytalk, melodic contours play another role: they are tied to interactional contexts and give infants the first categorical messages to help them conceptualize the most relevant interactional situations (Papoušek, Papoušek and Bornstein 1985). For instance, parents use cuckoocalls when trying to achieve visual contact with infants, rising high-pitch contours when encouraging infants' participation in dialogues, bell-shape contours when rewarding infant smiles or new achievements in vocal and motor skills, or slowly falling low-pitch contours when soothing upset infants (Papoušek and Papoušek 1984, 1989).

Innovative studies have recently discovered another important predisposition for perception and processing of rapid acoustic chains similar to those in speech. Infants are obviously capable of segregating coherent acoustic elements (pitch modulations), discriminating them from the complex stream of acoustic background, and grouping them into holistic complexes on the base of similarity or proximity (Demany 1982; Fassbender 1989; Thorpe and Trehub 1989). It is not yet known whether this capacity is innate and specific to human infants, but it is in function in 1.5 to 5-month-olds at the latest (Fassbender 1989) and thus may be relevant to the exchange of melodic messages. The effect of parental contours on infant behavior has recently been demonstrated in the first experimental verification (Papoušek et al. 1990); encouraging contours increased and discouraging contours decreased infant visual attention to identical pictures of strangers.

With the infant's advancing age and vocal competence, parents adequately change teaching strategies and contents while following infant real progress rather than chronological age. Step by step, parents intuitively support the development of those prerequisites in both vocalization and cognition that are necessary for the prominent, species-specific achievement of human infancy — the acquisition of speech.

The interrelation between infant developmental progress and nonconscious adjustment in parental strategies can be illustrated with changes related to the differentiation of brain hemispheres. Prior to the age of approximately 8 months, infants can process and store relatively complex procedural but not yet declarative information; brain structures also allow processing of complex visual perception including the physiognomy of faces (de Schonen and Mathivet 1989). Until then, parents very seldom encourage the use of declarative messages, such as naming. Their teaching instructions mostly concern procedural skills and include displays of exaggerated facial expressions and prosodic melodies.

The onset of brain functions allowing verbal interchanges coincides with the appearance of reduplicated syllables in infant vocalization. Such syllables seem to act as cue signals for a new parental strategy: a strikingly increased use of declarative information with attempts to utilize every reduplicated syllable as a potential proto-word with some attributed lexical meaning. Similar parallelisms between infantile and parental repertoires of nonconscious behaviors strongly indicate innateness, due to coevolution of behavioral counterparts, as is true about behaviors of a high adaptive relevance (Papoušek 1989).

The hypothesis on innateness of intuitive parental behaviors is additionally reinforced by their universality and early emergence during ontogeny. Although the number of comparative studies is still limited, they evidence equal distribution of individual components of intuitive parental behaviors across parental sex and culture. For instance, the set of melodic contours in parental babytalk is the same not only in mothers and fathers (Papoušek and Papoušek 1984), but also in mothers using stress and tonal languages as demonstrated in cross-cultural comparisons of German, Caucasian American, and Mandarin Chinese mothers (Papoušek and Papoušek 1987). In narrative Mandarin Chinese speech, prosodic tone determines differences in lexical meaning of words. In spite of this, mothers use melodic contours in babytalk in the same form and manner as mothers speaking German or English.

In general, infancy researchers have described forms and the developmental process of early integrative and communicative abilities in human infants. However, they have also elucidated caretakers' competence for guiding and supporting the infant abilities. Accumulated data raise the question of human specificity in observed abilities.

The specificity cannot be looked for in the early beginnings of learning capacities. Basic forms of learning have been shown to start very early also in other animals. Operant conditioning in head turning, similar to what Siqueland and Lipsitt (1966) analyzed in human neonates, was also demonstrated in newborn rats by Johanson and Hall (1979). In cognitive development, young chimpanzees parallel human infants and children in all aspects with the exception of internal representation based upon verbal abstractions (Chevalier-Skolnikoff 1982). However, no animal parallel has yet been found to the early development of crucial requisites for the acquisition of speech, including an adequate vocal tract, complex neural structures (Lieberman 1984), and specific guidance by caretakers (Papoušek and Papoušek 1987). In this sense, humans seem to be both pre-cocious and unique.

Humanity Development at Risk

Intrinsic motivation for successful communication is still far from being measurable; however, to observers of parent-infant dialogues, it looks strong and is associated with a pleasurable and desirable experience. It is doubtless a substantial part of bonding. Equally effective may be the loss of communication or the inability to establish dialogic interchanges with a relevant social environment.

The present authors assume that such motivational aspects play an important role not only in the course of parent-infant interactions, but also in more general abilities to cope adaptively with various life conditions (Papoušek and Papoušek 1979). A favorable course of parent-infant interactions can generally increase the capability of interacting partners to resist various risk factors — biological, physical, or socio-cultural — and compensate for other occasional losses or failures. For instance, a healthy infant can successfully motivate a juvenile mother to overcome her rejection of unwanted motherhood, the loss of her lover, the opposition in her environment, etc.

On the contrary, interactional failures — often due to the lack of communication — can dangerously decrease the resistance against risk factors and, moreover, cause a vicious circle which may lead to developmental retardation in the child or to maladaptive parental tendencies including child neglect or child abuse. Altruism, which characterizes parental love in particular and humanity in general, may turn into aggression, and the reversal may originate in mere failures in communication. At the beginning of a vicious circle, the failures may be hardly visible and yet far easier to correct and overcome.

The role of communicative disorders in the history and therapy of psychiatric patients beyond the age of infancy has long been acknowledged and utilized. Conversely, the role of preverbal communication has not been understood long enough to find a sufficient clinical application. Moreover, specifically human aspects of communicative disorders cannot be studied in animal models. Further difficulties result from the complexity and diffuse character of lesions which have caused early developmental disorders.

The first clinical applications of concepts on early communicative disorders still lack experimental and statistical analyses. Nevertheless, a few comments on them may facilitate further projects and direct clinical attention to points of potential cooperation. The comments to be presented here are based upon valuable contributions from several centers where clinicians and therapists have tried to apply the concepts on preverbal interventions for several years. Particularly relevant experience has been accumulated at the Child Development Center in Hamburg (Director Dr. Inge Flehmig), the Rehabilitation Center in Landstuhl/Pfalz (Director Prof. Dr. Andreas Fröhlich), and the Child Center of the Maximilian University in Munich, Dept. of Social Pediatrics (Director Prof. Dr. Hubertus von Voss, successor to Prof. Dr. Theodor Hellbrügge).

Clinicians should keep in mind the twofold role of communication in preverbal interactions, namely, fulfillment of the need to be together and communicate with someone, on the one hand, and formation of the most adequate method for providing preverbal subjects with age-specific "educational materials," on the other. Earlier in this presentation, the two roles were explained in relation to preverbal infancy. Clinical experience has evidenced, however, that preverbal means of communication may also be effective beyond infancy age, for instance, in older children whose communicative level still corresponds to that of preverbal infants. Following the principles of preverbal support, therapists have been able to establish communication and strikingly increase motivation for further dialogues in retarded children beyond the age of 6 years.

The twofold role of communication explains the close and bilateral interrelationships between communicative and other disturbances in mental development. For instance, a primary social deprivation not only causes a defect in communication in otherwise healthy infants, but also a secondary mental retardation due to missing support for learning and cognitive abilities. In another case, a hearing defect in the infant can secondarily cause social isolation and, therefore, result in mental retardation. Or, conversely, a primary muscular hypotony with a decreased expressiveness in facial and vocal signalling can cause deficient communication, parental neglect, and secondary impairment of originally intact intellectual predispositions in infants. It is generally known that older children have frequently been treated as mentally retarded or behaviorally disturbed, although the primary defect originally concerned only the production of speech sounds (Martin 1981; Amorosa, to be published).

Thus, infants with intact mental predispositions can still become mentally retarded or deviated if environmental circumstances cause interactional failures and communicative difficulties. A mere reduction of maternal availability, such as in one of nature's experiments — the twins — may cause a mild retardation in speech development in the absence of other pathogenic factors (Bornstein and Ruddy 1984). Early detection of primary communicative defects in infants and therapeutic guidance in parent-infant interactions may, therefore, help prevent both impairment of speech acquisition and secondary retardation in other integrative capacities.

Conversely, if a primary disorder impairs mental development, proper guidance in interactional communication can not only fulfill the child's need for communication, but also preserve communication as an effective channel for delivery of preverbal educational material. The present understanding of preverbal forms of interactive communication confirms and extends former ethological findings on the role of nonverbal mother-child communication in the development of language (Mahoney 1975).

Although communicative and integrative disorders can interrelate in many directions, clinical experience has indicated the following combinations which deserve attention from the view of the discussed topics:

- *Missed Experience in the Initial Communication.* Sometimes one or both parents discover the first chance of interacting with the child rather late. Fathers, in particular, may be absent for various reasons and may miss the opportunity to orchestrate intuitive predispositions for parenting in accordance with the newborn's individuality. Similar difficulties may arise if the premature newborn has to be isolated due to intensive medical care, if the mother is not available due to perinatal complications, or if parents adopt an older infant. Most parents overcome such difficulties; however, some parents may be discouraged by initial failures and become unable to develop their predispositions for intuitive parenting without assistance, particularly if the infant keeps responding to them as strangers.

- *Initial Discouragement Due to Infant Handicaps.* Infant responsivity and communicative expressiveness may temporarily be reduced because of postpartum difficultes, such as muscular hypotony or increased sleepiness due to hyperbilirubinemia. Prior to infant recovery, parents' intuitive predispositions for communication may decrease as a consequence of unsuccessful attempts to initiate interchanges, of absent feedback signals from the infant, or of deviant forms in infant behavior and vocalization which are difficult to cope with. Without help, parental competence may be inhibited and fail at the time when the infant recovers and might be capable of the first interchanges.

- *Mismatch Between Parental and Infantile Predispositions.* In some cases, parental tendencies — adaptive under other conditions — may appear to be inappropriate and cause communicative failures. For instance, the infant's perceptual thresholds may rise due to various nervous disorders. The infant would then still respond to stimuli of increased intensities; however, the parent may tend to use careful and tender stimulation under the impression of being confronted with a sick and fragile infant. A thorough assessment of partial nervous handicaps helps disclosure of the reasons for mismatch and the choice of adequate forms of therapy.

- *Major Delay in the Need for Preverbal Forms of Communication.* Some children, retarded children in particular, cannot acquire speech during the first several years. In this period, they lose the features of babyishness which elicit intuitive caretaking, including a preverbal support for speech acquisition. Yet they still need the type of support which parents or caretakers are otherwise unintentionally capable of giving to preverbal infants. These children may be in a particularly disadvantageous situation: they lack elicitors of preverbal support, and at the same time their parents may lack the original competence due to frustrations from preceding efforts. This problem raises the question of whether intuitive forms of preverbal support can be intentionally incorporated into therapeutic measures and will be discussed later.

Thus far, available clinical experience has already confirmed that the knowledge and clinical application of formerly explained principles of intuitive parental interventions can improve communicative development and prevent the origin of dangerous vicious circles. Several aspects have appeared particularly relevant.

First, it has become evident that diagnostic procedures should include a systematic assessment of prerequisites for preverbal communication on the side of both the child patient and the caretaker. This assessment can hardly be based on any fast and simple test; it should include direct observations of interacting partners. The presence of disorders other than communicative ones should not distract attention from the level of communicative interchanges or else the diagnosis would be incomplete, and secondary failures in communication might weaken therapeutic measures.

Second, preventive care for proper development of communication or a therapy for detected communicative disorders should be regularly incorporated into therapeutic plans. A careful guidance of preverbal parent-infant interactions is a necessary part of such plans.

Third, clinical attempts to utilize intuitive forms of caretaking have evidenced that human predispositions of this sort can be elicited in the absence of infant cue signals and intentionally applied in therapy. As explained earlier in this presentation, parents can hardly control intuitive caretaking behaviors rationally or display them in the absence of infants. Fernald and Simon (1984) convincingly documented this in relation to the use of motherese.

However, a rational control is not entirely impossible; it can at least start an infant-caretaker interchange which then continues functioning as soon as the infant responds to the caretaker's efforts. The first signs of attention and feedback signals in the child seem to prime intuitive predispositions in the caretaker for further interchanges. The intentional start may thus open a way for a chain of unintentional interchanges. Experienced therapists can, in fact, find the most effective modes of communication in individual cases faster than parents and their encouraging examples can help parents regain self-confidence and motivate them for further efforts.

The existence of a biologically founded system of preverbal teaching may also raise the question of whether one of the possible "ideological frames" of early human rearing may be especially justifiable because of its biological origins. It is true that the needs of modern cultures may have outdated evolutionary relics in behavioral tendencies. It may be equally true, however, that the present alarming phenomena — overpopulation, world wars, or ecological disasters — signal dangerous deviations from predispositions, selected in the course of thousands of generations, and a necessity to disclose and correct such deviations.

Any attempt to answer this extremely difficult question can still be only speculative and brings us to the border between knowledge and belief. The younger generation of scientists should be aware of such questions and of the need to answer them. If a correction appears to be necessary, the intuitive forms of parental teaching interventions may still remain in the center of attention as natural vehicles for corrective messages during the proliferative period of human life. They may still be safer, easier, and less utopistic than other suggested ways, including genetic manipulation or a change from the parental role to sophisticated artificial substitutes. The present scientific generation should perhaps more carefully watch the growing danger that a flood of commercial educational aids for rearing superbabies might eliminate the parental role before its potential is fully understood. The development of humanity seems to face the danger of a crude dehumanization, and infancy researchers should not merely be witness to this.

References

Amorosa H (to be published) Disorders of vocal signalling in children. In: Papoušek H, Jürgens U, Papoušek M (eds) Nonverbal vocal communication: comparative and developmental approaches. Cambridge University Press, Cambridge

Bornstein MH, Ruddy M (1984) Infant attention and maternal stimulation: prediction of cognitive and linguistic development in singletons and twins. In: Bouma H, Bouwhuis E (eds) Attention and performance. Erlbaum, London, pp 433-445

Chevalier-Skolnikoff S (1982) A cognitive analysis of facial behavior in Old World monkeys, apes, and human beings. In: Snowdon CT, Brown CH, Petersen MR (eds) Primate communication. Cambridge University Press, Cambridge, pp 303-368

Darwin C (1871) The descent of man. Murray, London

Demany L (1982) Auditory stream segregation in infancy. Infant Behav. Develop 5:261-276

de Schonen S, Mathivet E (1989) First come, first served: a scenario about the development of hemispheric specialization in face recognition during infancy. Cah Psychol Cognit 9:3-44

Fassbender C (1989) Auditory grouping and segregation processes in infancy (doctoral dissertation). Free Univ (Dep Educat Sci) Berlin

Fernald A, Simon T (1984) Expanded intonation contours in mothers' speech to newborns. Dev Psychol 20:104-113

Frisch K von (1965) Tanzsprache und Orientierung der Bienen (in German). Springer, Berlin Heidelberg New York

Gardner RA, Gardner BT (1969) Teaching sign language to a chimpanzee. Science 165:664-672

Harris PL (1983) Infant cognition. In: Haith M, Campos JJ (eds) Infancy and developmental psychobiology, vol 2.Handbook of child psychology. Wiley, New York, pp 689-782

Johanson IB, Hall WG (1979) Appetitive learning in one-day-old rat pups. Science 205:419-421

Kawai M (1963) On the newly acquired behaviors of the natural troop of Japanese monkeys on Koshima Island. Primates 4:113-115

Kestermann G (1982) Gestik von Säuglingen: Ihre kommunikative Bedeutung für erfahrene und unerfahrene Bezugspersonen (in German) (doctoral dissertation). Univ Dep Biol, Bielefeld

Konner M (1982) Biological aspects of the mother-infant bond. In: Emde RN, Harmon RJ (eds) The development of attachment and affiliative systems. Plenum, New York, pp 137-159

Konner MJ, Worthman C (1980) Nursing frequency, gonadal function, and birth spacing among !Kung hunter-gatherers. Science 207:788-791

Lawick-Goodall J van (1967) My friends the wild chimpanzees. National Geographic, Washington

Lieberman P (1984) The biology and evolution of language. Harvard University Press, Cambridge

Lovejoy CO (1981) The origin of man. Science 211:341-350

Mahoney GJ (1975) Ethological approach to delayed language acquisition. Am J Ment Defic 80:139-148

Martin JAM (1981) Voice, speech and language in the child: development and disorder. Springer, Wien New York

Meltzoff AN, Moore MK (1983) Newborn infants imitate adult facial gestures. Child Dev 54:702-709

Papoušek H (1967) Experimental studies of appetitional behavior in human newborns and infants. In: Stevenson HW, Hess EH, Rheingold HL (eds) Early behavior: comparative and developmental approaches. Wiley, New York, pp 249-277

Papoušek H (1977) Entwicklung der Lernfähigkeit im Säuglingsalter (in German). In: Nissen G (ed) Intelligenz, Lernen und Lernstörungen. Springer, Berlin Heidelberg New York, pp 75-93

Papoušek H, Papoušek M (1978) Interdisciplinary parallels in studies of early human behavior: from physical to cognitive needs, from attachment to dyadic education. Int J Behav Develop 1:37-49

Papoušek H, Papoušek M (1979) Care of the normal and high risk newborn: a psychobiological view of parental behavior. In: Harel S (ed) The at risk infant (Int Congr Series 492:368-371). Excerpta Medica, Amsterdam

Papoušek H, Papoušek M (1982) Integration into the social world: survey of research. In: Stratton PM (ed) Psychobiology of the human newborn. Wiley, London, pp 367-390

Papoušek H, Papoušek M (1984) Learning and cognition in the everyday life of human infants. Adv Study Behav 14:127-163

Papoušek H, Papoušek M (1987) Intuitive parenting: a dialectic counterpart to the infant's integrative competence. In: Osofsky J (ed) Handbook of infant development (2nd edn). Wiley, New York, pp 669-720

Papoušek H (1989) Coevolution of supportive counterparts in caretakers: a potential contribution to the hemispheric specialization during early infancy. Cah Psychol Cognit 9:113-117

Papoušek H, Papoušek M (to be published) Early interactional signalling: the role of facial movements. In: Kalverboer AF, Hopkins B, Geuze RH (eds) A longitudinal approach to the study of motor development in early and later childhood. Cambridge University Press, Cambridge

Papoušek M, Papoušek H (1981) Musical elements in the infant's vocalization: their significance for communication, cognition and creativity. In: Lipsitt LP, Rovee-Collier CK (eds) Advances in infancy research, vol.1. Ablex, Norwood, pp 163-224

Papoušek M, Papoušek H, Bornstein MH (1985) The naturalistic vocal environment of young infants: on the significance of homogeneity and variability in parental speech. In: Field T, Fox N (eds) Social perception in infants. Ablex, Norwood, pp 269-297

Papoušek M, Papoušek H (1987) Models and messages in maternal speech to presyllabic infants in tone and stress languages. Presentation at the 6th Biennial Meetings Soc Res Child Develop, April, Baltimore

Papoušek M, Papoušek H (1989) Stimmliche Kommunikation im frühen Säuglingsalter als Wegbereiter der Sprachentwicklung (in German). In: Keller H (ed) Handbuch der Kleinkindforschung. Springer, Berlin Heidelberg New York, pp 465-489

Papoušek M, Bornstein MH, Nuzzo C, Papoušek H, Symmes D (1990) Infant responses to prototypical melodic contours in parental speech. Infant Behav Dev 13:539-545

Rheingold HL, Adams JL (1980) The significance of speech to newborns. Dev Psychol 16:397-403

Rovee-Collier C (1987) Learning and memory in infants. In: Osofsky J (ed) Handbook of infant development (2nd ed). Wiley, New York, pp 98-148

Rovee-Collier CK, Lipsitt LP (1982) Learning, adaptation, and memory in the newborn. In: Stratton P (ed) Psychobiology of the human newborn. Wiley, New York, pp 147-190

Schoetzau A, Papoušek H (1977) Mütterliches Verhalten bei der Aufnahme von Blickkontakt mit dem Neugeborenen (in German). Z Entwicklungspsychol Pädagog Psychol 9:1088-1089

Seyfarth RM, Cheney DL, Marler P (1980) Vervet monkeys alarm calls: semantic communication in a free-ranging primate. Anim Behav 28:1070-1094

Siqueland ER, Lipsitt LP (1966) Conditioned head-turning in human newborns. J Exp Child Psychol 3:356-376

Solkoff N, Cotton C (1975) Contingency awareness in premature infants. Percept Mot Skills 41:709-710

Thorpe LA, Trehub SE (1989) Duration illusion and auditory grouping in infancy. Dev Psychol 25:122-127

4 Analysis of Fine Motor Problems in Children with Specific Developmental Disorders of Speech and Language

H. Amorosa, M. Noterdaeme

Introduction

As background for a discussion of fine motor problems in children with specific developmental disorders of speech and language, an explanation seems necessary about why such problems are of interest in child psychiatry. And this in turn necessitates a brief discussion of the relationship between speech/language disorders and psychiatric disorders in children.

The distribution of psychiatric diagnoses in children differs from that in adults. In both of the major classifications of mental disorders, the ICD-10 (in preparation) and DSM-III-R, special sections for disorders beginning in childhood or adolescence highlight this fact. In ICD-10 these sections are mental retardation (F7), disorders of development (F8), and behavioral and emotional disorders beginning in childhood and adolescence (F9). Moreover, in a study of all out-patient facilities serving children with psychiatric and developmental disorders in three counties in Germany, Remschmidt and Walter (1989) showed that specific emotional disorders, conduct disorder, and the special syndromes, all included in section F9 of ICD-10, constitute the major portion of psychiatric diagnoses made for children and adolescents. A large percentage of the children seen in these outpatient facilities have specific developmental disorders of speech and language, of motor coordination, or of both, coded in section F8 of the ICD-10. A combination of psychiatric problems and one or more developmental disorders is very common.

Psychiatric Disorder and Language Disorder

Several studies have shown that about half of the children with speech or language disorders have a psychiatric diagnosis (Stevenson and Graham 1985; Cantwell and Baker 1985). In a study of our own we observed 24 children between 4;6 and 8;0 years of age with unintelligible speech, normal intelligence, and normal hearing. Nine of these children (37%) also had a psychiatric diagnosis — 5 of them hyperkinetic syndrome of childhood (ICD-9, 314) and 4 of them a disturbance of emotions specific to childhood and adolescence (ICD-9, 312; Amorosa et al. 1986b). There is no agreement about why there is this coexistence of psychiatric symptoms and speech and language disorders. A common third factor such as minimal brain dysfunction (MCD) has often been discussed.

We saw a significant increase in behavioral disorders in those children with speech/language disorders who were also diagnosed as having MCD, a diagnosis based on abnormalities in the neurological examination according to Touwen (1982), a pathological EEG, and a history of high risk for early brain damage. Behavioral abnormalities did not contribute to the diagnosis. The children with both a psychiatric disorder and a diagnosis of MCD were almost exclusively boys with hyperactivity (ICD-9, 314); Berger et al. 1990). However, Esser et al. (1983) found no correlation between MCD, as they defined it, and psychiatric disorders in a group of 8-year-old children with speech and language disorders.

Most studies that address the question of the interrelation of psychiatric symptoms and speech/language disorders with third factors, especially brain damage or brain dysfunction, have used global measurements such as "psychiatric diagnosis," "neurologically abnormal," and "risk factors for early brain damage in the history of the child." These global categories are insufficient for the assessment of the role of brain damage. Studies of brain development in vertebrates have shown that the concept of brain damage used does not capture the complexity of the processes induced by interference with the normal development of the brain.

The level of development of the brain at the time of damage is an important predictor for later behavioral deficits (Isaacson and Spear 1984). For example, Largo et al. (1986) found a high correlation between problems with language development and nonoptimal perinatal signs but no correlation with signs of prenatal problems. These findings suggest that it is important to specify the time of occurrence associated with risk factors.

Findings on functional deficits also depend on the level of development at the time of assessment. In longitudinal studies of infants at risk (Touwen et al. 1982; Hadders-Algra et al. 1986), major abnormalities were found when the children were seen as toddlers, but learning disabilities, and especially speech and language disorders, were often detected only after the children had reached school age.

Another important aspect is the task that is investigated. We know from positron emission tomography (PET) studies that different areas of the brain are involved in such seemingly closely related tasks as repetitive and successive finger movements. Repetitive touching of the thumb with the index finger does not lead to an increase in metabolism in the supplementary motor area, whereas successive touching with all four fingers does (Orgogozo and Larsen 1979; Roland et al. 1980). If the general term "neurologically abnormal" is used, important differences in the type of brain disorder could be overlooked.

Consequently it seems important to analyze specific functions of the brain in much more detail than heretofore to collect information on specific patterns of deficit before conclusions can be drawn about common factors underlying the psychiatric and developmental disorders that occur together in so many children.

In the following some results are presented of studies performed at the children's department of the Max Planck Institute of Psychiatry on motor functions in children with specific developmental disorders of speech and language. This diagnostic category is used for children with abnormalities of speech and language development only when the deficit cannot be attributed either to low IQ or to hearing loss. Some of the children with this diagnosis are so severely affected that they are unintelligible to strangers well into their school years. Often their utterances are short, with incorrect word order and grammatical markers. And some of the children have problems not only with producing but also with understanding language.

Problems with motor coordination have often been reported in the group of children with speech/language disorders, but systematic studies are rare and frequently fine and gross motor functions have not been separated. Very few studies include speech as one type of fine motor task.

Fine Motor Coordination

There were two reasons why we focused our attention on fine motor functions. First, in children with speech and language disorders fine motor development is not age appropriate. Second, the organization of control of the hands and of speech is very similar (Evarts 1981), in both cases involving large parts of the brain. Areas in the precentral and frontal cortex, the thalamus, and the cerebellum are involved in the control of both systems. These areas are considerably larger in man than in primates.

The cortex, especially the precentral area, seems to be important for individuation and fractionation (Evarts 1984), factors important for the speed and accuracy of speech and finger movements. The supplementary motor area together with the lateral cerebellum plays a role in planning and automatizing sequences of movements, whereas the intermediate cerebellum mediates incoming sensory input for the updating of ongoing movements. Deficits in either function will lead to problems in complex motor tasks, but for different reasons.

The areas involved in speech and hand control have different developmental schedules. One would assume that damage to the developing organism at different stages would have differential effects on later performance on fine motor tasks. At the same time, one would expect different cognitive and behavioral disorders to be associated with the resulting functional deficit.

Studies on Hand Motor Control

We have been interested in determining whether specific fine motor functions of the hands are impaired or whether there is a more general delay in all functions. In a study of 21 children with specific developmental disorders of speech and language between 7 and 13 years of age (Bäumler 1989), we compared the children's performance on a fine motor test to that of a control group of children with normal speech and language development matched for age and sex. The test *(Leistungsserie nach Schoppe)* is based on factors described by Fleishman (1972) as being important for fine motor performance.

The scores of the children with speech/language disorders were not uniformly depressed in all subtests. There was a significant interaction effect between group and hand. The children in the experimental group differed little from those in the control group in their performance with the left hand, but their performance with the right hand was significantly worse. Another interesting finding is related to the children's performance profiles for the subtests. In the control group the best results were on the tapping task, whereas in the experimental group the worst results were usually on this subtest.

We can therefore conclude that problems of fine motor coordination are specific and do not indicate a general delay. The first result suggests that the typical improvement of the right hand during the preschool and school years (Wolff and Hurwitz 1976) does not occur in the group of children with speech and language disorders. The improvement of the right hand is indicative of the ability to isolate or individuate movements for specific tasks and to regulate the force, e.g., fractionate the movement, both of which functions are cortically represented (Kuypers 1982; Phillips and Porter 1977; Evarts 1984).

The second result, the poor performance on the fast tapping task, indicates a similar deficit. The speed of tapping can be increased by moving the fingers only, rather than the whole hand. But children with developmental disorders of speech and language very often use the arm and shoulder in addition. They cannot isolate the movements sufficiently. In a similar group of patients, Noterdaeme et al. (1988) also observed this insufficient individuation of movements. Tapping speed is also dependent on precise temporal coordination of the actions of agonist and antagonist. The lateral cerebellum probably plays an important role here.

The results reported are differences in group means. Interindividual variability in the experimental group was higher than in the control group in all studies, which suggests that problems of fine motor coordination of the hands are not uniform in the group of children with specific developmental disorders of speech and language.

Our studies on hand motor control suggest that as a group children with specific developmental disorders of speech and language have problems with individuation and fractionation of movements and with the precise temporal coordination of agonist and antagonist. The group is not homogeneous, and dysfunctions are seen in varying combinations in different children. In a longitudinal study of finger movements now in progress we are following the time course of each movement.

We hope this study will give us more information on individual performance and allow inferences about possible impairment of cortical, subcortical, or cerebellar functions.

Studies on Speech Motor Control

An impairment of speech motor control cannot be detected by observing simple movements of the tongue or lips, as is usually done in clinical studies. Instead, procedures must be used that allow the study of speech movements during speaking without interfering with the speech act itself. Acoustic analysis of tape-recorded utterances is a technique that has been used to analyze disorders of speech movements in adults with dysarthria and dyspraxia, but only rarely to study speech disorders in children.

Changes in the acoustic signal are due to changes in the vocal tract, caused by movements of the articulators, the larynx, or the speech breathing system. If speech tasks are selected carefully, changes in the acoustic signal will allow inferences about specific aspects of the underlying movements. In digitized utterances, defined segments can be analyzed in terms of duration, energy distribution and intensity changes. Since tape recordings of simple speech tasks can be used, acoustic analysis is well suited for work with children.

Fricatives are sounds produced with a narrow constriction at some point in the vocal tract through which air escapes, producing a noise that lasts at least 100 ms. These sounds require movements that are much more fractionated than those required for stop consonants (Hardcastle 1976) and a delicate balance between agonist and antagonist muscles. Our acoustic analysis of fricative production in children with developmental speech and language disorders showed that such children have problems not only establishing the correct position of the articulators but also keeping the articulators in a stable position. For the initial movement to be executed correctly, fractionation and fine coordination of agonist and antagonist forces is necessary, whereas maintaining the position of the articulators over time requires precise timing of modulated force changes (Schäfersküpper et al. 1986; Winner 1990). The children had problems similar to those described for hand movements, showing deficits on tasks requiring fractionation and precise temporal coordination of agonist and antagonist.

In the study already cited of 24 children between 4;6 and 8;0 years of age with unintelligible spontaneous speech we analyzed the production of simple syllable repetitions such as /papapa/, /tatata/, and /kakaka/ and the syllable string /pataka/. The children in the experimental group spoke more slowly and showed more variability in syllable duration, energy distribution, and intensity changes than the children with normal speech development matched for age (Amorosa 1989). The fast repetition of syllables requires the individuation of movements: For example, the syllable /ta/ can be repeated faster when only the tongue tip is moved, not the tongue body or the jaw. The repetition becomes less variable when automatized movement sequences are used. Both the individuation of movements and the automatizing were less well developed in the group of children with specific developmental speech and language disorders.

A second result of the study was that a significant portion of the children with unintelligible speech were unable to produce the syllable string /pataka/ several times correctly in succession. This inability was unrelated to the speed with which the children were able to repeat simple syllables (Thron, unpublished data). Again, the automatizing of sequences of simple movements was affected. The children often were able to repeat the sequence /pataka/ a few times under conscious control, but failed when they had to continue to do so, or if they were asked to speed up.

The results reported are group results. In the studies on speech movements discussed here both the inter- and intraindividual variability were significantly higher in the experimental group than in the control group, which suggests that the children were heterogeneous with regard to type of disorder.

Discussion

The results reported here together with those from studies we have done on the speech breathing system and the phonatory system (Amorosa et al. 1986a; Amorosa et al. 1990) are a clear indication of problems in fine motor control of speech and hand movements in children with specific developmental disorders of speech and language. The findings are in agreement with clinical descriptions. Moreover, they show that deficits in fine motor control in children with specific developmental disorders of speech and language can be attributed to several different aspects of movement control: the individuation, fractionation, coordination of agonist and antagonist forces, and automatizing of movement sequences. In complex motor tasks deficits in any of these areas can lead to decreases in performance. But only simple tasks allow differentiation among different deficits, and this differentiation is necessary if conclusions are to be drawn about brain-behavior relationships.

The interindividual variations in performance in our experimental groups suggest that the underlying deficits and hence the brain regions involved are different in different children. We postulate that these differences in underlying deficits indicate differences in the time or type of interference with brain development or differences in the response of the brain to such interference or both. If we use the concept of the brain as a self-organizing system (e.g., Singer 1987; von der Malsburg and Singer 1988), such responses to unusual conditions have an important effect on later behavior. In such a self-organizing system genetic information sets border conditions but sensory input and attentional processes are also important determinants of the self-organizing process. We can expect that even small changes in the system or in experience can lead to major changes in outcome. A similar concept of a self-organizing and self-optimizing system has been postulated for the development of the sound system of a language (Lindblom et al. 1983). Two important factors contribute to this development, factors of fine motor control and those of sound discrimination.

Both the brain and the fine motor behavior of the hands and speech develop as complex integrated systems that interact during pre- and postnatal development. If we could gain a better understanding of these interactions and the resultant fine motor behavior it might then be easier to explain the occurrence of different types of behavior disorders in children with developmental speech and language disorders.

References

Amorosa H (1989) Die Untersuchung kindlicher Sprechbewegungsstörungen mit Hilfe der akustischen Analyse, Habilitation (postdoctoral thesis). University of Munich, Munich

Amorosa H, von Benda U, Dames M, Schäfersküpper P (1986a) Deficits in fine motor coordination in children with unintelligible speech. Eur Arch Psychiatry Neurol Sci 236:26- 30.

Amorosa H, von Benda U, Wagner E (1986b) Die Häufigkeit psychiatrischer Auffällig-keiten bei 4- bis 8jährigen mit unverständlicher Spontansprache. Z Kinder Jugend-psychiatr 14: 289-295

Amorosa H, von Benda U, Wagner E (1990) Voice problems in children with unintelligible speech as indicators of deficits in fine motor coordination. Folia Phoniatr 42:64-70

Bäumler C (1989) Untersuchung über Störungen der Feinmotorik bei sprachentwick-lungsgestörten Kindern, Dissertation (doctoral dissertation). University of Munich, Munich

Berger F, Amorosa H, Scheimann G (1990) Psychiatrische Auffälligkeiten bei sprachauffäl-ligen Kindern mit und ohne Minimale Zerebrale Dysfunktion. Z Kinder Jugendpsychiatr 18:71-77

Cantwell DP, Baker L (1985) Psychiatric and learning disorders in children with speech and language disorders: a descriptive analysis. In: Gadow KD (ed) Advances in learning and behavioral disabilities, vol 4. JAI, Greenwich, pp 29-47

Esser G, Lehmkuhl G, Schmidt M (1983) Die Beziehung von Sprechstörungen und sprach-lichem Entwicklungsstand zur zerebralen Dysfunktion und psychiatrischen Auffälligkeiten bei 8-jährigen Grundschülern. Sprache Stimme Gehör 2:59-62

Evarts EV (1981) Analogies between central motor programs for speech and for limb movements. In: Grillner S, Lindblom B, Lubker J, Persson A (eds) Speech motor control. Pergamon,Oxford, pp 19-41

Evarts EV (1984) Hierarchies and emergent features in motor control. In: Edelman GM, Gall WE, Cowan WM (eds) Dynamic aspects of neocortical function. Wiley, New York, pp 557-579

Fleishman EA (1972) Structure and measurement of psychomotor abilities. In: Singer RN (ed) The psychomotor domain — movement behaviour. Philadelphia, pp 78-106

Hadders-Algra M, Touwen BCL, Huisjes HJ (1986) Neurologically deviant newborns: neurological and behavioral development at the age of six years. Dev Med Child Neurol 28:569-578

Hardcastle WJ (1976) Physiology of speech production. Academic, London, p.157

Isaacson RL, Spear LP (1984) A new perspective for the interpretation of early brain damage. In: Finger S, Almi CR (eds) Early brain damage, vol 2, neurobiology and behavior. Academic, Orlando, pp 73-98

Kuypers HGJM (1982) A new look at the organization of the motor system. In: Kuypers HGJM, Martin GF (eds) Anatomy of descending pathways to the spinal cord. Elsevier, New York, pp 381-403

Largo RH, Molinari L, Pinto LC, Weber M, Duc G (1986) Language development of term and preterm children during the first five years of life. Dev Med Child Neurol 28:333-350

Levelt WJM (1989) Speaking: from intention to articulation. Bradford, London, p. 592

Lindblom B, MacNeilage P, Studdert-Kennedy M (1983) Self-organizing processes and the explanation of phonological universals. Linguistics 21:181-203

Noterdaeme M, Amorosa H, Ploog M, Scheimann G (1988) Quantitative and qualitative aspects of associated movements in children with specific developmental speech and language disorders and in normal pre-school children. J Hum Movement Studies 15:151-169

Orgogozo JM, Larsen B (1979) Activation of the supplementary motor area during voluntary movement in man suggests it works as a supramotor area. Science 206:847-850

Phillips CG, Porter R (1977) Corticospinal neurones: their role in movement. Academic, New York, p.435

Remschmidt H, Schmidt M (1986) Multiaxiales Klassifikationsschema für psychiatrische Erkrankungen im Kindes- und Jugendalter nach Rutter, Shaffer und Sturge, 2nd edn. Huber, Bern, p.168

Remschmidt H, Walter R (1989) Evaluation kinder- und jugendpsychiatrischer Versorgung. Enke, Stuttgart, p.362

Roland PE, Larsen B, Lassen NA, Skinhoj E (1980) Supplementary motor area and other cortical areas in organization of voluntary movements in man. J Neurophysiol 43:118-136

Schäfersküpper P, Amorosa H, von Benda U, Dames M (1986) Spektrale Energieverteilungen des /s/-Lautes bei sprachentwicklungsgestörten Kindern. Folia Phoniatr 38:36-42

Singer W (1986) The brain as a self-organizing system. Eur Arch Psychiatry Neurol Sci 236:4-9

Singer W (1987) Activity-dependent self-organization of synaptic connections as a substrate of learning. In: Changeux JP, Konishi M (eds) The neural and molecular bases of learning. Wiley, New York, pp 301-336

Stevenson J, Graham P (1985) Behaviour problems and language abilities at three years and behavioural deviance at eight. J Child Psychol Psychiatry 26:215-230

Touwen B (1982) Die Untersuchung von Kindern mit geringen neurologischen Funktionsstörungen. Thieme, Stuttgart, p.186

Touwen B, Lok-Meijer T, Huisjes H, Olinga A (1982) The recovery rate of neurologically deviant newborns. Early Hum Dev 7:131-148

von der Malsburg C, Singer W (1988) Principles of cortical network organization. In: Rakic P, Singer W (eds) Neurobiology of neocortex. Wiley, New York, pp 96-100

Winner A (1990) Ein akustisches Analyseverfahren zur Untersuchung von Artikulationsbewegungen bei der Produktion stimmloser Frikative von sprachlich unauffälligen und sprachentwicklungsgestörten Kindern. Dissertation (doctoral dissertation). University of Munich, Munich

Wittchen H-U, Saß H, Zaudig M, Koehler K (1989) Diagnostisches und statistisches Manual psychischer Störungen — DSM-III-R. Beltz, Weinheim, p.530

Wolff PH, Hurwitz I (1976) Sex differences in finger tapping: a developmental study. Neuropsychologia 14:35-41

World Health Organization (1978) Mental disorders: glossary and guide to their classification in accordance with the ninth revision of the international classification of diseases. WHO, Geneva

5 What Is Old and What Is New in the Genetics of Endogenous Psychoses?

E. Zerbin-Rüdin

The genetic problem of psychiatric disorders is currently being tackled from many angles, with various methods, and in different populations. The endogenous psychoses are being approached by methods of molecular genetics as well as of Mendelian genetics and quantitative biometric genetics. Research strategies at the physiological, anatomical, biochemical, and molecular level supplement studies at the behavioral level. Reports are widely scattered and the results are not infriquently contradictory. What follows is a brief survey of some of the main lines of research and some of the principal results.

Behavioral, Clinical Level

The most certain results are still at quite a superficial clinical and phenomenological level. The good old familial risk figures for the schizophrenias and affective psychoses worked out for the first time by Rüdin (1916) and his school (e.g.,Schulz 1932) at the Deutsche Forschungsanstalt für Psychiatrie (now the Max Planck Institute for Psychiatry) have been confirmed by many subsequent family studies, some of them quite recent (for surveys see, e.g., Zerbin-Rüdin 1980a,b; Dunner et al. 1988). The family data have been supplemented by the results of twin and adoption studies.

The best predictor for both schizophrenic and affective psychoses is to be the monozygotic twin of a patient: The risk for schizophrenia is about 60%-80% and for affective psychosis about 70%. To be the sibling or offspring of a patient still has a high predictive value: The morbidity risk is 10%-15% for schizophrenia and 10%-20% for the affective psychoses.

It is clear that different genetic factors play a role in the schizophrenias and the affective psychoses, but what they are is still unknown. Mendelian ratios cannot be recognized in the families, and the concordance rates in the monozygotic twins are far from 100%.

It was hoped that Mendelian ratios would emerge by "lumping" (i.e., including borderline cases and marginal or related disorders in the endogenous psychoses) or by "splitting" (i.e.,excluding marginal and atypical groups from the core groups). But the use of these techniques has not made the genetic situation any clearer.

- *Lumping:* Some twin studies have suggested that traits such as schizoidia or untreated minor depression might be abortive manifestations of endogenous psychoses. However, these traits are so frequent in the general population and they occur so often in individuals with no family history of psychosis that it is premature, if not unrealistic, to assume that they are all related genetically to the endogenous psychoses. Some of them may be, but most are probably not.

- *Splitting:* Some quantitative and qualitative differences in the family data for various clinical subgroups have emerged. In the schizophrenias, for instance, the familial morbidity risk decreases from the hebephrenic, to the catatonic, to the paranoid forms, and the clinical picture of probands and secondary cases is similar in many, but not all, cases. But the differences observed do not suffice to suggest genetic heterogeneity. Therefore, criteria on which to base other subdivisions are being sought, e.g., early versus late onset of illness, paranoid versus nonparanoid forms, productive versus nonproductive symptomatology.

In the affective psychoses, Angst (1966), Perris (1966) and Winokur and Clayton (1967) uncovered some genetic differences between unipolar (depressive) and bipolar (manic-depressive) forms. However, the hope that a clear-cut genetic dichotomy would emerge from an increasing amount of data was not borne out. Therefore, the most recent and most widely accepted hypothesis is that unipolar and bipolar psychoses have at least part of their genetic basis in common. Multifactorial causation and multithreshold models are favored. Based on these models a continuous scale of liability to affective illness is postulated, the liability being determined by genetic and environmental factors in continuous variation with two or more thresholds. Illness will result when liability is greater than a threshold value. If the first threshold is exceeded, i.e., if a certain number of factors are present, the result is a unipolar psychosis; surpassing a second threshold gives rise to a bipolar psychosis, and surpassing a third to schizoaffective psychosis.

Multifactorial threshold models are helpful because they demonstrate how complex the etiology of psychiatric illness is. However, they also oversimplify the situation because they take into consideration the quantity but not the quality of contributing factors and they allow for additive effects only, but not for interacting and epigenetic effects. All of the models fit some of the empirical data only, and the same empirical data have been analyzed and interpreted in different ways, which has given rise to contradictory conclusions. As long as the presumed factors or some of them are not identified, the models are hypothetical and of limited value.

As is well known, the American DSM-III (Diagnostic and Statistical Manual of Mental Disorders, 3rd edition), as opposed to the ICD-9 (Mental Disorders: Glossary and Guide to Their Classification in Accordance with the Ninth Revision of the International Classification of Diseases), has dropped the time-honored term "endogenous psychosis" and has given up the traditional dichotomy of endogenous depression versus non-endogenous, nonpsychotic, neurotic, reactive depression. American authors have tried to support or refute the new concept and also other diagnostic systems by using family data. To put it very simply: If a classification allows placement of patients and their affected relatives in the same diagnostic categories, it is correct, i.e., it is "true." If it does not, it is not "true," it is not in agreement with reality. Papers have been published with titles such as "DSM III schizophrenia: Is there evidence for familial transmission?" (Tsuang et al. 1985). The authors' conclusion is yes. In depression the findings favor the new concept less clearly. When studying papers like "The validation of the concept of endogenous depression. A family study approach" (Andreasen et al. 1986) or "The validity of four definitions of endogenous depression" (Zimmerman et al. 1986) the reader, especially the European reader, is sometimes inclined to draw conclusions different from those the authors have reached.

In earlier times the family data suggested that the schizoaffective psychoses belonged to the schizophrenias, whereas today they suggest a relationship with the affective psychoses. This shift can be explained in part by the different methods of ascertaining the probands. Formerly schizoaffective probands were selected from among patients presenting with schizophrenic symptomatology but not fitting the Kraepelinian definition adequately; today they come from patients fulfilling standardized diagnostic criteria for affective disorder, but also showing schizophrenic symptoms. All studies agree that the familial risk for homotypical secondary cases is very low, but that the global risk for various psychiatric disorders is quite high. To be sure, the schizoaffective psychoses are heterogeneous. Besides cases related genetically to either the schizophrenias or the affective psychoses, a small group breeding true may exist. Genetically mixed schizoaffective psychoses with schizophrenia and affective psychosis occurring separately in the maternal and paternal lines are very rare (Zerbin-Rüdin 1986).

For many decades psychiatric geneticists endeavored to prove a close relationship between schizophrenia on the one hand and schizoidia and other personality disorders on the other — in vain. Today they are searching for genetic relationships between the affective psychoses and subaffective disorders, anxiety and panic reactions, anorexia and bulimia, neuroses, and alcoholism (Zerbin-Rüdin 1988). All of these disorders are to some degree controlled by genes, but the views on whether, and if so to what extent, they are related genetically differ widely. As an example, Table 1 shows the conflicting results on depression, anorexia, and

Table 1. Familial relations between depression and eating disorders

The morbidity risk for depression in the relatives of anorectic (A) and/or bulimic (B) patients is increased:	
In all A	Winokur et al. 1980; Rivinus et al. 1984; Gershon et al. 1984
Only when A themselves are depressed	Biederman et al. 1985
More when A is bulimic than when nonbulimic	Strober et al. 1982
Not at all in normal weight B	Stern et al. 1984
At the same rate in A, AB, and normal weight B	Hudson et al. 1983

bulimia. As long as there are no conclusive findings to the contrary, it seems appropriate not to consider affective psychoses and the other disorders mentioned as varying manifestations of the same genetic basis.

Winokur et al. (1971) proposed a subdivision of depression into pure depression and spectrum depression, with the genes in spectrum depression expressing themselves as depression in the women only, and as alcoholism or sociopathy in the men. This conclusion is debatable because the methodology of the study is open to serious question. As a general rule, disorders with different clinical pictures have a higher probability of being genetically different than of springing from identical genes. Quite often even phenomenologically identical disorders are genetically heterogeneous.

Intermediate Level

It can be assumed that neuropsychological and neurophysiological traits are somewhat closer to the genetic basis than behavioral traits. Deficits in attention and association, deviations in the galvanic skin response, and anomalies of eye movements have been observed frequently in schizophrenic patients, but have been studied only rarely in the relatives. Thus the family data are sparse and not unequivocal.

Griesinger and Kraepelin considered schizophrenia to be a brain disease, and in the course of time a multitude of neuropathological findings were described (e.g., Vogt and Vogt 1952). Dilated ventricles were noted as early as 1927 by Jacobi and Winkler (1927). However, many different cellular changes were seen, and taken together they provided no evidence for any specific and obligatory structural abnormality in schizophrenia. Therefore the neuropathological approach fell somewhat into disuse, the more so as the new antipsychiatry movement took little heed of neuropathology.

At present neuropathology is gaining increasing attention again, especially under developmental aspects (Kerwin 1989; Lewis 1989). Weinberger (1987) proposed that "schizophrenia is a neurodevelopmental disorder in which a fixed brain lesion from early in life interacts with certain normal maturation events that occur much later." Thus very early brain lesions are thought to give rise to abnormal development in various brain areas and, finally, to schizophrenia.

Another hypothesis is that pre- and perinatal traumata such as gestational and obstetric complications produce minor brain damage and, provided genetic liability for schizophrenia is present, schizophrenia. As a third possibility, early brain damage or anatomical anomalies may be the basis for sporadic, nonfamilial, nongenetic schizophrenia (Reveley et al. 1984).

Russian authors especially suspected that immunological mechanisms play an important role in the etiology of schizophrenia and found brain antibodies and antithymic immune factors in schizophrenic patients and their nonaffected relatives in proportions close to Mendelian ratios (Koliaskina et al. 1980; Vartanian et al. 1978). However, other research groups were unable to reproduce these findings.

Propping (1989) speculated that a considerable proportion of the schizophrenias are symptomatic, i.e., they are possible but not cogent manifestations of various biochemically defined genetic disorders. This is the view of a biochemist rather than of a psychiatrist.

The most promising candidates in the chorus of suspected etiological factors for schizophrenia are neurochemical and endocrine variables, especially the neuro-transmitters. For the time being researchers are busy (a) defining the normal range of activity of these substances, (b) finding out whether, and if so when, decreased or increased activity is abnormal and specific for some psychiatric disorder, and (c) working out whether, and if so how, this activity is under genetic control. Considering the present state of knowledge, it is not yet promising checking nonaffected relatives whenever patients have any abnormal findings. When this was done in the past the findings in the relatives were usually negative; obviously the deviations were state dependent and not trait dependent. There have been some promising attempts, however. For example, Bondy and Ackenheil (1987) found that the binding capacity of lymphocytes for the dopamine antagonist spiperone was increased not only in schizophrenic patients but also in about 50% of their nonaffected relatives. Confirmation is needed. The same is true for the following finding: When exposed to bright light depressed patients and some of their relatives react with increased suppression of melatonin (Goldin 1988).

Chromosomal and Molecular Level

Nowadays geneticists do not think so much in terms of genes as in terms of DNA sequences, and psychiatric geneticists rarely speak of genes for schizophrenia or affective psychoses, but mostly of genetic vulnerabilities, liabilities, and predictors. A novel strategy to identify or localize the parts of DNA responsible for or contributing to vulnerabilities for psychiatric disorders is the search for biological markers, vulnerability markers, and linkage markers.

Vulnerability markers usually have a share in the process of illness and are under genetic control. Possible markers are, for example, neurotransmitters, other endogenous peptides, and immunological and endocrine factors. In the affective psychoses more than ten variables have been tested for their usefulness as vulnerability markers — to no avail (Gershon et al. 1983). Neither has the search for vulnerability markers in schizophrenia been successful.

Linkage markers are traits with known chromosomal localization that occur together with the trait of interest more often than by chance. They do not have any inner relationship with it, but are situated next to it in the DNA helix and thus label it. They must be present before and after onset of illness and in remission.

Color blindness, Xg blood group, and glucose-6-phosphatase deficiency have been used as linkage markers for affective psychoses. They are located on the X chromosome and were expected to prove an X-chromosomal mode of transmission. However, as color blindness and Xg blood group are situated on opposite ends of the X chromosome, the claimed linkage with both of them is hardly possible. Moreover, father-son transmissions are not uncommon, although they should not occur in X-linked transmission. Thus X-chromosomal inheritance exists in some families only, if at all (Zerbin-Rüdin 1987a)! Linkage of schizophrenia with the HLA complex was suggested and studied repeatedly, but could not be proven.

The most recent strategy uses DNA probes or restriction fragment length polymorphisms (RFLPs) as linkage markers. With this method Huntington's disease was localized on chromosome 4 (Gusella et al. 1983). In the late 1980s the discovery of genetic markers for bipolar psychosis on chromosome 11 and for schizophrenia on chromosome 5 was sensational. But unfortunately it turned out to be an error. The findings could not be reproduced and methodological flaws were demonstrated in the original reports (Edwards and Watt 1989; Detera-Wadleigh et al. 1989). Nevertheless the method is most promising (Bulyzhenkov et al. 1990).

Summary

State of Knowledge. At the behavioral level the empirical familial morbidity risk figures for endogenous psychoses have been established. Further research along traditional lines is useless. Beyond doubt, genetic factors are involved, but they are as unknown as are contributing environmental factors. The mode of transmission is simply unknown; arguing about it will not help. Quantitative biometric methods have served us well in the past, but now seem to have nothing more to offer (Zerbin-Rüdin 1983, 1985).

Current Research Strategies. At the superficial behavioral level clinical subgroups other than the classical ones are being tried out and checked for their genetic characteristics. Studies at the neuropsychological, neurophysiological, neurochemical, and immunological level are expected to bring us closer to the genetic basis. In the schizophrenias neuroanatomical research has been revived and symptomatic schizophrenias are being studied. In the affective psychoses possible genetic relations to subaffective disorders, alcoholism, anxiety, panic disorder, anorexia, and bulimia are being looked for.

"I came to realize the importance of descending from the top...down to the more analyzable molecular level. Now, of course, the challenge is to climb...from the molecular bottom up again to the analysis of the complex phenotype" (Bodmer 1981) to do justice to the individual as a whole and to nongenetic influences. Genetic psychiatry research at the clinical and phenotypic level has not become superfluous. Without it one might be in the position of the six blind wise men from East India who groped at an elephant: Each described meticulously certain circumscribed parts of the animal, but they were still unable to recognize the elephant as a whole.

References

Andreasen NC, Scheftner W, Reich TH, Hirschfeld RMA, Keller MB (1986) The validation of the concept of endogenous depression. A family study approach. Arch Gen Psychiatry 43:246-251

Angst J (1966) Zur Ätiologie und Nosologie endogener depressiver Psychosen. Monogr Gesamtgeb Neurol Psychiatr. Springer, Berlin Heidelberg New York

Biederman J, Rivinus T, Kemper K, Hamilton D, MacFadyen J, Harmatz J (1985) Depressive disorders in relatives of anorexia nervosa patients with and without a current episode of nonbipolar major depression. Am J Psychiatry 142:1495-1497

Bodmer WF (1981) The William Allan reward address: gene clusters, genome organization, and complex phenotypes. When the sequence is known, what will it mean? Am J Hum Genet 33:664-682

Bondy B, Ackenheil M (1987) 3H-Spiperone binding sites in lymphocytes as possible vulnerability marker in schizophrenia. J Psychiatr Res 21:521-529

Bulyzhenkov V, Christen Y, Prilipko L (eds) (1990) Genetic approaches in the prevention of mental disorders. Springer, Berlin Heidelberg New York

Detera-Wadleigh SD, Goldin LR, Sherrington R, Encio I, de Miguel C, Berrettini W, Gurling H, Gershon ES (1989) Exclusion of linkage to 5q11-13 in families with schizophrenia and other psychiatric disorders. Nature 340:391-393

Dunner DL, Gershon ES, Barret JE (eds) (1988) Relatives at risk for mental disorder. Am Psychopath Assoc Series. Raven, New York

Edwards JH, Watt DC (1989) Caution in locating the gene(s) for affective disorder. Psychol Med 19:273-275

Gershon ES, Nurnberger JI, Nadi NS, Berrettini WH, Goldin LR (1983) Current status in genetic research in affective disorders. In: Angst J (ed) The origins of depression: current concepts and approaches, Dahlem Workshop. Springer, Berlin Heidelberg New York, pp 187-204

Gershon ES, Schreiber JL, Hamovit JR (1984) Clinical findings in patients with anorexia nervosa and affective illness in their relatives. Am J Psychiatry 141:1419-1421

Goldin LR (1988) Biological variables as predictors in relatives at risk. In: Dunner DL, Gershon ES, Barrett JE (eds) Relatives at risk for mental disorder. Am Psychopath Assoc Series. Raven, New York, pp 1-8

Gusella JF, Wexler NS, Conneally PM, Naylor SL, Anderson MA, Tanzi RE, Watkins PC, Ottina K, Wallace MR, Sakaguchi AY, Young AB, Shoulson I, Bonilla E, Martin JB (1983) A polymorphic DNA marker genetically linked to Huntington's disease. Nature 306:234-238

Hudson JI, Pope HG, Jonas JM, Yurgelun-Todd D (1983) Family history study of anorexia nervosa and bulimia. Br J Psychiatry 142:133-138

Jacobi W, Winkler H (1927) Encephalographische Studien an chronisch Schizophrenen. Arch Psychiatr Nervenkr 81:299-332

Kerwin RW (1989) How do the neuropathological changes of schizophrenia relate to pre-existing neurotransmitter and aetiological hypothesis? Psychol Med 19:563-567

Koliaskina G, Tsutsulkovskaya M, Domashneva I, Maznina T, Kielholz P, Gastpar M, Bunney W, Rafaelsen O, Heltberg J, Coppen A, Hippius H, Hoecherl B, Vartanian F (1980) Antithymic immune factor in schizophrenia.   Neuropsychobiology 6:349-355

Lewis SW (1989) Congenital risk factors for schizophrenia. Psychol Med 19:5-13

Perris C (1966) A study of bipolar (manic depressive) and unipolar recurrent depressive psychoses. Acta Psychiatr Scand [Suppl] 194: 15-44

Propping P (1988)Psychiatrische Genetik. Springer, Berlin Heidelberg New York

Reveley AM, Reveley MA, Murrey RM (1984) Cerebral ventricular enlargement in non-genetic schizophrenia: a controlled twin study. Br J Psychiatry 144:89-93

Rivinus TM, Biederman J, Herzog DB (1984) Anorexia nervosa and affective disorders: a controlled family history study. Am J Psychiatry 141:1414-1418

Rüdin E (1916) Studien über Vererbung und Entstehung geistiger Störungen. I. Zur Vererbung und Neuentstehung der Dementia praecox. Monogr Gesamtgeb Neurol Psychiatr. Springer, Berlin

Schulz B (1932) Zur Erbpathologie der Schizophrenie. Z Ges Neurol Psychiatr 143:175-298

Stern SL, Dixon KL, Nemzer E, Lake MD, Sansone RA, Smeltzer DJ, Lanz S, Schrier SS (1984) Affective disorder in the families of women with normal weight bulimia. Am J Psychiatry 141:1224-1227

Strober M, Salkin B, Borroughs J, Morell W (1982) Validity of the bulimia restrictor distinction in anorexia nervosa: parental personality characteristics and familiy psychiatric morbidity. J Nerv Ment Dis 170:345-351

Tsuang MT, Kendler KK, Gruenberg AM (1985) DSM III schizophrenia: is there evidence for familial transmission? Acta Psychiatr Scand [Suppl] 319:77-83

Vartanian FE (1978) Neurochemical and immunological components. In: Schizophrenia. National Foundation, New York

Vogt C, Vogt O (1952) Altérations anatomiques de la schizophrénie et d'autres psychoses dites fonctionelles. J Neuropathol Exp Neurol 11:211-213

Weinberger DR (1987) Implications of normal brain development for the pathogenesis of schizophrenia. Arch Gen Psychiatry 44:660-669

Winokur G, Cadoret RJ, Dorzab J, Baker M (1971) Depressive disease. A genetic study. Arch Gen Psychiatry 24:135-144

Winokur G, Clayton P (1967) Family history studies. I. Two types of affective disorders separated according to genetical and clinical factors. In: Wortis J (ed) Recent advances in biological psychiatry 9. Plenum, New York, pp 35-50

Winokur A, March V, Mendels J (1980) Primary affective disorder in relatives of patients with anorexia nervosa. Am J Psychiatry 137:695-698

Zerbin-Rüdin E (1980a) Psychiatrische Genetik. In: Kisker KP, Meyer JE, Müller C, Strömgren E (eds) Grundlagen und Methoden der Psychiatrie, Teil 2, Psychiatrie der Gegenwart, (2nd edn, vol 1/2). Springer, Berlin Heidelberg New York, pp 545-618

Zerbin-Rüdin E (1980b) Genetics of affective psychoses. In: Van Praag HM, Lader MH, Rafaelsen OJ, Sachar EJ (eds) Handbook of biological psychiatry, part III. Dekker, New York pp 35-58

Zerbin-Rüdin E (1983) Schizophrenien-Somatosehypothese und Genetik. In: Gross G, Schüttler R (eds) Empirische Forschung in der Psychiatrie. Schattauer, Stuttgart, pp 55-64

Zerbin-Rüdin E (1985) Wo steht die genetische Schizophrenieforschung heute? In: Pflug B, Foerster K, Straube E (eds) Perspektiven der Schizophrenie-Forschung. Fischer, Stuttgart, pp 47-61

Zerbin-Rüdin E (1986) Schizoaffective and other atypical psychoses: the genetical aspect. In: Marneros A, Tsuang MT (eds) Schizoaffective psychoses. Springer, Berlin Heidelberg New York, pp 225-231

Zerbin-Rüdin E (1987a) Genetik. In: Kisker KP, Lauter H, Meyer JE, Müller C, Strömgren E (eds) Affektive Psychosen, Psychiatrie der Gegenwart (vol 5). Springer, Berlin Heidelberg New York, pp 137-164

Zerbin-Rüdin E (1987b) Psychiatric genetics and psychiatric nosology. J Psychiatr Res 21:377-383

Zerbin-Rüdin E (1988) Beiträge der genetischen Forschung zur Klassifikation affektiver Störungen. In: von Zerssen D, Möller HJ (eds) Affektive Störungen. Springer, Berlin Heidelberg New York, pp 29-45

Zimmerman M, Coryell W, Pfohl B, Stangl D (1986) The validity of four definitions of endogenous depression. Arch Gen Psychiatry 43:234-244

6 Systems Theory of Psychosis: "Filtering", Comparison, Error Correction, and Its Defects

H.M. Emrich

> Nothing is known — everything is imagined
> G. Leopardi, in Fellini's *La voce della luna*

Introduction

One of the greatest unresolved problems in psychiatry is how to explain the pathogenesis of schizophrenia. On the one hand psychiatric genetics data demonstrate the existence of genetic/constitutional factors — on the other, no clear Mendelian rules of transmission can be demonstrated. There is a great variability of symptomatology and penetrance of the illness, and the disorder can be mimicked by many organic brain processes, e.g., different types of encephalitis, tumors, and drugs, especially psychotomimetics such as phencyclidine (PCP). Finally, also in healthy persons extreme situations such as sensory and sleep deprivation can precipitate psychotic symptomatology. Interestingly, schizophreniform psychoses appear to be confined to humans, indicating that it is especially the nature of the human mind which is disturbable by this type of illness. Therefore, to some extent, schizophrenic psychoses may be interpreted as having a quasi "intimate relation" to something which is highly characteristic for the human mind — like a negative template which mirrors the original. It is proposed here that this speciality of the human mind is its capability creatively to construe, stabilize and appropriately adapt "fictional realities."

Humans live within a highly elaborate and in a to some extent "artificial" self-made world, represented within a phenomenon which we call "consciousness." To be "conscious" in an awake state may be defined as to compare an internal construct of fictional "reality" ("world model" according to W. Prinz) with real sensory data (Emrich 1990). (Interestingly, also higher animal species, according to this definition, have "consciousness" and create fictional realities; however, these are probably less elaborate and "creatively" disposable, and, in particular, animals lack "self-consciousness"* — at least as far as we know.) Hence — since conscious experiences are normally (in the awake state) driven by sensory data — consciousness and perception are intimately connected; however, also in dreams, daydreams, and phantasies we appreciate special types of "consciousness" and then apparently make use of internally generated "percepts" which interact with internal world models. Thus, sensory perception has to be regarded as representing one typical part of the conscious life which, however, appears to be an especially easily explorable example of consciousness, since basic features of consciousness-generating systems can be analyzed here.

Three-Component Model of Perception and Consciousness

The three-component model of perception assumes that perception is principally made up of three components: firstly, sensory input ("sensualistic" component); secondly, the internal production of concepts ("constructivistic" component); and thirdly control ("censor" component). It also assumes that the special interaction between these three components is responsible for a biologically fruitful and efficacious conscious internal representation of the external world during perception, and that equilibria between these three components may be disturbed during psychosis.

The constructivistic component can also be termed "phantasy component," "hypotheses-generating component," or "conceptualization component." Its representation in the present model takes into account the fact that processing of data is possible only on the basis of a conceptualization which has to be applied to data, before a successful interpretation is possible. Historically, this component goes back to the philosophies of G. Vico, I. Kant, J.G. Fichte, H. Bergson, and others and has recently reappeared in the "constructivism" of, e.g., Watzlawick (1985) and von Glasersfeld (1985). The "censor" function can also be termed "correcting" function and may be qualified as partially due to an "erasing" system and partially to a "suppressing" or "rejecting" system. Also consciousness obviously is a derivative of such a heterogeneity of origins (cf. Bisiach 1988): interactional processes are responsible for its realization (e.g., environmental, bodily, emotional, and cognitive factors) and, apparently, here a great difficulty arises: the more elaborate and complicated such a "private conscious world" is, the more prominent two problems become, which interact in an intrinsic antinomy: on the one hand the fictional reality has to be so flexible that it can be adapted to

---

* In humans apparently a metarepresentation of consciousness takes place which, as Frankfurt (1976) has shown, has the consequence that "second-order volitions" are possible, i.e., evaluations of one's wishes, desires, and proposals — processes which can be performed only by highly developed "censorship" systems.

the changing requirements of the external world; on the other hand this private world has to be stabilized so far that it is not continuously in danger of losing its stability, i.e., to "decompensate," that means that both the flexibility of creativity and — on the other hand — the stability of the subjective world are required. For a fulfillment of these two opposed requirements, intricate equilibria between neuronal networks have to be established, and disturbances of such ("vulnerable") equilibria may manifest themselves as "psychotic" states.

Filtering and Psychosis

According to Broadbent's classical model of filtering (Broadbent 1958), selective attention is performed by the functioning of a "selective filter" which operates in combination with a channel for sensory data with a limited transmission capacity ("p-channel"). As a consequence of the finding that schizophrenic patients show impairments of selective attention, Chapman and Chapman (1973) proposed a filter defect as a major pathogenetic principle of schizophrenic psychoses. Such a filter defect, however, cannot explain the pathogenesis of hallucinations in psychotic patients, since a loosening of selective attention would not make clear how not externally originated sensory data may get into the perceptual system. The original Broadbent filter can only explain hallucinations if one assumes that the "filter" is also adapted to internally generated data, i.e., "conceptualizations." It has to be admitted that — due to the fact that conceptualization was not at all implemented in the original version of Broadbent's filter model — a second version was later proposed by Broadbent (1971), which includes "pigeonholing" as the determinant factor of "filtering." But also if one applies this second-generation filter model to the problem of the pathogenesis of schizophrenia, it remains unclear why, on the one hand, selective attention is impaired within psychoses (filter impairment) and, on the other, pigeonholing-driven conceptualization is strengthened (hallucinations). Thus, an alternative view of the disturbance of interaction of subcomponents of perceptual — and in general conscious-generating — processes has to be envisaged (censorship model, see below).

Creativity and Psychosis

Die Phantasie in meinem Sinn
Ist dießmal gar zu herrisch
Fürwahr, wenn ich das alles bin
So bin ich heute närrisch.
J.W. v. Goethe, *Faust I*, Idealist

The relationship between creativity and madness has often been stressed in the past in discussions as to the possible mode of pathogenesis of psychotic behavior. Pioneers in this regard have been authors such as Lombroso, Lange-Eichbaum, and others [for a review cf. Emrich (1990)], but also the famous existentialistic author Gottfried Benn collected a sample of typical cases in this regard, and Karl Jaspers' interest in this field is documented in his book: Strindberg and van Gogh (1922). Goethe, probably for several reasons, was very much engaged in the field of imagination, phantasy, and daydreams, on the one hand, obviously, since he personally had a lot of experiences with such phenomena, which were, according to his statements (e.g., in *Dichtung und Wahrheit*) very vivid in himself, and on the other, since he was strongly interested in the possible mechanisms of how mental events are created [cf.,e.g., his term *"Gedankenfabrik"* (i.e., "factory of thoughts") in Faust I] and, what kind of relationship is established between imagination and abnormal mental life (see the poem above).

Goethe was "modern" not only insofar as he envisaged the possibilities of gene technology ("homunculus" idea; cf. Manfred Eigen's lecture at the CINP 1988, Munich), he also made concrete proposals regarding artificial intelligence: *"Zur Anschauung gesellt sich die Einbildungskraft, diese ist zuerst nachbildend, die Gegenstände nur wiederholend. Sodann ist sie produktiv, indem sie das Angefaßte belebt, entwickelt, erweitert, verwandelt"*: "Perception is associated with imagination. This operates firstly depicting and only repeats the objects. Later on it is productive by vitalizing the touched by developing, extending, and transforming it." From these sentences one may derive that Goethe was already aware of the possibility of the production of new conceptualizations of possible world models by derivatization, and that creative acts may be fulfilled by competition between proposals in the sense of M. Heisenberg's idea of a "lottery of proposals," which he conceptualizes as a source of "intention" (in the sense of "goals"; cf. Marcel 1988), using the term "initial activity." Such a competition between more or less suitable proposals of possible world models may also legitimize Edelman's view of "Neural Darwinism" (Edelman 1987), which is realized by competition and selection of neuronal "intentional" conceptualizations, and this part of Edelman's idea is, as far as I see, not touched by Crick's critical paper "Neural Edelmanism" (Crick 1989).

From a theory about creativity several definitions may result as to the functioning of mental life. If, for example, creativity is defined as the ability to handle world models in such a way that derivative possible world models (variants) can be construed, then "thinking" may be regarded as the ability to handle and compute these models in such a way that the possible realistic consequences are internally represented. The little poem by Goethe, cited above, gives an ironic proposal regarding the function of phantasy in mental life and its implications regarding possibilities of becoming crazy: "Phantasy in my mind is really too dominant today. Indeed, if I am all of this I am presently crazy." In a sense, these sentences may be regarded as containing a whole theory about the possible mode of origin of madness: if the activity of my phantasy is too dominant, then the question arises as to whether I really might be "everything" which appears in my mind and then I am apparently crazy ("*wenn ich das alles bin, dann bin ich heute närrisch*"). This interpretation of Goethe's text refers also to another relationship which might be regarded as important in the context of belletristic literature in relation to a theory of psychoses, namely, the unity of person. As early as pre-Freudian, preanalytical "dynamic psychiatry" (cf. Ellenberger 1970), which existed under the influence of Mesmerism in the nineteenth century, the unity of person became a problem, and double persons, e.g., the Medardus/Menardus figure in E.T.A. Hoffmann's book "*Die Elixiere des Teufels,*" were created. An especially impressive example of this is Mr. Goljädkin in Dostoyevski's book "The Double Person," which one can read from two perspectives: on the one hand one may interpret the emerging two identities as split products of an originally integral ego, the disruption of which results from a disease process (this is the common view), but alternatively one may envisage the two new identities of Mr. Goljädkin as being due to an uncovering of an originally preexisting dividedness of the ego.

If this latter concept contains some truth, the question arises as to how the "glue," normally producing the illusion of "the unity of the ego," is realized. The concept to be proposed here is that "correcting- and adapting"-processors are the relevant systems which cope with the original dividedness of persons into substructures. These processors, however, should also play a functional role in perception and other consciousness-generating processes, since also here integrative illusions play an important role. A method to make such processes observable is the examination of complex illusionary perceptions and their disturbances in psychotic states.

Binocular Depth Inversion-Illusion and Its Disturbance in Schizophrenia

The phenomenon of depth inversion is documented impressively in the Haunted Mansion at Disneyland in California, where visitors see a pair of human faces that appear to rotate precisely as they walk by. In reality, these faces are three-dimensional outside-in (hollow) masks, which are perceived incorrectly as normal faces. This illusion of "depth inversion" had been investigated by von Helmholtz and

Mach in the nineteenth century; questions as to its basic mechanisms have been reconsidered by Gregory (1973). It has been demonstrated, especially in experiments by Yellott (1981), that stereoscopic visual experience is the result of "a process in which the brain tests hypotheses about the three-dimensional shape of objects against the evidence provided by their retinal images." Binocular depth inversion does not occur under all conditions with hollow three-dimensional objects, but in those instances "with an overwhelmingly improbable real form so that it looks normal only when it is seen inverted in depth" (see also Wolf 1987). Mental preconceptions appear to measure the sensory input in a critical way, creating visual experience, and this interaction is conceptualized by unconscious perceptual learning. From this point of view, binocular depth inversion can be regarded as representing an indicator of the "correcting processor" (censorship), mentioned above.

The three-component hypothesis of perception, as presented above, gives rise to the idea that the equilibrium between a constructivistic and a correcting processor function is disturbed in psychosis. Thus, if the correction of preconceptions is impaired in psychosis and if the processor, which is relevant for visual perception, were disturbed in the way predicted above, an impaired binocular depth inversion should be observed in psychotic patients. Such experiments have in fact been performed (Emrich 1988) using a stereoscopic projection device and linearly polarized light: 40 schizophrenic patients (20 productive and 20 nonproductive), were investigated in comparison with 20 healthy volunteers. All the normal probands saw the three-dimensional hollow faces as normal (not hollow) human faces, when the glasses were exchanged (i.e., the information for the right eye was projected to the left eye and vice versa), whereas the schizophrenics were unable to perform this binocular depth inversion completely: they all observed hollow faces in these experiments, at least partially. The extent of this effect was dependent on the productivity of the psychosis, i.e., from the extent of the presence of actual hallucinatory and/or delusional experiences.

This finding appears to support the idea that schizophrenic psychoses are not primarily due to a deficiency of a "filter" which protects the brain from an overload of information arising from the outer world, but results from a deficiency of an active correcting processor which interacts with both internal conceptualization and external sensory input (i.e., the results indicate a deficiency in "correction" of the sensory data (Emrich 1988).

Though developed independently, this concept has some analogy to Huxley's (1954) interpretation of the mode of action of psychedelic drugs, developed under the influence of Bergson and Broad, which states that these psychotogenic compounds tend to weaken an internal censoring function, which is relevant for perception.

Also Malenka et al. (1982) observed central error in the correcting behavior of motor control in schizophrenic patients. The view of the basic deficiency in psychosis, elaborated here, appears to be in line with the concepts both of Huxley (1954) and of Malenka et al.(1982), insofar as it is assumed that internal correcting systems are deficient or in imbalance, in relation to conceptualization during a psychotic state (cf. also Frith's important contributions in this regard (Frith 1987; Frith and Done 1988, 1989).

Neurobiology of Censorship

During the recent past the concept of "modularity of mind" has become dominant in the field of concepts about the organizational structure of mind (Fodor 1983; Gazzaniga 1985). The main idea is that — in contrast to the classical concepts of neuropsychology (which also influenced Freud), in which a linear computation is exerted, finally coming to a conscious result in one dimension (other parts of mental representation remain "subconscious") — the processing in the brain is a "parallel" one. The different mental representations are performed by different "modules" which can interact with each other but cannot change their qualitative character, i.e., many of them cannot be translated into "language": i.e., they are influential but not recognizable and thus remain "paraconscious." (They cannot also by themselves become parts of "world models.")

An important module in this concept is Gazzaniga's "interpretor," a module which coordinates and integrates the computations (the "votes") of other modules, and the result of such an "interpretor"-related computation apparently has the subjective quality of being "granted," being "true," being "real." This system obviously exerts what the above mentioned "censorship" has to be attributed to. The function of this system is to stabilize "reality fictions" and one may — as a result of the present considerations as well as from the impaired inversion-illusion in psychosis — anticipate that especially this system is disturbed or to an increased extent "vulnerable" in psychosis. To be more precise: in hallucinations one may argue that it is the equilibrium between "conceptualizations" and "censorship" which is disturbed by relative censorship impairment.

How might such a system be realized neurobiologically? Censorship certainly has great demands regarding long-term memory, since the question of what is "plausible," "senseful," "biologically meaningful at present," can only be decided on the basis of a history of experiences of failures and successes which are stored over longer periods. Thus, hippocampal structures may play a prominent role herein. As Sonntag (1990) has recently summarized, hippocampal structures may work as "comparators" (Gray and Rawlins 1986; Olton 1989) and calculate meaningful expectations in relation to sensory input. Recently, neurochemical data on GABA in the hippocampus have been acquired which are in line with this concept (Bischoff 1986). Interestingly, dopamine also plays a functional role herein (Bischoff 1986), a finding which may explain the therapeutic effects of antidopaminergic (neuroleptic) compounds.

Thus the censorship systems, described above, may be characterized as such "comparators," a concept which fits into the idea that to have "consciousness" means to "compare" world models with actual (sensory or imagined) intentional data. Comparison of actual data with sets of acquired world models: this definition may thus turn out to be an adequate description of the function of "censorship," which is to stabilize "reality fictions": and it is this that appears to be so highly developed in human mental life and what also appears to be so vulnerable and obviously impaired during psychotic states: consciousness.

References

Bisiach E (1988) The (haunted) brain and consciousness. In: Marcel AJ, Bisiach E (eds) Consciousness in contemporary science. Clarendon, Oxford, pp 101-120

Bischoff S (1986) Mesohippocampal dopamine system: characterization, functional and clinical implications. In: Isaacson RL, Pribram KH (eds) The hippocampus, vol 3. Plenum, New York, pp 1-32

Broadbent DE (1958) Perception and communication. Pergamon, New York

Broadbent DE (1971) Decision and stress. Academic, London

Chapman LJ, Chapman JP (1973) Disordered thought in schizophrenia. Meredith, New York

Crick F (1989) Neural edelmanism. Trends Neurosci 12: 240-248

Edelman GM (1987) Neural darwinism: the theory of neuronal group selection. Basic Books, New York

Ellenberger HF (1970) The discovery of the unconscious. Penguin, London

Emrich HM (1988) Zur Entwicklung einer Systemtheorie produktiver Psychosen. Nervenarzt 59: 456-464

Emrich HM (1990) "... und fliegt über die Grenzen der Vernunft". Die Rolle der Phantasie bei Psychosen. Universitas 45: 28-38

Fodor JA (1983) The modularity of mind. MIT, Cambridge

Frankfurt HG (1976) Conditions of personhood. In: Rorty AO (ed) The identities of persons. University of California Press, Berkeley

Frith CD (1987) The positive and negative symptoms of schizophrenia reflect impairments in the perception and initiation of action. Psychol Med 17: 631-648

Frith CD, Done DJ (1988) Towards a neuropsychology of schizophrenia. Br J Psychiatry 153: 437-443

Frith CD, Done DJ (1989) Experiences of alien control in schizophrenia reflect a disorder in the central monitoring of action. Psychol Med 19: 356-363

Gazzaniga MS (1985) The social brain. Basic Books, New York

Glasersfeld E von (1985) Konstruktion der Wirklichkeit und des Begriffs der Objektivität. In: Schriften der C.F.v.-Siemens-Stiftung (vol 10) Einführung in den Konstruktivismus. Oldenbourg, München, pp 1-26

Gray JA, Rawlins JNP (1986) Comparator and buffer memory: an attempt to integrate two models of hippocampal functions. In: Isaacson RL, Pribram KH (eds) The hippocampus (vol 4). Plenum, New York, pp 159-201

Gregory RL (1973) The confounded eye. In: Gregory RL, Gombrich EH (eds) Illusion in nature and art. Freeman, Oxford, pp 49-96

Heisenberg M (1989) A neurobiologists view of intentionality and perception. Presentation at the congress on "Biological aspects of Non-psychotic disorders". Book of abstracts, Jerusalem, p 199

Huxley A (1954) The doors of perception. Chatto and Windus, London

Jaspers K (1922) Strindberg und van Gogh. Barth, Leipzig

Malenka RC, Angel RW, Hampton B, Berger PA (1982) Impaired central error-correcting behavior in schizophrenia. Arch Gen Psychiatry 39: 101-107

Marcel AJ (1988) Phenomenal experience and functionalism. In: Marcel AJ, Bisiach E (eds) Consciousness in contemporary science. Clarendon, Oxford, pp 121-158

Olton DS (1989) Mnemonic functions of the hippocampus: single unit analyses in rats. In: Chan-Palay V, Köhler C (eds) The hippocampus: new vistas. Liss, New York, pp. 411-424

Sonntag R (1990) Schizophrenia, working memory, and evolutionary biology: mechanisms of psychopathobiology. (to be published)

Watzlawick P (1985) Wirklichkeitsanpassung oder angepaßte "Wirklichkeit". In: Schriften der C.F.v.-Siemens-Stiftung (vol 10) Einführung in den Konstruktivismus. Oldenbourg, München, pp 69-83

Wolf R (1987) Der biologische Sinn der Sinnestäuschung. Biol Zeit 17:33-49

Yellott JI Jr (1981) Binocular depth inversion. Sci Am 245:118-125

Part II: Psychiatric Neuropharmacology and Neurochemistry

7 Peptides as Neuronal Signalling Molecules

W. Zieglgänsberger, H.-U. Dodt, R.A. Deisz, H. Pawelzik

Introduction

Neuropeptides form a major class of messenger substances in nervous systems. Current research suggests that neuropeptides play a key role in synaptic signalling and allow specific subsystems of the brain to communicate. In addition to the classical synaptic mechanisms, information transfer can also occur via the extracellular space (Agnati et al. 1986a,b). Neuropeptides are considered to be major candidates for such integrative actions and long-term changes in neuronal excitability which alter behavior, mood, and mental processes as well as endocrine and autoregulatory functions (Fuxe et al. 1988). The mechanisms underlying the physiological role of neuropeptides in the mammalian peripheral (North 1986) and central (Bloom 1984, 1988) nervous system (CNS) remain to be elucidated.

What Role Do Neuropeptides Play in Neuronal Signalling Mechanisms?

The mere presence of neuropeptides in neuronal elements does not necessarily warrant their involvement in intercellular signalling. However, the specific distribution in the neuropile, the Ca^{2+}-dependent release, and the distinct actions that some neuropeptides exert on neurons of the mammalian CNS do give credence to the belief that synaptic and nonsynaptic intercellular communication may, in part, be peptidergic in nature. The slow time course of their actions, the mismatch between their site of release and the location of their receptors on (a) the soma-dendritic membrane, (b) presynaptic terminals, (c) glia, and (d) blood vessels suggest a more diffuse site of action in addition to a clearly targeted action through conventional synaptic contacts. There is evidence that highly selective receptors for neuropeptides are not restricted to subsynaptic areas but are distributed over the entire soma-dendritic membrane of central neurons (Herkenham 1987). Recently it has been reported (Sontheimer et al. 1988; Marrero et al. 1989; Usowicz et al. 1989) that, in addition to receptors for neuropeptides, astrocytes

(type II), a glia cell type almost exclusively found in the white matter, also express
L-glutamate receptors. Furthermore, the molecular structure of a binding protein
for kainate has been characterized on glial membranes (Gregor et al. 1989). This
neuron/glia interaction occurs in a part of the CNS which was always considered
to be involved mainly as a passive participant in the information transfer. The role
of glia receptors in intercellular signaling remains to be determined.

Mode of Action of Neuropeptides in the CNS

A few of the hitherto characterized actions of neuropeptides on neuronal targets
are assumed to be modulatory, i.e., peptides alter the response of a target neuron
to a classical neurotransmitter without interfering with neuronal excitability by a
shift in membrane permeability (Siggins and Gruol 1986). The intercellular
communication may transiently be altered by these signal molecules which are co-
released from either the same or adjacent terminals (Nicoll 1988). Pre- and
postsynaptic interactions between neuropeptides and classical neurotransmitters,
for example monoamines or amino acids, have been demonstrated in various
neuronal systems (Bloom 1988). Although the mechanism of differential release
of co-existing neuropeptides and neurotransmitter(s) is still unknown, it has been
suggested that high frequency stimulation preferentially releases neuropeptides,
most probably from dense-core vesicles. The findings reported here also ten-
tatively suggest that low frequency versus high-frequency stimulation of neocortical interneurons releases different neurotransmitters or different combinations of
these substances. However, the physiological significance of the multiplicity of
messengers through co-transmission is still unknown, and the multiplicity of
messengers and receptors certainly complicates the interpretation of synaptic
activity and receptor responses. A major breakthrough would be the development
of more selective receptor antagonists which might be able to probe the actions of
the various components of the response.

Neuropeptides influence transmembrane ion fluxes at pre- and postsynaptic sites
as well as intracellular enzyme activity through G-protein coupled mechanisms. It
has been shown that neuropeptides can increase the intracellular Ca^{2+}-con-
centration and trigger the Ca^{2+}-dependent metabolic cascades, as well as intracellular mechanisms involving cAMP, inositol phosphate or other second messenger
systems through activation of voltage- and ligand-gated Ca^{2+} channels or mobili-
zation of Ca^{2+} from intracellular stores (Berridge 1987; Chuang De-Maw 1989).
After this release neuropeptides are not taken up again but are degraded by
relatively unspecific peptidases located in the extracellular environment. Peptidase
inhibitors which prolong the actions of neuropeptides may gain therapeutic potential (a) when neuropeptides have finally been tailored which can cross the blood-
brain barrier or (b) when it has become possible to enhance the action of tonically
active peptide-releasing neurons.

Opioid Peptides

The opioidergic innervation of neocortical neurons is mainly derived from pro-enkephalin A and pro-enkephalin B (-dynorphin) precursors. Like most neuropeptides, the pro-enkephalin A and pro-enkephalin B derived opioid peptides are not contained in neuronal projection systems but function as neurotransmitters or neuromodulators of locally restricted interneurons. Only the pro-opiomelanocortin (POMC) projection system, which originates mainly from the nucleus arcuatus and the mediobasal hypothalamus, gives rise to a large number of collaterals. Although no afferent fibers have been demonstrated, POMC-derived opioid peptides may contribute to opioid actions, e.g., in neocortical neurons through mechanisms which do not involve synaptic contacts (Agnati et al. 1986a) (see below).

Although the three opiate receptor subtypes have not yet been cloned, purification and affinity labelling of the receptors support the concept that μ-, δ- and κ-opiate receptors are discrete molecular entities. This concept was initially derived from binding and activity profiles, from different sensitivity of the agonists to naloxone, as well as from the protection and inactivation kinetics. At present, the structure of the opiate receptor is unknown but will probably resemble other inhibitory receptors coupled to G-proteins (Simonds 1988). These receptors are characterized by their seven transmembrane helices and a large cytoplasmatic loop.

The fragments of POMC and pro-enkephalin A have affinities mainly to the μ- and δ-binding sites, while those of pro-enkephalin B (-dynorphin) have affinities mainly to the κ-binding site. Only the synthetic compounds display almost exclusive binding at one site; all the endogenous opioid peptides bind to more than one type of binding site. The different levels of the various receptor subtypes in a brain area will most likely be a decisive factor in determining the final response of the target cell to the opioids — exogenous and endogenous (Mansour et al. 1987; Tempel and Zukin 1987; Harlan et al. 1987). There is evidence that the μ- and δ-subtypes of the opiate receptor are co-expressed on various neurons (see below).

The predominantly inhibitory effects of opioid peptides on spontaneous or chemically evoked neuronal discharge activity are qualitatively similar throughout the mammalian central and peripheral nervous systems (Zieglgänsberger 1986; Siggins and Gruol 1986; Deisz et al. 1988). Some major exceptions to the usually depressant action exist, such as the naloxone-reversible excitatory responses seen in the majority of hippocampal pyramidal cells. The bulk of the extracellular and intracellular data support a disinhibitory mechanism of action for the single-unit excitatory effects of these opioid peptides in the hippocampus. In these neurons the excitation may actually be indirect, resulting from a primary inhibitory effect on neighboring (inhibitory) GABAergic interneurons leading to excitation by disinhibition (Zieglgänsberger et al. 1979). Pyramidal cells of the hippocampus show in vitro little or no direct transmembrane effects of morphine or opioid peptides. Most studies on the hippocampal slice indicate that the enkephalins and β-endorphin primarily reduce the size of recurrent and feedforward inhibitory postsynaptic potentials (IPSPs) in both CA1 and CA3 cell groups, thus supporting a disin-hibitory mechanism (Siggins and Zieglgänsberger 1981).

The inhibition by opiate agonists is generally stereo-specific, blocked by nalo-xone, and reduced during tolerance development following long-term ad-ministration of opiates. These findings suggest the involvement of the empirically defined opiate receptors. The past decade has seen an increase in intracellular studies leading to a better understanding of the mechanisms of opioid function. Similar to other neuropeptides, opioid peptides can trigger several mechanisms at different sites. As many as four mechanisms involving pre- and postsynaptically located receptors have been postulated to account for the depressant effects of opioids on central and peripheral mammalian neurons (Zieglgänsberger 1986; Siggins and Gruol 1986).

A synopsis of histochemical, ultrastructural, and electrophysiological data suggests a preferential postsynaptic interaction between opioid peptides and transmitters released from adjacent terminals. The substantial decrease in opiate binding following deafferentation and the finding that opioids can reduce release of synaptic transmitters suggest an additional presynaptic site of action which might involve the blockade of voltage-sensitive Ca^{2+} channels. The final outcome of release of endogenous opioids may thus depend upon the local circuitry as well as the strategic location of the receptor subtypes. Unfortunately, the difficulty in recording from presynaptic terminals in the mammalian CNS generally precludes direct examination of the actual mechanisms involved. In a study in neuroblastoma * glioma hybrid cells (NG 108-15), we used the tight-seal whole-cell variant of the patch-clamp technique to analyze the functional coupling of opiate receptors to voltage-dependent Ca^{2+} channels. As previously shown for the relatively unselective agonist D-Ala^2-D-Leu^5-enkephalin (Hescheler et al. 1987), both μ- (D-Ala^2-NMe-Phe^4-Gly^{5}ol) (DAGO) and δ-selective (D-Pen^2-D-Pen^5-enke-phalin) (DPDPE) agonists reversibly reduced voltage-dependent Ca^{2+} currents. The increase in intracellular Ca^{2+} following depolarizing pulses was measured with an intracellular fluorescence technique (FURA II). Since the action of the δ-preferring agonist DPDP could be antagonized in some cells with a receptor selective opioid antagonist (ICI 174,864) without altering the effect of the μ-preferring agonist DAGO it is suggested that both μ- and δ-receptors are co-expressed and probably linked to the same effector system (Zieglgänsberger and Neher, unpublished data). These results are in accordance with previous investigations reporting the activation of a pertussis-toxin-sensitive G protein (Go) as an essential step in mediating the inhibition of voltage-activated Ca^{2+} channels by opioids (Hescheler et al. 1987). Also studies performed in cultured dorsal root ganglia neurons, which could provide insights into the presynaptic effects of opioid peptides, revealed that opioid agonists reduce Ca^{2+} influx. In these neurons (derived from either chick or rat neonates), none of the opioid peptides tested altered membrane potentials, but they did reduce the duration of the action potential. This is presumably due to an enhancement of some K^+ conductance, e.g., Ca^{2+}-dependent K^+ or the delayed rectifier conductance. Dorsal root ganglion cells obtained by rapid isolation from adult rats do not show this opiate effect on action potential duration. It seems possible that either the relevant (somatic) opiate receptors disappear entirely with maturity or that they migrate down the axons to the terminals in the spinal cord (Zieglgänsberger 1986; Siggins and Gruol 1986; Williams and Zieglgänsberger 1981).

The coupling of the κ-receptors to voltage-dependent Ca^{2+} channels is suggested from several investigations in different preparations (Macdonald and Werz 1986). The molecular events that take place subsequent to the activation of the opiate receptor subtypes have not yet been elucidated in detail. A series of findings obtained in various sites in the CNS showed that opioid peptides induce hyper-polarization and that the increased conductance involves K^+ channels (North et al. 1987). More recent data suggest that the K^+ channels involved in the opioid-in-duced hyperpolarization are the same voltage-dependent (inwardly rectifying) channels activated by several other inhibitory transmitters (e.g., muscarinic receptors, $GABA_B$ receptors, α_2-adrenoreceptors), and that such activation (Christie and North 1988) involves a pertussis-toxin-sensitive GTP-binding protein (McFadzean 1988; Williams et al. 1988). Since the effects of the inhibitory agonists are nonadditive, it is suggested that the agonists open the same population of potassium channels and inhibit cell firing through an increase in potassium conductance and consequent hyperpolarization. In newborn rats, currents through single channels were activated by DAGO (Miyake et al. 1989). The unitary inward currents showed conductances of approximately 45 pS. An intimate coupling between the receptor and the potassium channel was suggested by these studies. It was postulated that μ-opiate-receptors, α_2-adrenoreceptors and probably also somatostatin receptors are directly coupled to potassium channels through GTP-binding proteins in the membrane. Interestingly, in the rat substantia nigra zona compacta the principal cells, which are by far the majority of cells encountered in that area, are hyperpolarized by dopamine and the $GABA_B$ agonist baclofen whereas μ- and δ-opiate receptor agonists have no effect (Lacey et al. 1989).

Potassium channels are widely distributed in the nervous tissue and are ubi-quitous membrane proteins. However, in various sites in the CNS, opioid peptides do not change the membrane potential or membrane resistance (Lacey et al. 1989) but decrease the magnitude and rate of rise of the excitatory postsynaptic potentials (EPSPs) (Deisz et al. 1988). Postsynaptic modulation of the actions of excitatory amino acid transmitters which mediate these EPSPs (Monaghan et al. 1989) was one of the first described actions of opioid peptides and opiate alkaloids on central neurons (Siggins and Gruol 1986). In a recent study, we investigated the actions of the μ- and δ-receptor specific opioid peptides DAGO and DPDP in neocortical neurons of the rat (see Fig. 1) employing intracellular recording including single electrode voltage clamp techniques. Despite the fact that neocortical neurons have potassium conductances (voltage independent and inwardly rectifying), these neurons are not hyperpolarized by opiates. Applications of either agonist caused small invariable changes in membrane potential which were difficult to separate from slow spontaneous fluctuations ($\pm$ 2 mV). Current voltage relationships revealed minor, if any, changes. At the same time the EPSPs evoked by low stimulus intensities were reduced, on the average, by 50%. At higher stimulus

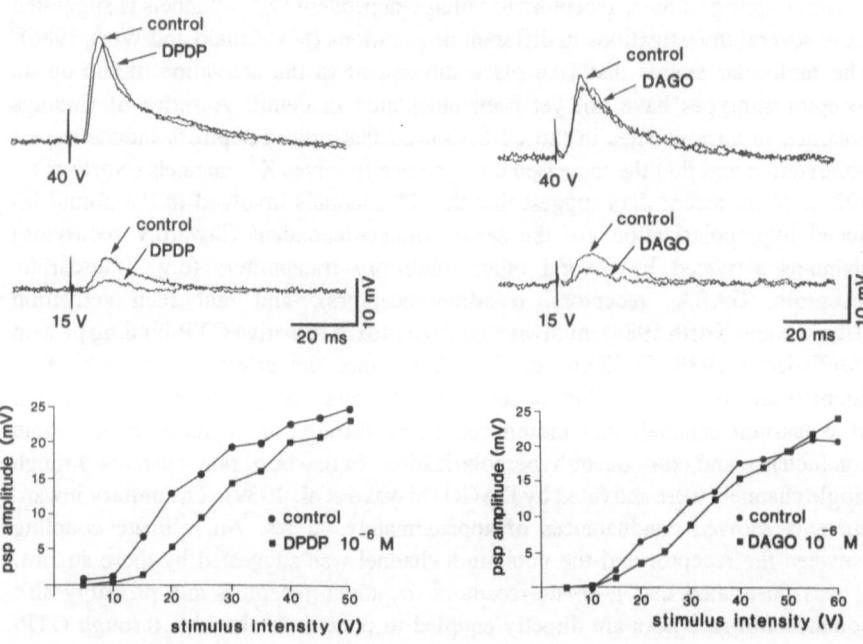

Fig.1. Both DPDP and DAGO (10^{-6} *M*) reduce evoked EPSPs of neocortical neurons. *Upper* and *middle traces* show original recordings whereas the *lower part* shows the I/O curves. Note that the depression of EPSPs is more pronounced at low stimulus intensities. *Methods:* Most of the information gathered so far about the actions of neuropeptides in the CNS has been derived from extracellular recording of single unit activity in combination with iontophoretic or pneumatic administration of drugs from multibarreled micropipettes in regions containing a high density of specific binding sites (Siggins and Gruol 1986). The establishment of in vitro preparations of the mammalian CNS has introduced interesting possibilities in the analysis of neuropeptide actions. In the present study intracellular recordings were made from neurons in layers II and III of the dorsomedial frontal neocortex of Sprague-Dawley rats (for further details see Howe et al. 1987). The study includes 62 intracellular recordings [membrane potential, -80.9 mV ± 9.7mV (SD); input resistance, 29.6 MΩ ± 4.1MΩ (SD); action potential amplitude, 100.7 mV ± 9.0 mV (SD)]. Drug testing was started 30-40 min after impalement. DPDP, DAGO, VIP, adrenergic agonists (isoprenaline, phenylephrine) and the opiate antagonist naloxone were added to the perfusion medium or were applied by pressure (10-100 kPa) from micropipettes filled with the diluted solutions (10^{-8}-10^{-5} *M*). The action of the neuropeptides persisted in Ca^{2+}-free/high-Mg^{2+} medium, suggesting that they were mediated through postsynaptically located receptors. High performance liquid chromatography (HPLC) techniques were employed to control the integrity of the neuropeptides. They appeared to be unchanged after contact with the slices when used in the superfusion medium (concentrations: 10^{-6} and 10^{-7} *M*).

intensities the attenuation of the postsynaptic transients became less pronounced. Both DAGO and DPDP applied either iontophoretically or added to the perfusion medium attenuated the depolarizing responses to iontophoretically applied L-glutamate. Single electrode voltage-clamp measurements showed that opioids reduced the inward currents triggered by synaptic stimulation and by iontophoretic application of L-glutamate (or quisqualate). The blocking effect of opioids on L-glutamate-induced depolarizations was still present when the synaptic transmission was blocked by high Mg^{2+} and low Ca^{2+} concentrations in the perfusion medium, suggesting a postsynaptic site of action. It was postulated that the opiates interfere with the chemically excitable cationic channels permeable to Na^+ and K^+ which are also opened by synaptically released excitatory transmitters. It is concluded from these results that the predominant effect of opioid peptides on neocortical neurons is a selective modulation of non-N-methyl-D-aspartate (NMDA) responses. In contrast to L-glutamate (and quisqualate) evoked depolarizations, the NMDA-induced depolarizations and inward currents were either not influenced or reduced only slightly by opioids. The depolarizations, elicited by NMDA, were blocked by D-2-amino-5-phosphonovaleric acid (APV), which, at the concentrations employed (5-50 μM), did not affect L-glutamate-induced depolarizations. In agreement with other studies, it was shown that NMDA and L-glutamate-induced inward currents are triggered through the activation of different receptors, are carried by a different ionic composition, and show different ion and voltage sensitivities. NMDA receptor activation leads to an inward current which increases with more depolarized holding potentials and is carried to a great extent by Ca^{2+} ions entering along with Na^+ ions. This current is markedly potentiated by removal of Mg^{2+} ions (for reviews see Monaghan et al. 1989; Cotman et al. 1988). In contrast to the repetitive firing induced by L-glutamate, due to the voltage sensitivity of the NMDA response, regenerative currents are induced which increase with depolarization and induce burst-like firing patterns. This latter effect is exploited to differentially activate interneurons (see Fig. 2). Besides the four main L-glutamate receptor subtypes [NMDA, AMPA (α-amino-3-hydroxy-5-methyl-4-isoxazolepropionic acid), kainate, 2-amino-4-phosphono-butyrate], a fifth receptor has been characterized which is coupled to a G protein. This receptor subtype may prove to be of particular interest since it may provide the trigger for intracellular metabolic actions which are also affected by other signalling molecules (Monaghan et al. 1989). Most recently a cDNA clone from a rat forebrain cDNA library was isolated which encodes a functional L-glutamate receptor (Hollmann et al. 1989). It has been shown that this protein forms an ion channel but bears only slight resemblance to other members of the ligand-gated channel superfamily characterized by four transmembrane regions. It remains to be elucidated whether these receptor subtypes constitute a novel class of ligand-gated channels.

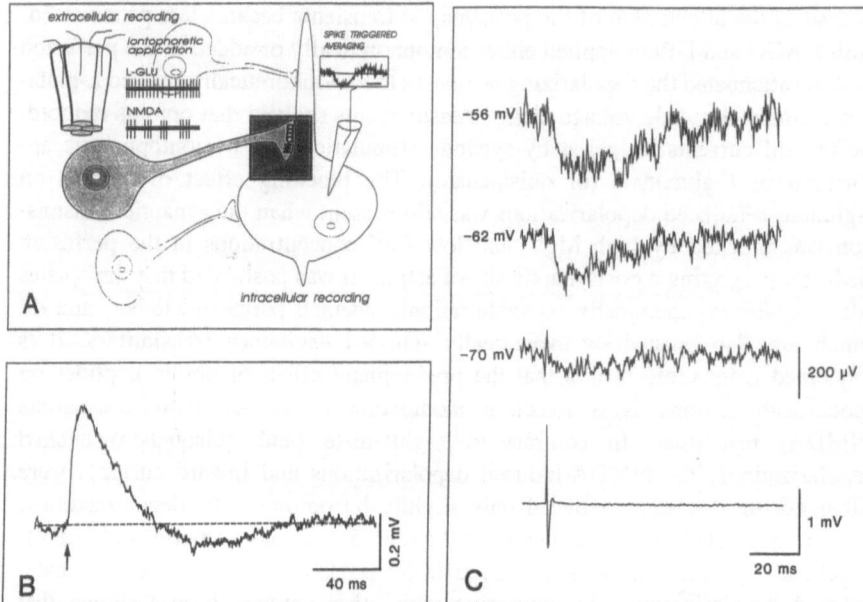

Fig. 2. A, Scheme of the experimental setup for spike-triggered averaging. The discharge activity of an extracellularly recorded neuron was evoked by or enhanced by iontophoretic application of either L-glutamate or NMDA from a multibarreled micropipette and was used to trigger the averaging of intracellular potentials of pyramidal neurons. L-glutamate most commonly evoked repetitive discharges, whereas NMDA evoked high-frequency burst discharges. The responses of the target neuron to the two different discharge patterns evoked in the neighboring neuron were compared. In 84 intracellularly and 272 extracellularly recorded neurons 26 single-axon synaptic connections were revealed. In 23 cases action potentials of the presynaptic cell resulted in depolarization of the target cell with an average amplitude of 188 ± 114 μV and a latency to peak of 5-25 ms. Only three purely inhibitory connections were found.
B, Averaged record of a spike-triggered postsynaptic potential. The depolarizing potentials were followed by hyperpolarizing potentials (in 11 out of 23 neurons) with a time-to-peak of about 60 ms and amplitudes of 34 ± 21 μV. The time-to-peak of these potentials lies between the time-to-peak of fast ($GABA_A$, 20 - 25 ms) and slow ($GABA_B$, 150-250 ms) inhibitory postsynaptic potentials in neocortical pyramidal cells. Thus this potential may represent a novel synaptic component which can only be revealed by spike-triggered averaging. The *arrow* indicates the occurrence of the extracellularly recorded spike generated by the presynaptic neuron.
C, Voltage dependence of an averaged single-axon inhibitory postsynaptic potential. Current injection changes the conventional IPSP and the postsynaptic transient in the same manner. The reversal potential was in the same range (-70 - -75 mV). The lowest trace shows the averaged extracellularly recorded spike of the presynaptic neuron. Activation of interneurons with different frequencies lacked clearly distinct responses. Attempts to separate peptidergic components by blockade of the $GABA_A$ component by bicuculline have been made. The neuropeptide(s) involved in the remaining response are currently being investigated (Pawelzik et al. unpublished data)

Vasoactive Intestinal Polypeptide in the Neocortex

In a comparable sample of neurons in which the above-described opioid actions were studied, intermediate synaptic stimuli evoked APV-sensitive synaptic components. These NMDA-mediated synaptic components were increased in a number of neurons by exogenously applied vasoactive intestinal polypeptide (VIP) as well as norepinephrine (NE). VIP is contained in neocortical bipolar inter-neurons with radially directed processes branching in cylinders about 30 μm in diameter (Morrison et al. 1984) and with somata distributed in laminae II and III (Magistretti and Morrison 1985). In addition to afferent terminals from inter-neurons containing VIP, the pyramidal neurons in these laminae receive nor-adrenergic synaptic afferents which are composed of fine axons and are organized predominantly in a plane parallel to the pial surface (Parnavelas and Papadopoulos 1989). The cell bodies of this highly divergent trajectory are located in the locus coeruleus. Ample evidence suggests that their activation produces potent and specific forms of conditional actions on their target neurons. When tested on basal discharge activity, NE and VIP appear to be mainly inhibitory (Ferron et al. 1985). On the other hand, NE may function as an "enabler", i.e., it enhances the responsiveness of target neurons to other excitatory and inhibitory synaptic inputs which may be active simultaneously (Bloom 1988). Current research suggests that the convergence of NE and VIP on neocortical neurons might create metabolic hot spots on neocortical neurons by acting synergistically to increase cAMP levels (Magistretti and Schorderet 1984, 1985; Magistretti and Morrison 1988). As both VIP and NE were shown to increase the excitability of pyramidal cells to synaptic inputs, the response of a well-defined cortical domain could selectively be altered. Long-lasting VIP responses and event-related NE effects could provide the basis for the induction of neuronal plasticity in exactly defined cortical columns.

References

Agnati LF, Fuxe K, Merlo Pich E et al. (1986a) Aspects of the integrative capacities of the central nervous system: evidence for "volume transmission" and its possible relevance for receptor-receptor interactions. In: Fuxe K, Agnati LF (eds) Receptor-receptor interactions: a new intramembrane integrative mechanism. Macmillan, London, pp 236-249

Agnati LF, Fuxe K, Zoli M, Ozini I, Toffano G, Ferraguti F (1986b) A correlation analysis of the regional distribution of central enkephalin and β-endorphin immunoreactive terminals and of opiate receptors in adult and old male rats. Evidence for the existence of two main type of communication in the central nervous system: the volume transmission and the wiring transmission. Acta Physiol Scand 128: 201-207

Berridge MJ (1987) Inositol triphosphate and diacylglycerol: two interacting second messengers. Ann Rev Biochem 56: 159-193

Bloom FE (1984) General features of chemically identified neurons. In: Björklund A, Hökfelt T (eds) Handbook of chemical neuroanatomy, vol 2. Biomedical Elsevier, pp 1-22

Bloom FE (1988) Neurotransmitters: past, present, and future directions. FASEB J 2: 32-41

Christie MJ, North RA (1988) Agonists at μ-opioid, M_2-muscarinic and $GABA_B$-receptors increase the same potassium conductance in rat lateral parabrachial neurones. Br J Pharmacol 95: 896-902

Chuang De-Maw (1989) Neurotransmitter receptors and phosphoinositide turnover. Ann Rev Pharmacol Toxicol 29: 71-110

Cotman CW, Monaghan DT, Ganong AT (1988) Excitatory amino acid neurotransmission: NMDA receptors and Hebb-type synaptic plasticity. Ann Rev Neurosci 11: 61-80

Deisz RA, Madamba S, Moore S, Siggins GR, Sutor B, Zieglgänsberger W (1988) Regulation of neuronal excitability by opioid peptides: intracellular analysis in several brain regions. In: Illes P, Farsang C (eds) Regulatory role of opioid peptides. VCH Press, Weinheim New York, pp 147-164

Dodt H-U, Zieglgänsberger W (1990) Visualizing unstained neurons in living brain slices by infrared DIC-videomicroscopy. Brain Res 537:333-336

Ferron A, Siggins GR, Bloom FE (1985) Vasoactive intestinal polypeptide acts synergistically with norepinephrine to depress spontaneous discharge rate in cerebral cortical neurons. Proc Natl Acad Sci U.S.A. 82: 8810-8812

Fuxe K, Agnati LF, Hartstrand A, Cintra A, Aronsson M, Zoli M, Gustafson J-A (1988) Principles for the hormone regulation of wiring transmission and volume transmission in the central nervous system. In: Ganten D, Pfaff D (eds) Current topics in neuroendocrinology, vol 8. Springer, Berlin Heidelberg New York, pp 1-53

Gregor P, Mano I, Maoz I, McKoewn M, Teichberg VI (1989) Molecular structure of the chick cerebellar kainate-binding subunit of a putative glutamate receptor. Nature 342: 689-691

Harlan RE, Shivers BD, Romano QJ, Howells RD, Pfaff DW (1987) Localization of preproenkephalin mRNA in the rat brain and spinal cord by in situ hybridization. J Comp Neurol 258:159-184

Herkenham H (1987) Mismatches between neurotransmitter and receptor localization in brain: observations and implications. Neuroscience 23: 1-38

Hescheler J, Rosenthal W, Trautwein W, Schultz G. (1987) The GTP-binding protein, G_o, regulates neuronal calcium channels. Nature 325: 445-447

Hollmann M., O'Shea-Greenfield A., Rogers S.W., Heinemann S (1989) Cloning by functional expression of a member of the glutamate receptor family. Nature 342: 643-648

Howe JR, Sutor B, Zieglgänsberger W (1987) Baclofen reduces postsynaptic potentials of rat neocortical neurones by an action other than its hyperpolarizing action. J Physiol 384: 539-569

Lacey MQ, Mercuri NB, North RA (1989) Two cell types in rat substantia nigra zona compacta distinguished by membrane properties and the actions of dopamine and opioids. J Neurosci 9:1233-1241

Macdonald RL, Werz MA (1986) Dynorpin A decreases voltage-dependent calcium conductance of mouse dorsal root ganglion neurones. J Physiol (Lond) 377: 237-249

Magistretti PJ, Morrison JH (1985) VIP neurons in the neocortex. Trends Neurosci 8: 7-8

Magistretti PJ, Morrison JH (1988) Noradrenaline and vasoactive intestinal peptide-containing neuronal systems in neocortex: functional convergence with contrasting morphology. Neuroscience 24:367-378

Magistretti PJ, Schorderet M (1984) VIP and noradrenaline act synergistically to increase cyclic AMP in cerebral cortex. Nature 308: 280-284

Magistretti PJ, Schorderet M (1985) Norepinephrine and histamine potentiate the increases in cyclic adenosine 3',5'-monophosphate elicited by vasoactive intestinal polypeptide in mouse cerebral cortical slices: mediation by α_1-adrenergic and H_1-histaminergic receptors. J Neurosci 5:363-368

Mansour A, Khachaturian H, Lewis ME, Akil H, Watson SJ (1987) Autoradiographic differentiation of mu, delta, and kappa opioid receptors in the rat forebrain and midbrain. J Neurosci 7: 2445-2464

Marrero H, Astion ML, Coles JA, Orkand RK (1989) Multiple conductance channels in type-2 cerebellar astrocytes activated by excitatory amino acids. Nature 339:378-380

McFadzean I (1988) The ionic mechanisms underlying opioid actions. Neuropeptides 11:173-180

Miyake M, Christie MJ, North RA (1989) Single potassium channels opened by opioids in rat locus coeruleus neurons. Proc Natl Acad Sci USA 86: 3419-3422

Monaghan DT, Bridges RJ, Cotman CW (1989) The excitatory amino acid receptors: their classes, pharmacology, and distinct properties in the function of the central nervous system. Ann Rev Pharmacol Toxicol 29: 365-402

Morrison JH, Magistretti PJ, Benoit R, Bloom FE (1984) The distribution and morphological characteristics of the intracortical VIP-positive cell: an immunohistochemical analysis. Brain Res 292: 269-282

Nicoll RA (1988) Neurotransmitter regulated ion channels. Science 241: 545-555

North RA (1986) Mechanisms of autonomic integration. In: Bloom FE (ed) Handbook of physiology, vol on intrinsic regulatory systems of the brain. The American Physiological Society, Bethesda, Maryland, pp 115-153

North RA, Williams JT, Surprenant AM, Christie MJ (1987) μ and δ receptors belong to a family of receptors that are coupled to potassium channels. Proc Natl Acad Sci USA 84: 5487-5491

Parnavelas JG, Papadopoulos GC (1989) The monoaminergic innervation of the cerebral cortex is not diffuse and nonspecific. Trends Neurosci 12: 315-320

Siggins GR, Gruol DL (1986) Synaptic mechanisms in the vertebrate central nervous system. In: Bloom FE (ed) Handbook of physiology, vol on intrinsic regulatory systems of the brain. The American Physiological Society, Bethesda, Maryland, pp 1-114

Siggins GR, Zieglgänsberger W (1981) Morphine and opioid peptides reduce inhibitory synaptic potentials in hippocampal pyramidal cells in vitro without alteration of membrane potential. Proc Natl Acad Sci USA 78: 5235-5239

Simonds WF (1988) The molecular basis of opioid receptor function. Endocr Rev 9: 200-212

Sontheimer H, Kettenmann H, Backus KH, Schachner H (1988) Glutamate opens Na^+/K^+ channels in cultured astrocytes. Glia 1: 328-336

Tempel A, Zukin RS (1987) Neuroanatomical patterns of the mu, delta, and kappa opioid receptors of rat brain as determined by quantitative in vitro autoradiography. Proc Natl Acad Sci U.S.A. 84: 4308-4412

Usowicz MM, Gallo V, Cull-Candy SG (1989) Multiple conductance channels in type-2 cerebellar astrocytes activated by excitatory amino acids. Nature 339: 380-383

Williams JT, North RA, Tokimasa T (1988) Inward rectification of resting and opiate-activated potassium currents in rat locus coeruleus neurons. J Neurosci 8: 4299-4306

Williams JT, Zieglgänsberger W (1981) Mature spinal ganglion cells are not sensitive to opiate receptor mediated actions. Neurosci Lett 21: 211-216

Zieglgänsberger W (1986) Central control of nociception. In: Bloom FE (ed) Handbook of physiology, vol on intrinsic regulatory systems of the brain. The American Physiological Society, Bethesda, Maryland, pp 581-645

Zieglgänsberger W, French ED, Siggins GR, Bloom FE (1979) Opioid peptides may excite hippocampal pyramidal neurons by inhibiting adjacent inhibitory interneurons. Science 205: 415-417

8 Physiological Role of ß-Nerve Growth Factor and Its Possible Pathophysiological Implication in the Central Nervous System

R.Hellweg, C.Hock, H.D.Hartung

Nerve Growth Factor: Classical Retrograde Messenger Between Peripheral Target Tissues and Their Innervating Neurons

Beta-nerve growth factor (NGF) is a well-known 26-kDa homodimeric protein, whose physiological functions are well established in the peripheral nervous system. There NGF has been shown to be essential for the ontogenetic development and maintenance of specialized properties of the sympathetic and neural crest-derived sensory neurons (for reviews, see Greene and Shooter 1980; Thoenen and Barde 1980; Levi-Montalcini 1987). Under physiological conditions, this neurotrophic factor is produced and released in limiting amounts by tissues densely innervated by NGF-sensitive neurons (Korsching and Thoenen 1983a; Heumann et al. 1984; Shelton and Reichardt 1984). Following release, NGF is bound by an NGF receptor on the surface of these neurite terminals, internalized and then transported together with NGF receptors (Korsching and Thoenen 1983b; Palmetier et al. 1984; Johnson et al. 1987; Raivich and Kreutzberg 1987). This apparently occurs in the form of an NGF-NGF receptor complex, which is transported retrogradely to the neuronal perikarya in sympathetic and primary sensory ganglia,where it exerts most of its neurotrophic effects by still unknown second-messenger mechanisms (for reviews, see Thoenen et al. 1985,1987a; cf. Levi et al. 1988). The function of NGF as a retrograde messenger between peripheral target tissues and their innervating neurons was also recognized from previous observations demonstrating that any restriction of the availability of NGF to the perikarya of NGF-responsive neurons results in serious impairments of their function (Thoenen and Barde 1980; Johnson et al. 1986; Thoenen et al. 1987b): during limited periods of embryonic development administration of anti-NGF antibodies or interruption of the retrograde axonal transport of NGF results in a degeneration of the corresponding neurons. In fully differentiated neurons interference with the availability of NGF by the same procedures results consistently in an impairment of specialized functions, such as a reduction in the synthesis of enzymes involved in the neuron-specific transmitter formation (Thoenen and Barde 1980; Thoenen and Edgar 1985; Thoenen et al. 1985) and/or in a reduced formation of neuron-specific peptides in sensory neurons (Schwartz et al. 1982; Otten 1984). However, although NGF is the best characterized neurotrophic factor so far, little is known about its role in the pathogenesis of any disease(s). Very recently we provided initial evidence that NGF may play a pathophysiological role in diabetic neuropathy (Hellweg and Hartung 1990; Hellweg et al. 1991). Moreover, NGF and the expression of its receptor may play a crucial role during peripheral nerve regeneration (see Raivich et al. 1990 for recent review).

Increasing Evidence for a Physiological Role of NGF in the Central Cholinergic Nervous System

In contrast, evidence for a physiological role of NGF in the central nervous system (CNS) has accumulated gradually only during most recent years (for reviews, see Thoenen et al. 1987 a,b; Whittemore and Seiger 1987; Ebendal 1989). After it had been demonstrated that central catecholaminergic neurons neither respond to NGF nor express NGF receptors (Konkol et al. 1978; Schwab et al. 1979), the cholinergic neurons of the mammalian basal forebrain nuclei have been shown to bind NGF with high selectivity and to transport it retrogradely from their fields of projection (such as hippocampus and cortex) to the corresponding cholinergic perikarya (such as septal region and nucleus basalis of Meynert) (Schwab et al. 1979; Seiler and Schwab 1984). These neurons respond to NGF with elevated levels of choline acetyltransferase (ChAT) activity, the enzyme responsible for the synthesis of the cholinergic neurotransmitter acetylcholine (Honegger et al. 1982; Gnahn et al. 1983; Hefti et al. 1985; Cavicchioli et al. 1989; Fusco et al. 1989). In analogy to the periphery there is a close correlation between the levels of NGF-mRNA and the density of innervation by NGF-sensitive neurons in their fields of projection (Korsching et al. 1985; Large et al. 1986; Whittemore et al. 1986). Even within a given brain region, such as the hippocampus, the differences in the density of cholinergic innervation are reflected by corresponding differences in NGF levels (Korsching et al. 1985). Further evidence supporting the physiological role of NGF for the cholinergic neurons of the basal forebrain system was gained from the observation that there is a closely coordinated increase in NGF and ChAT levels during specific periods of early postnatal development (Large et al. 1986; Auburger et al. 1987).

Immunological Neutralization of Central NGF: Final Proof for Its Physiological Role for Central Cholinergic Neurons

However, these observations support the notion of a physiological function of NGF in the central cholinergic basal forebrain system only within the limits of conclusiveness of correlated phenomena [see Thoenen et al. (1987a) as for further discussion]. If NGF should have a physiological role in the development of these central cholinergic neurons which is similar to that in peripheral sympathetic or sensory neurons, it would be expected that the administration of anti-NGF antibodies does result in a decrease of the number of cholinergic neurons in the basal forebrain nuclei during a restricted period of their ontogenetic development and also in a reduction of their ChAT levels when these are fully differentiated. Analogous to the peripheral nervous system, where the survival effect of NGF is most prominent at the time when the outgrowing axons just reach their target tissues, it had to be assumed that the cholinergic basal forebrain neurons are particularly sensitive to anti-NGF antibodies during the early postnatal period (see Thoenen et al. 1987a,b). However, neither intracerebroventricular (i.c.v.) nor intracortical injection of polyclonal anti-NGF antibodies from birth to the 7th postnatal day had any effect on ChAT levels in the hippocampus, cortex, and septum of young rats (Gnahn et al. 1983). Additional efforts to influence ChAT levels in basal forebrain neurons by i.c.v. injection of affinity-purified Fab fragments of anti-NGF antibodies every 2nd day from birth to the 14th postnatal day were also without effect (Thoenen et al. 1987b). The Fab fragments used were shown to block the biological activity of NGF *in vitro* and, according to their size, should better penetrate into the brain tissue than intact IgG antibodies. However, it has recently been reported that i.c.v. injection of polyclonal anti-NGF antibodies decreased ChAT activity in different brain regions of rat pups (Vantini et al. 1989). But this effect was transient since ChAT activity returned to normal values within 25 days after birth (Vantini et al. 1989).

Thus, no study has so far shown that specific removal or neutralization of endogenous NGF by immunological means causes alterations in adult NGF-sensitive neurons of the CNS so that these negative results can be taken as evidence against a physiological role of NGF. However, the validity of the anti-NGF antibody experiments is questionable in view of the limited penetration of antibodies injected into the brain (cf. Springer and Loy 1985; Thoenen et al. 1987a,b). We investigated, therefore, the *in vivo* relationship between NGF and the central cholinergic basal forebrain system by intrauterine injection of hybridoma cells which released monoclonal antibodies directed against NGF (cf. Rohrer et al. 1988). We chose the prenatal approach of anti-NGF treatment because the blood-brain barrier in the rodent basal forebrain does not close before the end of gestation (see Risau and Wolburg 1990 for recent review). Thus, the antibodies released by the hybridoma cells should penetrate into the brain tissue. Six weeks after birth, i.e., when the neurons of the forebrain cholinergic system are fully differentiated in rats (cf. Large et al. 1986; Auburger et al. 1987), we measured (according to Fonnum 1975) decreased ChAT activity levels of 13% and 30% in the prenatally anti-NGF treated hippocampus and cortex, respectively ($p < 0.001$ each as compared with sham operated controls), and found that ChAT activity levels were unchanged in the olfactory bulb, septal region, striatum, brain stem, and cerebellum (Hellweg et al., manuscript in preparation). Since we were able to demonstrate that prenatal neutralization of endogenous NGF results in cholinergic deficits in young adult rat brain, our results finally proved a physiological role for NGF in the CNS. Thus, it is generally accepted that NFG is produced in the cholinergically innervated target areas to act as a retrograde trophic factor in the forebrain cholinergic system, also in adulthood.

Cholinergic Dysfunction in the Aging CNS and Its Implication for the Pathophysiology of Senile Dementia: Is This Due to Alterations in Central NGF Levels?

In the following we would like to address the question of whether alterations in endogenous NGF and ChAT activity levels play a pathophysiological role in the aging CNS and its cognitive capacities. With special respect to the topic of this symposium, we will try to evaluate whether and how results obtained experimentally in rodents may also be relevant for man, particularly for the pathophysiology of senile dementia (Alzheimer's disease). It should be emphazised, however, that some of the conclusions drawn are still a matter of speculation and thus require further investigation. Taking this *caveat* into account, speculative conclusions may be allowed on the occasion of an interdisciplinary symposium, since they possibly open the way for new concepts in the understanding or even therapy of diseases of the CNS.

In various neocortical, hippocampal, and striatal regions an age-dependent decline in acetylcholine synthesis (Vijayan 1977; Strong et al. 1980; Gibson and Peterson 1981; Sims et al. 1982; Dravid 1983; Rama Sastry et al. 1983; Springer et al. 1987), acetylcholine release (Rama Sastry et al. 1983; Gilad et al. 1987), and high-affinity choline uptake (Sherman et al. 1981; Gilad et al. 1987) has been observed in rodents. Evidence is increasing that also the morphology of the cholinergic basal forebrain system, including the striatal regions, deteriorates with advancing age in rodents (Hornberger et al. 1985; Altavista et al. 1988; Fischer et al. 1989).

These observations are interesting in view of the increasing evidence that the cholinergic basal forebrain neurons play an important role in memory, learning, and other cognitive processes (Deutsch 1971; Bartus et al. 1982). These functions are considered to be affected during aging. Brain aging, however, is not a uniform process. This heterogeneity is exemplified by the marked variation in behavioral impairments seen between individuals of the same aged rat population (Gage and Björklund 1986; Fischer et al. 1987, 1989). But recently, evidence has been provided that all major cholinergic cell groups in the rat forebrain undergo degenerative changes with age, and that the most severe changes are found in those rats displaying the most profound spatial learning impairments (Fischer et al. 1989; Koh et al. 1989).

The relationship of the integrity of the cholinergic basal forebrain system to the cognitive functions may also be valid for humans. Alzheimer's disease, which is characterized by a progressive loss of memory and of other cognitive functions, is associated with the degeneration of the cholinergic forebrain system (for review see Hefti and Weiner 1986 and Butcher and Woolf 1986). Although other transmitter systems are also affected (cf. Thoenen et al. 1987), it seems that the loss and/or atrophy of cholinergic neurons is the most consistent neuropathological finding in Alzheimer's disease (Terry and Davies 1980; Coyle et al. 1983; Pearson et al. 1983; Arendt et al. 1984; Perry 1988; Reinikainen et al. 1988) and that the impairment of acetylcholine synthesis is the earliest sign of the disease (Francis et al. 1985) and is highly correlated with cognitive impairments (Perry et al. 1978, 1981, 1985).

Since i.c.v. NGF treatment can, at least partially, prevent degenerative changes in the cholinergic basal forebrain system and reverse learning deficits in a subpopulation of aged rats (Fischer et al. 1987) and also in young adult rats with lesions of the cholinergic septohippocampal pathway (Hefti et al. 1984; Will and Hefti 1985; Hefti 1986; Williams et al. 1986; Kromer 1987), it has been suggested that NGF may play a role in the loss of cognitive ability and decline of cerebral cholinergic function seen in aging and/or Alzheimer's disease (see Hefti 1983; Hefti and Weiner 1986). As Koh and Loy (1988) have pointed out, degeneration of basal forebrain neurons may be caused by the lack of target-derived NGF, reduced responsiveness to NGF, reduced NGF transport, or failure of coupling to "second messenger" systems. But no direct evidence has so far been found for the involvement of NGF in normal aging of the human brain and/or in the pathophysiology of Alzheimer's disease (Goedert et al. 1986; but cf. Whittemore and Seiger 1987; Ebendal 1989).

Levels of NGF and ChAT in the Brain of Cognitively Impaired Aged Rats

In collaboration with Dr. W. Fischer and Prof. A. Björklund (University of Lund, Dept. of Medical Cell Research, Lund, Sweden) and Prof. F. H. Gage (University of California, Dept. of Neurosciences, San Diego, La Jolla, California, United States), we have determined levels of NGF (according to Hellweg et al. 1989a) and ChAT activity in young nonimpaired and aged subpopulations of Sprague-Dawley rats with either slight or severe spatial learning impairments, which were assessed by the Morris water maze test (see Morris 1984 and Fischer et al. 1989). In order to distinguish age-related phenomena from alterations due to specific learning impairments, we have compared young nonimpaired with aged slightly impaired and with aged severely impaired rats. Moreover, we addressed the question of whether our biochemical data are correlated with the degree of spatial learning and memory impairments in the aged rats.

We found no support for the hypothesis that reduced endogenous NGF levels in aged rat brain could account for the severe learning impairments seen in a subpopulation of aged Sprague-Dawley rats. On the contrary, NGF levels were significantly ($p < 0.05$) increased by up to 30% in some aged brain regions, notably the cortex, septal region, olfactory bulb, and cerebellum as compared with the young controls (for details, see Hellweg et al. 1990).

The significant but moderate increase in NGF levels which has been observed in our study with unmanipulated, but learning-impaired aged rats and even after nearly complete cholinergic deafferentation of the hippocampus by fimbria-fornix transection (cf. Björklund and Stenevi 1981) in other studies with young adult rats (Gasser et al. 1986; Korsching et al. 1986; Weskamp et al. 1986; Lärkfors et al. 1987) speaks in favor of a stringent regulation of NGF production and/or NGF utilization. The elevated NGF levels could be due to augmented NGF synthesis, e.g., by reactive gliosis. At least *in vitro*, astroglial cells are capable of producing NGF (and other growth factors) (Lindsay 1979). Moreover, after transection of the fimbria-fornix (comprising the major cholinergic input to the hippocampus; Björklund and Stenevi 1981) an increase in weights of the hippocampus and neocortex to maximally 122 % of sham-operated controls, possibly resulting from glial scar formation, has been reported (Lärkfors et al. 1987). Thus, an ongoing, age-dependent gliosis may well explain the increased NGF levels in the affected areas. In this context, it is interesting to note that interleukin-1 levels in Alzheimer's disease temporal lobe homogenates are elevated, as are the levels of S-100 and glial fibrillary acidic protein, two proteins reportedly elevated in reactive astrocytes (Griffin et al. 1989). These recent data suggest that the astrogliosis in Alzheimer's disease may be promoted by elevation of interleukin-1 (Griffin et al. 1989). Since interleukin-1 has been shown to increase NGF synthesis in the CNS (Spranger et al. 1990), it may be speculated that the elevated NGF levels observed in our study might be due to an elevation in interleukin-1 in the affected brain regions, thereby leading to reactive gliosis. Alternatively, it seems possible that the elevated NGF levels could be due to impaired removal of NGF by degenerating neurons. This possibility is supported by the fact that after transection of the fimbria-fornix increased NGF levels, but no changes in NGF-mRNA levels, have been observed in the hippocampus (Korsching et al. 1986; Weskamp et al. 1986; Lärkfors et al. 1987; Whittemore et al. 1986). Interestingly, however, the elevation of NGF content after transection of the septohippocampal pathway was even more pronounced in the septum (Gasser et al. 1986; Weskamp et al. 1986), where normally only low levels of NGF-mRNA are detectable (Korsching et al. 1985; Whittemore et al. 1986). Thus, the elevated NGF levels observed in our study may, in the target regions, be primarily due to a combination of increased production and accumulation of NGF due to the reduced removal by normal retrograde axonal transport, whereas the increase in the cell body-rich septal area may be primarily due to increased local synthesis, perhaps as a result of reactive gliosis (see Gage et al. 1988 for further discussion).

Moreover, ChAT activity was significantly decreased by about 20 % in the striatum and brain stem of the aged rat group as compared with the young controls ($p < 0.05$). The only significant difference in levels of ChAT activity between the two behaviorally defined aged groups was observed in the striatum (-20 % compared with the severely impaired animals, $p < 0.05$). On the other hand, ChAT activity was increased in the cerebellum in the aged group by maximally 30 % ($p < 0.05$; in detail, see Hellweg et al. 1990). The parallel increase in both NGF content and ChAT activity in the cerebellum has not been observed before (cf. Korsching et al. 1985) and is somewhat surprising since adult rat cerebellum was thought to contain no cholinergic neurons as revealed by negative immunohistochemistry for ChAT (Gould and Butcher 1987). But ChAT activity has been demonstrated in the cerebellum of aging mice (Vijayan 1977) and, recently, receptors for NGF have also been demonstrated in adult rat cerebellum (Taniuchi et al. 1986; Pioro and Cuello 1988). On the contrary, changes in levels of NGF and ChAT activity observed in the aging striatum and brain stem were not correlated, suggesting an independent mechanism.

Lacking Correlation of Biochemical Data to the Degree of Spatial Learning and Memory Impairment in Aged Rats

The observed changes, both in NGF and ChAT levels, did not correlate with the spatial learning performance within the aged rat group (Hellweg et al. 1990) despite the severe degenerative changes at the cell body level which have been observed in all major cholinergic cell groups in the aged rat forebrain and which are substantial enough to severely impair the function of the affected neurons (Fischer et al. 1989). This indicates that the NGF changes observed in our animal model probably reflect aging phenomena rather than a special mechanism of learning impairments. But particularly in studies including old Alzheimer's disease cases there is generally a degree of overlap between values from Alzheimer's disease and from control brains that is inconsistent with the behavioral differences between a terminal Alzheimer's disease case and a normally functioning old person (Coleman and Flood 1987).

Age-Dependent Cholinergic Atrophy Due to Reduced Responsiveness to NGF Rather Than to Lack of the Trophic Factor

Thus, age-dependent cholinergic neuron atrophy and cell loss in the forebrain is likely to occur even in the presence of increased NGF levels in the target regions. Interestingly, a marked reduction in NGF receptor immunoreactivity in the aged rat forebrain (Koh and Loy 1988; Gómez-Pinilla et al. 1989), which is correlated with spatial memory impairment (Koh et al. 1989), has been reported recently. This may be taken to suggest that the aging forebrain cholinergic neurons have a reduced capacity to bind and transport NGF from their targets. Such reduced NGF transport could explain the overall tendency toward increased NGF levels in the cholinergically innervated targets and also explain why the receptor-deficient neurons undergo atrophic changes in the presence of maintained NGF tissue levels (Hellweg et al. 1990). This seems to be inconsistent with the observation that exogenous NGF, administered intraventricularly via minipump, can reduce the age-dependent cholinergic atrophy (Fischer et al. 1987). But it should be considered that NGF levels administered in these experiments are most probably considerably larger than those present in the brain tissue *in vivo* (Hellweg et al. 1990). In this way administered NGF has been shown to induce its own (low affinity) receptor on intact, cholinergic neurons in the basal forebrain nuclei (Cavicchioli et al. 1989; Higgins et al. 1989). On the contrary, the expression of the (low-affinity) NGF receptor is reduced in the basal forebrain cholinergic neurons of aged Long-Evans rats (Koh and Loy 1988), and the reduction in NGF receptor immunoreactivity was highly correlated with the degree of spatial learning impairment (Koh et al. 1989). This seems to be consistent with the idea that the age-dependent cholinergic neuron atrophy is due to reduced responsiveness to NGF rather than to a lack of the trophic factor (Hellweg et al. 1990). As in our study, Koh and Loy (1988) observed a wide variability in the population of aged rats, which suggests that NGF receptor loss may be an ongoing process. Such degenerative changes may then occur over a long period before there is any detectable cell loss in aging animals. Also in man, the changes in brain function found in normal aging, benign senescent forgetfulness, and Alzheimer's disease can be seen as a continuum, possibly reflecting a single underlying process (Brayne and Calloway 1988; for review, see Coleman and Flood 1987).

Sustained or Increased NGF Levels in the Aged Brain May Be Important for a Compensatory Increase in ChAT Activity in Remaining Functional Neurons

Although sustained or increased NGF levels in the aged brain appear unable to prevent age-dependent cholinergic neuron atrophy, they may play a role in the compensatory changes associated with this process (Hellweg et al. 1990). Fischer et al. (1989) have shown that the ChAT activity levels in the target regions (such as cortex and hippocampus) are only marginally affected even in severely impaired aged rats, despite the fact that their cell body regions have undergone substantial atrophic changes and cell loss. This suggests a compensatory increase in ChAT activity in the remaining functional neurons. Since NGF is known to increase ChAT activity in the forebrain cholinergic neurons, both in adults and during development (Gnahn et al. 1983; Cavicchioli et al. 1989; Fusco et al. 1989), the sustained NGF levels in the aged brain could be important for the maintenance of cholinergic neurotransmission in a situation when the system is undergoing progressive degenerative changes (Hellweg et al. 1990).

Possible Neuropathological Implications of Age-Related NGF Increase: Abnormal Sprouting Response and Amyloid Formation

However, it may be allowed on the occasion of this symposium to play the devil's advocate for once and to speculate in a different direction. Our results are also consistent with the observation that sprouting responses occur in brains afflicted with Alzheimer's disease (Probst et al. 1983), which are similar to those seen in injured brains of rats (Geddes et al. 1985) and which could be triggered by accumulation and/or enhanced production of neuronotrophic factor(s) such as NGF. Accumulation of NGF which may lead to sprouting responses may not be a simple repairing of damaged circuits since neuronal atrophy and/or degeneration continues (cf. Fischer et al. 1989). Moreover, abnormal neurite sprouting occurs within senile plaques (Probst et al. 1983) and may be involved in the formation of this neuropathological hallmark in Alzheimer's disease brain (Nukina and Ihara 1983) in which dystrophic ChAT-positive processes surrounding the amyloid core have been observed (Armstrong et al. 1986). As one speculative explanation of our results, therefore, increased NGF levels in aged (learning impaired) rat brain may enhance abnormal neuronal metabolism as well as induce ChAT activity in degenerating and/or (still) undamaged cholinergic neurons. This would be consistent with the recent results obtained for synaptosomal high-affinity [^{3}H]choline uptake indicating that regions exhibiting cholinergic neuronal loss in Alzheimer's disease experience a profound upregulation of neuronal activity in remaining neurons (Slotkin et al. 1990). In consequence, neurons may be exhausted or become increasingly vulnerable to excitotoxic substances (cf. Geddes et al. 1985) leading to neuronal atrophy and/or degeneration (cf. Slotkin et al. 1990). Moreover, increased NGF levels may even give rise to synthesis of the ß-amyloid precursor protein (cf. Mobley et al. 1988), which is one of the major prerequisites for amyloid formation in an Alzheimer's diseased brain (reviewed in Glenner 1988 and Selkoe 1989), thereby possibly compromising the neurotrophic effects of NGF on central cholinergic neurons (cf. Marx 1990). It has been recently demonstrated in rat hippocampal cultures that NGF even potentiated the neurotoxicity of ß-amyloid by a factor of about 100 000 (Yankner et al. 1990). Thus, despite possible compensatory biochemical changes (as discussed in the former paragraph), cholinergic transmission may nevertheless remain impaired in the behaviorally deficient animals as well as in the Alzheimer's diseased brain (see Fischer et al. 1989 and Hoyer 1988, respectively, for further discussion).

Alzheimer's Disease: A Dynamic Process of Functional Compensation Finally Changing into Decompensation

Based on results of quantitative studies of neuronal changes in brain aging and Alzheimer's disease (as reviewed by Coleman and Flood 1987), Arendt and Bigl (1987) suggested that Alzheimer's disease "represents a neuronal degeneration to an extent which lies beyond the functional compensatory capacity of the brain rather than a loss of the plastic capacity itself." This hypothesis would be consistent with our results in aged learning impaired rats in so far that in brain regions which are important for learning abilities, levels of NGF and/or ChAT activity were sustained or increased possibly reflecting compensatory and/or adaptive changes which are still present but functionally insufficent under condition(s) beyond the capacity of compensation. This may be particularly the case in our severely impaired aged rats as well as in the fully developed stage of Alzheimer's disease as discussed by Arendt and Bigl (1987). Thus they concluded that the understanding of the pathomechanism of degenerative disorders as a dynamic process of functional compensation which finally changes into decompensation might help to develop strategies to prevent or at least to ameliorate the loss of brain function (Arendt and Bigl 1987).

Streptozotocin-Induced Impairment of Cerebral Glucose Utilization: A Model for the Study of Early Pathological Events in Senile Dementia?

For this purpose it is mandatory to know more about the early events in aging and/or cognitive impairments. Prof. S. Hoyer and coworkers (University of Heidelberg, Dept. of Pathochemistry and General Neurochemistry, Heidelberg, FRG) have observed that a single i.c.v. injection of streptozotocin (STZ) in a subdiabetogenic dosage impairs the passive avoidance learning of adult rats within 2 - 3 weeks (Mayer et al. 1990) and results in a decreased cerebral uptake of glucose as well as an increased release of lactate from the brain without changes in cerebral arteriovenous differences of oxygen and carbon dioxide content (Nitsch et al. 1989). These findings do not reflect an unspecific decrease in general brain metabolism due to already degenerated neurons (which should also cause changes in oxygen and carbon dioxide consumption) but are consistent with a specific and early impairment of cerebral glucose utilization (Hellweg et al. 1989b), which resembles alterations measured in early-onset Alzheimer's disease (Hoyer et al. 1988). In collaboration with Prof. Hoyer's group we are investigating whether NGF and ChAT activity levels in the basal forebrain system of adult rats are altered by i.c.v. injection of STZ. In preliminary experiments (see Hellweg et al. 1989b) we found that on day 7 after injection (d7) NGF content was significantly decreased in the septal region by 30%, whereas on d21 NGF content was significantly increased in the hippocampus and cortex by about 35% as compared with controls. The reduction in NGF content in the basal forebrain after i.c.v. application of STZ, which was followed by an elevation of NGF levels in the cholinergic target regions, suggests an impaired retrograde axonal transport of NGF. This could account for the decreased ChAT activity levels (by maximally 15%) in the hippocampus measured in the preliminary experiments, whereas ChAT activity levels in the remaining STZ-treated brain regions were only marginally affected (Hellweg et al. 1989b) as it was observed in cognitively impaired aged rats (Fischer et al. 1989; Hellweg et al. 1990). The elevated NGF levels on d21 may also be due to an altered NGF synthesis, e.g., by reactive gliosis, possibly reflecting compensatory mechanisms as discussed above. Thus, alterations in central NGF levels of aged learning-impaired rats (as described above) resemble, in many respects, those in adult rats after i.c.v. STZ treatment. In contrast to the aged rat brain, in which the pathophysiology of aging had probably started long before the investigation, our current approach provides for detailed investigations of the early events that may lead to severely learning-impaired brain function, thus providing a model for the study of senile dementia. We suggest that the impairment of passive avoidance learning observed in rats after STZ injection is due to the perturbation of the cholinergic basal forebrain system (Hellweg et al. 1989b; Mayer et al. 1990). It remains to be investigated how these observations are related to the STZ-induced impairment of cerebral glucose metabolism (cf. Nitsch et al. 1989). Since STZ is known to destroy insulin-producing cells (such as in pancreatic islets) and to interfere with the insulin-insulin receptor-mediated glucose transport in adipocytes (see Garvey et al.

1989), it is reasonable to assume that there might be a similiar action of STZ in the brain (cf. Hoyer and Nitsch 1988; Nitsch et al. 1989). For the peripheral nervous system, we have recently shown that STZ-induced diabetes mellitus influences the production and/or transport of endogenous NGF (Hellweg and Hartung 1990), which consequently may account for some of the functional deficits known to occur in diabetic neuropathy, such as impaired catecholaminergic transmitter synthesis. The diabetes-induced changes in endogenous NGF levels do not seem to be due to permanent toxic effect(s) of the intraperitoneally injected STZ but rather to effect(s) of either lack of insulin and/or elevated glucose levels (Hellweg et al. 1991). In any case, the underlying mechanism(s) of the i.c.v. STZ-induced impairment of cerebral glucose metabolism should be investigated in detail to shed more light on the cascade of intracellular metabolic events which may contribute to cell damage also in dementia of the Alzheimer's type (for a proposal, see Hoyer, 1988; Hoyer and Nitsch 1988). These investigations may have implications for new interventions on the central (cholinergic) mechanism in Alzheimer's disease (cf. Hellweg et al. 1989b).

Conclusion

Although the physiological role of NGF in the peripheral sympathetic and neural crest-derived sensory and — more recently — also in the central cholinergic nervous system is well established, the involvement of NGF, or other trophic factor(s), in age-related neurodegenerative processes is unclear (for reviews, see Thoenen et al. 1987; Ebendal 1989). Our results presented indicate that brain NGF levels are maintained at normal or supranormal levels in aged rats with severe learning and memory impairments, and that the marked atrophy and cell loss in the forebrain cholinergic system, known to occur in the cognitively impaired aged rats, seems to be due to reduced responsiveness to NGF rather than to a reduced availability of NGF in the cholinergic target areas (Hellweg et al. 1990). Moreover, we provided initial evidence that the impairment of passive avoidance learning observed in adult rats after i.c.v. STZ treatment may be due to a perturbation of the cholinergic basal forebrain system in which alterations in central NGF levels resembled, in many respects, those in the cognitively impaired aged rats (Hellweg et al. 1989b). It remains to be investigated how these observations are related to the STZ- induced impairment of cerebral glucose metabolism which resembles alterations known to occur in early-onset Alzheimer's disease. Our results obtained so far suggest that we possibly have an appropriate animal model for the study of the early events leading to senile dementia, which may be well suited for a better pathophysiological understanding of the dynamic processes of functional compensation which finally changes into decompensation in degenerative disorders.

Acknowledgements. We thank Prof. H. Thoenen, in whose laboratory the experimental work of our "Guest Group of the Clinical Institute" was done, for his support. We thank Mrs. P. Schmid for excellent technical assistance, which has been supported by a grant of the Bundesministerium für Forschung und Technologie. We thank Mrs. C. Koll for secretarial assistance. C. Hock and H.-D. Hartung did this work as part of their Medical Doctoral Thesis at the Ludwig-Maximilians-Universität München. R. Hellweg was a fellow of the Krupp Foundation. We would like to thank Prof. H.M. Emrich and Prof. D. Ploog for their continuous and encouraging support.

References

Altavista MC, Bentivoglio AR, Crociani P, Rossi P, Albanese A (1988) Age-dependent loss of cholinergic neurons in basal ganglia of rats. Brain Res 455: 177-181

Arendt T, Bigl V, Tennstedt A, Arendt A (1984) Correlation between cortical plaque count and neuronal loss in the nucleus basalis in Alzheimer's disease. Neurosci Lett 48: 81-85

Arendt T, Bigl V (1987) Alzheimer's disease as a presumptive threshold phenomenon. Neurobiol Aging 8: 552-554

Armstrong DM, Bruce G, Hersh LB, Terry RD (1986) Choline acetyltransferase immunoreactivity in neuritic plaques of Alzheimer brain. Neurosci Lett 71: 229-234

Auburger G, Heumann R, Hellweg R, Korsching S, Thoenen H (1987) Developmental changes of nerve growth factor and its mRNA in the rat hippocampus: comparison with choline acetyltransferase. Dev Biol 120: 322-328

Bartus RT, Dean RL, Beer B, Lippa AS (1982) The cholinergic hypothesis of geriatric memory dysfunction. Science 217: 408-417

Björklund A, Stenevi U (1981) In vivo evidence for a hippocampal adrenergic neurotrophic factor specifically released on septal deafferentation. Brain Res 229: 403-428

Brayne C, Calloway P (1988) Normal ageing, impaired cognitive function, and senile dementia of the Alzheimer's type: a continuum? Lancet 4: 1265-1267

Butcher LL, Woolf NJ (1986) Central cholinergic systems: synopsis of anatomy and overview of physiology and pathology. In: Scheibel AB, Wechsler AF, Brazier MAB (eds) The biological substrates of Alzheimer's disease. UCLA Forum in Medical Sciences 27. Academic, Orlando, pp 73-86

Cavicchioli L, Flanigan TP, Vantini G, Fusco M, Polato P, Toffano G, Walsh FS, Leon A (1989) NGF amplifies expression of NGF receptor messenger RNA in forebrain cholinergic neurons of rats. Eur J Neurosci 1: 258-262

Coleman PD, Flood DG (1987) Neuron numbers and dendritic extent in normal aging and Alzheimer's disease. Neurobiol Aging 8: 521-545

Coyle JT, Price DL, de Long MR (1983) Alzheimer's disease: a disease of cortical cholinergic innervation. Science 219: 1184-1189

Deutsch JA (1971) The cholinergic synapse and the site of memory. Science 174: 788-794

Dravid AR (1983) Deficits in cholinergic enzymes and muscarinic receptors in the hippocampus and striatum of senescent rats: effect of chronic hydergine treatment. Arch Int Phamacodyn Ther 264: 195-202

Ebendal T (1989) NGF in CNS: experimental data and clinical implications. Prog Growth Factor Res 1: 143-159

Fischer W, Wictorin K, Björklund A, Williams LR, Varon S, Gage FH (1987) Amelioration of cholinergic neuron atrophy and spatial memory impairment in aged rats by nerve growth factor. Nature 329: 65-68

Fischer W, Gage FH, Björklund A (1989) Degenerative changes in forebrain cholinergic nuclei correlate with cognitive impairments in aged rats. Eur J Neurosci 1: 34-45

Fonnum F (1975) A rapid method for the determination of choline acetyltransferase. J Neurochem 24: 407-409

Francis PT, Palmer AM, Sims NR, Bowen DM, Davison AN, Esiri MM, Neary D, Snowden JS, Wilcock GK (1985) Neurochemical studies of early-onset Alzheimer's disease — possible influence on treatment. N Engl J Med 313: 7-11

Fusco M, Oderfeld-Nowak B, Vantini G, Schiavo N, Gradkowska M, Zaremba M, Leon A (1989) Nerve growth factor affects uninjured adult rat septohippocampal cholinergic neurons. Neuroscience 33: 47-52

Gage FH, Björklund A (1986) Cholinergic septal grafts into the hippocampal formation improve spatial learning and memory in aged rats by an atropine-sensitive mechanism. J Neurosci 6: 2837-2847

Gage FH, Olejniczak P, Armstrong DM (1988) Astrocytes are important for sprouting in the septohippocampal circuit. Exp Neurol 102: 2-13

Garvey WT, Huecksteadt TP, Birnbaum MJ (1989) Pretranslational suppression of an insulin-responsive glucose transporter in rats with diabetes mellitus. Science 245: 60-63

Gasser UE, Weskamp G, Otten U, Dravid AR (1986) Time course of the elevation of nerve growth factor (NGF) content in the hippocampus and septum following lesions of the septohippocampal pathway in rats. Brain Res 376: 351-356

Geddes JW, Monaghan DT, Cotman CW (1985) Plasticity of hippocampal circuitry in Alzheimer's disease. Science 230: 1179-1181

Gibson GE, Peterson C (1981) Brain acetylcholine synthesis declines with senescence. Science 213: 674-676

Gilad GM, Rabey JM, Tizabi Y, Gilad VH (1987) Age-dependent loss and compensatory changes of septohippocampal cholinergic neurons in two rat strains differing in longevity and response to stress. Brain Res 436: 311-322

Glenner GG (1988) Alzheimer's disease: its proteins and genes. Cell 52: 307-308

Gnahn H, Hefti F, Heumann R, Schwab M, Thoenen H (1983) NGF-mediated increase of choline acetyltransferase (ChAT) in the neonatal rat forebrain: evidence for a physiological role of NGF in the brain? Dev Brain Res 9: 45-52

Goedert M, Fine A, Hunt SP, Ullrich A (1986) Nerve growth factor mRNA in peripheral and central rat tissues and in the human central nervous system: lesion effects in the rat brain and levels in Alzheimer's disease. Mol Brain Res 1: 85-92

Gómez-Pinilla F, Cotman CW, Nieto-Sampedro M (1989) NGF receptor immunoreactivity in aged rat brain. Brain Res 479: 255-262

Gould E, Butcher LL (1987) Transient expression of choline acetyltransferase-like immunoreactivity in Purkinje cells of the developing rat cerebellum. Dev Brain Res 34: 303-306

Greene LA, Shooter EM (1980) The nerve growth factor: biochemistry, synthesis, and mechanism of action. Annu Rev Neurosci 3: 353-402

Griffin WST, Stanley LC, Ling C, White L, MacLeod V, Perrot LJ, White III CL, Araoz C (1989) Brain interleukin 1 and S-100 immunoreactivity are elevated in Down syndrome and Alzheimer disease. Proc Natl Acad Sci USA 86: 7611-7615

Hefti F (1983) Is Alzheimer disease caused by lack of nerve growth factor? Ann Neurol 13: 109-110

Hefti F, Dravid A, Hartikka J (1984) Chronic intraventricular injections of nerve growth factor elevate hippocampal choline acetyltransferase activity in adult rats with partial septohippocampal lesions. Brain Res 293: 305-311

Hefti F, Hartikka J, Eckenstein F, Gnahn H, Heumann R, Schwab M (1985) Nerve growth factor (NGF) increases choline acetyltransferase but not survival or fiber outgrowth of cultured fetal septal cholinergic neurons. Neuroscience 14: 55-68

Hefti F (1986) Nerve growth factor promotes survival of septal cholinergic neurons after fimbrial transection. J Neurosci 6: 2155-2162

Hefti F, Weiner WJ (1986) Nerve growth factor and Alzheimer's disease. Ann Neurol 20: 275-281

Hellweg R, Hock C, Hartung H-D (1989a) An improved rapid and highly sensitive enzyme immunoassay for nerve growth factor. Technique 1: 43-48

Hellweg R, Nitsch R, Hock C, Mayer G, Hoyer S (1989b) Changes of nerve growth factor levels in the central cholinergic system of aged learning-impaired rat resemble strep-tozotocin- induced impairments of brain glucose metabolism and learning abilities in adult rat. In: Kewitz H, Thomsen T, Bickel U (eds) Pharmacological interventions on central cholinergic mechanisms in senile dementia (Alzheimer's disease). Zuckschwerdt, München, pp 180-184

Hellweg R, Hartung H-D (1990) Endogenous levels of nerve growth factor (NGF) are altered in experimental diabetes mellitus: a possible role for NGF in the pathogenesis of diabetic neuropathy. J Neurosci Res 26: 258-267

Hellweg R, Fischer W, Hock C, Gage FH, Björklund A, Thoenen H (1990) Nerve growth factor levels and choline acetyltransferase activity in the brain of aged rats with spatial memory impairments. Brain Res 537: 123-130

Hellweg R, Wöhrle M, Hartung H-D, Stracke H, Hock C, Federlin K (1991) Diabetes mellitus-associated decrease in nerve growth factor levels is reversed by allogeneic pancreatic islet transplantation. Neurosci Lett 125:1-4

Heumann R, Korsching S, Thoenen H (1984) Relationship between levels of nerve growth factor (NGF) and its messenger RNA in sympathetic ganglia and peripheral target tissues. EMBO J 3: 3183-3189

Higgins GA, Koh S, Chen KS, Gage FH (1989) NGF induction of NGF receptor gene expression and cholinergic neuronal hypertrophy within the basal forebrain of the adult rat. Neuron 3: 247-256

Honegger P, Lenoir D (1982) Nerve growth factor (NGF) stimulation of cholinergic telencephalic neurons in aggregating cell cultures. Dev Brain Res 3: 229-238

Hornberger JC, Buell SJ, Flood DG, McNeill TH, Coleman PD (1985) Stability of numbers but not size of mouse forebrain cholinergic neurons to 53 months. Neurobiol Aging 6: 269-275

Hoyer S (1988) Glucose and related brain metabolism in dementia of Alzheimer type and its morphological significance. Age 11: 158-166

Hoyer S, Nitsch R (1988) Abnormalities in cerebral carbohydrate and related protein metabolism in dementia of Alzheimer type point to a deficiency of neuronal insulin receptor. In: Agnoli A, Cahn J, Lassen N, Mayeux R (eds) Senile dementias. Libbey, Paris, pp 131-136

Hoyer S, Oesterreich K, Wagner O (1988) Glucose metabolism as the site of the primary abnormality in early-onset dementia of Alzheimer type? J Neurol 235: 143-148

Johnson EM, Rich KM, Yip HK (1986) The role of NGF in sensory neurons *in vivo*. Trends Neurosci 1: 33-37

Johnson EM, Taniuchi M, Clark HB, Springer JE, Koh S, Tayrien MW, Loy R (1987) Demonstration of the retrograde transport of nerve growth factor (NGF) receptor in the peripheral and central nervous system. J Neurosci 7: 923-929

Koh S, Loy R (1988) Age-related loss of nerve growth factor sensitivity in rat basal forebrain neurons. Brain Res 440: 396-401

Koh S, Chang P, Collier TJ, Loy R (1989) Loss of NGF receptor immunoreactivity in basal forebrain neurons of aged rats: correlation with spatial memory impairment. Brain Res 498: 397-404

Konkol RJ, Mailman RB, Bendeich EG, Garrison AM, Mueller RA, Breese GR (1978) Evaluation of the effects of nerve growth factor and anti-nerve growth factor on the development of central catecholaminergic neurons. Brain Res 144: 277-285

Korsching S, Thoenen H (1983a) Nerve growth factor in sympathetic ganglia and corresponding target organs of the rat: correlation with density of sympathetic innervation. Proc Natl Acad Sci USA 80: 3513-3513

Korsching S, Thoenen H (1983b) Quantitative demonstration of the retrograde axonal transport of endogenous nerve growth factor. Neurosci Lett 39: 1-4

Korsching S, Auburger G, Heumann R, Scott J, Thoenen H (1985) Levels of nerve growth factor and its mRNA in the central nervous system of the rat correlate with cholinergic innervation. EMBO J 4: 1389-1393

Korsching S, Heumann R, Thoenen H, Hefti F (1986) Cholinergic denervation of the rat hippocampus by fimbrial transection leads to a transient accumulation of nerve growth factor (NGF) without change in mRNA[NGF] content. Neurosci Lett 66: 175-180

Kromer LF (1987) Nerve growth factor treatment after brain injury prevents neuronal death. Science 235: 214-216

Large TH, Bodary SC, Clegg DO, Weskamp G, Otten U, Reichardt LF (1986) Nerve growth factor gene expression in the developing rat brain. Science 234: 352-355

Lärkfors L, Strömberg I, Ebendal T, Olson L (1987) Nerve growth factor protein level increases in the adult rat hippocampus after a specific cholinergic lesion. J Neurosci Res 18: 525-531

Levi A, Biocca S, Cattaneo A, Calissano P (1988) The mode of action of nerve growth factor in PC 12 cells. Mol Neurobiol 2: 201-226

Levi-Montalcini R (1987) The nerve growth factor: thirty-five years later. EMBO J 6: 1145-1154

Lindsay RM (1979) Adult brain astrocytes support survival of both NGF-dependent and NGF-insensitive neurones. Nature 282: 80- 82

Marx J (1990) NGF and Alzheimer's: hopes and fears. Science 247: 408-410

Mayer G, Nitsch R, Hoyer S (1990) Effects of changes in peripheral and cerebral glucose metabolism on locomotor activity, learning and memory in adult male rats. Brain Res 532: 95-100

Mobley WC, Neve RL, Prusiner SB, McKinley MP (1988) Nerve growth factor increases mRNA levels for the prion protein and the ß-amyloid protein precursor in developing hamster brain. Proc Natl Acad Sci USA 85: 9811-9815

Morris R (1984) Developments of a water-maze procedure for studying spatial learning in the rat. J Neurosci Methods 11: 47-60

Nitsch R, Mayer G, Hoyer S (1989) The intracerebroventricularly streptozotocin-treated rat: impairment of cerebral glucose metabolism resembles the alterations of carbohydrate metabolism of the brain in Alzheimer's disease. J Neural Transm (P-D Sect) 1: 109-110

Nukina N, Ihara Y (1983) Immunocytochemical study on senile plaques in Alzheimer's disease. Proc Japan Acad 59: 288-292

Otten U (1984) Nerve growth factor and the peptidergic sensory neurons. Trends Pharmacol 7:307-310

Palmetier MA, Hartman BK, Johnson EM (1984) Demonstration of retrogradely transported endogenous nerve growth factor in axons of sympathetic neurons. J Neurosci 4: 751-756

Pearson RCA, Sofroniew MV, Cuello AC, Powell TPS, Eckenstein F, Esiri MM, Wilcock GK (1983) Persistence of cholinergic neurons in the basal nucleus in a brain with senile dementia of the Alzheimer's type demonstrated by immunohistochemical staining for choline acetyltransferase. Brain Res 289: 375- 379

Perry EK, Tomlinson BE, Blessed G, Bergmann K, Gibson PH, Perry RH (1978) Correlation of cholinergic abnormalities with senile plaques and mental test scores in senile dementia. Br Med J 25: 1457-1459

Perry EK, Blessed G, Tomlinson BE (1981) Neurochemical activities in human temporal lobe related to aging and Alzheimer-type changes. Neurobiol Aging 2: 251-256

Perry EK, Curtis M, Dick DJ, Candy JM, Atack JR, Bloxham CA, Blessed G, Fairbairn A, Tomlinson BE, Perry RH (1985) Cholinergic correlates of cognitive impairment in Parkinson's disease: comparisons with Alzheimer's disease. J Neurol Neurosurg Psychiatry 48: 413-421

Perry E (1988) Acetylcholine and Alzheimer's disease. Br J Psychol 152: 737-740

Pioro EP, Cuello AC (1988) Purkinje cells of adult rat cerebellum express nerve growth factor receptor immunoreactivity: light microscopic observations. Brain Res 455: 182-186

Probst A, Basler V, Bron B, Ulrich J (1983) Neuritic plaques in senile dementia of Alzheimer type: a Golgi analysis in the hippocampal region. Brain Res 268: 249-254

Raivich G, Kreutzberg GW (1987) Expression of growth factor receptors in injured nervous tissue. I. Axotomy leads to a shift in the cellular distribution of specific ß-nerve growth factor binding in the injured and regenerating PNS. J Neurocytol 16: 689-700

Raivich G, Hellweg R, Graeber MB, Kreutzberg GW (1990) The expression of growth factor receptors during nerve regeneration. Restor Neurol Neurosci 1: 217-223

Rama Sastry BV, Janson VE, Jaiswal N, Tayeb OS (1983) Changes in enzymes of the cholinergic system and acetylcholine release in the cerebra of aging male Fischer rats. Pharmacology 26: 61-72

Reinikainen KJ, Riekkinen PJ, Paljärvi L, Soininen H, Helkala E-L, Jolkkonen J, Laakso M (1988) Cholinergic deficit in Alzheimer's disease: a study based on CSF and autopsy data. Neurochem Res 13:135-146

Risau W, Wolburg H (1990) Development of the blood-brain barrier. Trends Neurosci 13: 174-178

Rohrer H, Hofer M, Hellweg R, Korsching S, Stehle AD, Saadat S, Thoenen H (1988) Antibodies against mouse nerve growth factor interfere in vivo with the development of avian sensory and sympathetic neurones. Development 103: 545-552

Schwab M, Otten U, Agid Y, Thoenen H (1979) Nerve growth factor (NGF) in the rat CNS: absence of specific retrograde axonal transport and tyrosine hydroxylase induction in locus coeruleus and substantia nigra. Brain Res 168: 473-483

Schwartz JP, Pearson J, Johnson EM (1982) Effect of exposure to anti-NGF on sensory neurons of adult rats and guinea pigs. Brain Res 244: 378-381

Seiler M, Schwab M (1984) Specific retrograde transport of nerve growth factor (NGF) from neocortex to nucleus basalis in the rat. Brain Res 300: 33-39

Selkoe DJ (1989) Biochemistry of altered brain proteins in Alzheimer's disease. Ann Rev Neurosci 12: 463-490

Shelton DL, Reichardt LF (1984) Expression of the ß-nerve growth factor gene correlates with the density of sympathetic innervation in effector organs. Proc Natl Acad Sci USA 81: 7951-7955

Sherman KA, Kuster JE, Dean RL, Bartus RT, Friedman E (1981) Presynaptic cholinergic mechanisms in brain of aged rats with memory impairments. Neurobiol Aging 2: 99-104

Sims NR, Marek KL, Bowen DM, Davison AN (1982) Production of [^{14}C]carbon dioxide from [U-^{14}C]glucose in tissue prisms from aging rat brain. J Neurochem 38: 488-492

Slotkin TA, Seidler FJ, Crain BJ, Bell JM, Bissette G, Nemeroff CB (1990) Regulatory changes in presynaptic cholinergic function assessed in rapid autopsy material from patients with Alzheimer's disease: implications for etiology and therapy. Proc Natl Acad Sci USA 87: 2452-2455

Spranger M, Lindholm D, Bandtlow C, Heumann R, Gnahn H, Näher-Noé M, Thoenen H (1990) Regulation of nerve growth factor (NGF) synthesis in the rat central nervous system: comparison between the effects of interleukin-1 and various growth factors in astrocyte cultures and *in vivo*. Eur J Neurosci 2: 69-76

Springer JE, Loy R (1985) Intrahippocampal injections of antiserum to nerve growth factor inhibit sympathohippocampal sprouting. Brain Res Bull 15: 629-634

Springer JE, Tayrien MW, Loy R (1987) Regional analysis of age-related changes in the cholinergic system of the hippocampal formation and basal forebrain of the rat. Brain Res 407:180-184

Strong R, Hicks P, Hsu L, Bartus RT, Enna SJ (1980) Age-related alterations in the rodent brain cholinergic system and behavior. Neurobiol Aging 1: 59-63

Taniuchi M, Schweitzer JB, Johnson EM (1986) Nerve growth factor receptor molecules in rat brain. Proc Natl Acad Sci USA 83: 1950-1954

Terry RD, Davies P (1980) Dementia of the Alzheimer type. Ann Rev Neurosci 3: 77-95

Thoenen H, Barde YA (1980) Physiology of nerve growth factor. Physiol Rev 60: 1284-1335

Thoenen H, Edgar D (1985) Neurotrophic factors. Science 229: 238-242

Thoenen H, Korsching S, Heumann R, Acheson A (1985) Nerve growth factor. In: Ciba Foundation Symposium 116, growth factors in biology and medicine. Pitman, London, pp 113-128

Thoenen H, Bandtlow C, Heumann R (1987a) The physiological function of nerve growth factor in the central nervous system: comparison with the periphery. Rev Physiol Biochem Pharmacol 109: 145-178

Thoenen H, Auburger G, Hellweg R, Heumann R, Korsching S (1987b) Cholinergic innervation and levels of nerve growth factor and its mRNA in the central nervous system. In: Dowdall MJ, Hawthorne JN (eds) Cholinergic mechanisms, vol 6, cellular and molecular basis of cholinergic function. Horwood, Chichester, pp 379-388

Vantini G, Schiavo N, Di Martino A, Polato P, Triban C, Callegaro L, Toffano G, Leon A (1989) Evidence for a physiological role of nerve growth factor in the central nervous system of neonatal rats. Neuron 3: 267-273

Vijayan VK (1977) Cholinergic enzymes in the cerebellum and the hippocampus of the senescent mouse. Exp Geront 12: 7-11

Weskamp G, Gasser UE, Dravid AR, Otten U (1986) Fimbria-fornix lesion increases nerve growth factor content in adult rat septum and hippocampus. Neurosci Lett 70: 121-126

Whittemore SR, Ebendal T, Lärkfors L, Olson L, Seiger A, Strömberg I, Persson H (1986) Developmental and regional expression of ß nerve growth factor messenger RNA and protein in the rat central nervous system. Proc Natl Acad Sci USA 83: 817-821

Whittemore SR, Seiger A (1987) The expression, localization and functional significance of ß-nerve growth factor in the central nervous system. Brain Res Rev 12: 439-464

Will B, Hefti F (1985) Behavioural and neurochemical effects of chronic intraventricular injections of nerve growth factor in adult rats with fimbria lesions. Behav Brain Res 17: 17-24

Williams LR, Varon S, Peterson GM, Wictorin K, Fischer W, Björklund A, Gage FH (1986) Continuous infusion of nerve growth factor prevents basal forebrain neuronal death after fimbria fornix transection. Proc Natl Acad Sci USA 83: 9231-9235

Yankner BA, Caceves A, Duffy LK (1990) Nerve growth factor potentiates the neurotoxicity of ß amyloid. Proc Natl Acad Sci USA 87:9020-9023

9 Anticonvulsants and Calcium Antagonists in the Treatment of Psychotic Disorders

M. Dose, H.M. Emrich

Based upon neuropharmacology, neurophysiology, biochemistry, and clinical experience, the "dopamine hypothesis" of schizophrenic and the "catecholamine hypothesis" of depressive psychoses represent an important part of the current knowledge about the etiology and pathophysiology of these psychiatric disorders. These hypotheses, however, are challenged by different findings, e.g., the antipsychotic effects of drugs such as lithium salts, anticonvulsants, and calcium (Ca^{2+}) channel blockers, which differ from "classical" neuroleptics and antidepressants in their chemical structure and pharmacology.

An integrative approach responds to this challenge by investigation of the clinical effects and the mode of action of such "atypical" drugs in order to contribute to the improvement of medical treatment and also to an understanding of psychotic disorders.

In this paper present knowledge about anticonvulsants and Ca^{2+} channel blockers in the treatment of different types of psychoses is summarized in order to speculate about a possible common mechanism of action of these psychotropic drugs.

Calcium Channel Blockers

Therapeutic effects of organic Ca^{2+} channel blocking substances which inhibit Ca^{2+} inward currents through Ca^{2+} channels of vertebrate neurons (Carbone and Lux 1984) were first reported in a manic patient who had developed side effects during lithium treatment and was treated with verapamil (Dubovsky and Franks 1983). The positive findings of this open trial have meanwhile been confirmed by controlled studies, which demonstrated the antimanic effects of verapamil (320-480 mg/day), which occurred with a delay of 5-7 days (Dose et al. 1985).

Prophylactic effects of verapamil were first reported in a manic-depressive patient who had frequently relapsed under lithium and was stabilized by constant verapamil medication for more than 1 year. However, in cardiac patients with no psychiatric history depression has been described following the use of the Ca^{2+} channel blocker nifedipine which resolved after its discontinuation.

The description of Ca^{2+} channel blocking effects of diphenylbutyl neuroleptics, which improve negative schizophrenic symptomatology (e.g., loss of drive, affective flattening, anhedonia), was followed by investigations of the use of Ca^{2+} channel blockers in schizophrenic patients. However, four studies in severely ill, chronic schizophrenic patients were unable to demonstrate therapeutic effects. In acute schizophrenic patients, verapamil (320 mg/day) has been demonstrated to be equally effective to neuroleptic treatment with haloperidol (10-40 mg/day) after 15-30 days of a controlled study (Price 1987).

In summary, the present evidence for antipsychotic effects of organic Ca^{2+} channel blockers is derived from a few controlled studies and — especially in schizophrenic psychoses — anecdotal reports which require further confirmation.

Anticonvulsants

The history of anticonvulsants as a remedy for affective and schizophrenic psychoses started in 1939 when psychotropic effects of diphenylhydantoin were observed in patients suffering from epileptic psychoses (Blair et al. 1939). Based upon this experience, antipsychotic effects of diphenylhydantoin in schizophrenic psychoses were investigated by several groups (Kalinowsky and Putnam 1943; Freyhan 1945; Kubanek and Rowell 1946) with conflicting results: half of the patients (especially with catatonic symptoms and excitement) responded well, while up to 50% were complete nonresponders. As a consequence — also due to the discovery of neuroleptics as antipsychotic medication — interest in psychotropic effects of anticonvulsants disappeared. A renaissance, however, occurred when psychotropic effects of carbamazepine were observed immediately after its establishment in the treatment of epileptic seizures (Dehing 1968). Today the acute antimanic and prophylactic effects of anticonvulsants such as carbamazepine and valproic acid alone or combined with lithium salts in affective psychoses are well established (Emrich et al. 1984). Adjunctive therapeutic effects of carbamazepine to the neuroleptic treatment of schizophrenic psychoses by which the dosages of neuroleptics and their extrapyramidal side effects could be significantly reduced have been observed in patients with (Hakola and Laulumaa 1982; Neppe 1983) and without (Dose et al. 1987) putative temporal lobe epilepsy as well as with (Klein et al. 1984) and without (Dose et al. 1987) manic excitement.

These findings, however, have up to now been reported only from a few controlled studies and need further confirmation in larger populations.

Theoretical Considerations of a Possible Mechanism of Action

Lithium and Calcium Channel Blockers

From a "classical" point of view, it is hard to understand how drugs like verapamil and carbamazepine should exert antipsychotic effects: neither do they act as postsynaptic dopamine-receptor antagonists like neuroleptics, nor do they directly affect catecholaminergic transmission by mechanisms similar to antidepressants (e.g., inhibition of reuptake). Organic Ca^{2+} channel blockers like verapamil inhibit Ca^{2+} (and slow Na^+) inward currents through a certain type of channel; their psychotropic effects may, therefore, be related to calcium-dependent mechanisms intrinsically determining neuronal activity. In this respect Ca^{2+} channel blockers share common physicochemical, neurophysiological, and pharmacological properties with lithium salts, for which a calcium-dependent mechanism of action is discussed (Aldenhoff and Lux 1982).

Lithium interacts with different peripheral calcium-dependent processes in humans (glucose metabolism, renal tubular ion transport, cardiac repolarization, release of thyroid hormones) and has been shown to alter the capability of dark adaptation of the human eye, which is suggested to be related to calcium-dependent processes (Ullrich et al. 1985; Emrich et al. 1990).

Biochemically lithium increases intracellular Ca^{2+} by an acute accumulation of inositol triphosphate promoting Ca^{2+} release from intracellular stores (van Calker and Greil 1988), which as a consequence reduces depolarization-induced Ca^{2+} inward currents. Ca^{2+} channel blockers such as verapamil possibly exert similar effects by inhibiting transmembrane inward currents.

Anticonvulsants

An involvement of Ca^{2+} in epileptogenesis is inferred from the fact that extracellular Ca^{2+} concentrations decrease during epileptiform activity in mammals (Heinemann et al. 1985) and that rhythmic discharges similar to epileptic activity are induced in hippocampal neurons at low extracellular Ca^{2+} concentrations. Epileptiform activity of this kind is prevented not only by anticonvulsants such as carbamazepine and valproic acid but also by inorganic and organic Ca^{2+} channel blockers, which may have their common mechanism of action in cell membrane stabilization. Supportive evidence for this hypothesis is lent by the finding that verapamil has anticonvulsant properties (Walden et al. 1986) and that neurotoxic effects of carbamazepine have been found to be potentiated by concomitant use of Ca^{2+} channel blockers (similar to the neurotoxic effects of lithium).

Calcium and Exitatory Amino Acids

The N-methyl-D-aspartate (NMDA) receptor, a specific subtype of an excitatory amino acid receptor (glutamate), has recently become a primary focus of attention. The NMDA receptor is linked to a Na^+/Ca^{2+} ion channel with an extraordinary Ca^{2+} conductance compared with other receptor-associated ion channels. Since a slow calcium-dependent process seems to be involved in excitotoxin-induced neuronal degeneration, it is possible that Ca^{2+} channel blockers as well as drugs which affect NMDA receptors contribute to the protection of nerve cells against excessive Ca^{2+} influx in the course of excitotoxin-mediated neuronal degeneration (Olney 1989).

A possible common denominator for the antipsychotic effects of such different drugs as lithium salts, Ca^{2+} channel blockers, and anticonvulsants, which do not fit into simplistic models of "single receptor or transmitter antagonists or agonists", may be an effect upon transmembrane Ca^{2+} currents: lithium — according to this hypothesis — by increasing intracellular Ca^{2+} delays cellular responses to external stimuli. Ca^{2+} channel blockers and anticonvulsants such as carbamazepine may have the same effect by inhibiting stimulus-induced neuronal Ca^{2+} inward currents. The consequence could be a reequilibration of disturbed balances between excitatory and inhibitory neuronal networks which clinically may result in antipsychotic effects. Such modulatory effects may at first sight be inferior to the immediate effects of "classical" antipsychotic drugs such as neuroleptics, since they do not occur in the short term but are rather delayed. However, the more "specific" a psychotropic drug interacts with certain transmitter substances and/or their receptors, the more unwanted side effects are to be expected, especially if these transmitters and/or receptors (e.g., dopamine receptors) are distributed across the whole brain and are not limited to certain brain areas such as the limbic cortex. Therefore, it appears promising for an integrative psychiatric approach to further investigate atypical psychotropic drugs with modulatory effects, which may not be too impressive at first sight, but perhaps are free of some of the unwanted effects which limit the usefulness of psychotropic drugs available today.

Acknowledgement. The authors gratefully acknowledge the personal care for and support of their scientific work by Prof. D. Ploog. At the same time we would like to thank all the patients, nurses, and colleagues who were involved in our clinical studies. Last but not least we thank our secretaries (Mrs. A. Wendl, H. Fehringer, and B. Kreutzer-Lampp) for their skillful assistance in data collecting and presentation.

References

Aldenhoff JB, Lux HD (1982) Effect of lithium on calcium-dependent membrane properties and on intracellular calcium-concentration in helix neurons. In: Emrich HM, Aldenhoff JB, Lux HD (eds) Basic mechanisms in the action of lithium. Excerpta Medica, Amsterdam, p 50

Blair D, Bailey KC, McGregor JS (1939) Treatment of epilepsy with epanutin. Lancet 2:363

Calker van D, Greil W (1988) Effects of lithium ions on the accumulation of inositol-phosphates in PC-12 cells and human granulocytes. In: Birch NJ (ed) Lithium: inorganic pharmacology and psychiatric use. IRL, Oxford, p 209

Carbone E, Lux HD (1984) A low voltage-activated, fully inactivating Ca channel in vertebrate sensory neurons. Nature 310:501-503

Dehing J (1968) Studies on the psychotropic action of tegretol. Acta Neurol Belg 68:895-905

Dose M, Emrich HM, Cording-Tömmel C, von Zerssen D (1985) Calcium antagonists in mania: a preliminary clinical report. In: Pichot P, Berner P, Wolf R (eds) Psychiatry: the state of the art, (vol 3). Plenum, New York, p 501

Dose M, Apelt S, Emrich HM (1987) Carbamazepine as an adjunct of antipsychotic therapy. Psychiatry Res 22:303-310

Dubovsky SL, Franks RD (1983) Intracellular calcium ions in affective disorders: a review and a hypothesis. Biol Psychiatry 18:781-797

Emrich HM, Okuma T, Müller AA (1984) Anticonvulsants in affective disorders. Excerpta Medica, Amsterdam

Emrich HM, Zihl J, Raptis C, Wendl A (1990) Reduced dark-adaptation: an indication of lithium's neuronal action in   humans. Am J Psychiatry 147:629-631

Freyhan FA (1945) Effectiveness of diphenylhydantoin in management of nonepileptic psychomotor excitement states. Arch Neurol Psychiatry 53:370-374

Hakola HPA, Laulumaa VA (1982) Carbamazepine in treatment of violent schizophrenics. Lancet 12:1358

Heinemann U, Franceschetti S, Hamon B, Konnerth A, Yaari Y (1985) Effects of anticonvulsants on spontaneous epileptiform activity which develops in the absence of chemical synaptic transmission in hippocampal slices. Brain Res 325:349-352

Kalinowsky LB, Putnam TJ (1943) Attempts at treatment of schizophrenia and other nonepileptic psychoses with dilantin. Arch Neurol Psychiatry 49:414-420

Klein E, Bental E, Lerer B, Belmaker RH (1984) Carbamazepine and haloperidol vs. placebo and haloperidol in excited psychoses. Arch Gen Psychiatry 41:165-170

Kubanek JL, Rowell RC (1946) The use of dilantin in the treatment of psychotic patients unresponsive to other treatment. Dis Nerv Syst 7:47-50

Neppe VM (1983) Carbamazepine as adjunctive treatment in nonepileptic chronic inpatients with EEG temporal lobe abnormalities. J Clin Psychiatry 44:326-331

Olney JW (1989) Excitatory amino acids and neuropsychiatric disorders. Biol Psychiatry 26:505-525

Price WA (1987) Antipsychotic effects of verapamil in schizophrenia. J Clin Psychiatry 9(2): 3-5

Ullrich A, Adamczyk J, Zihl J, Emrich HM (1985) Lithium effects on ophthalmological-electrophysiological parameters in young healthy volunteers. Acta Psychiatr Scand 72:113-119

Walden J, Speckmann E-J, Witte OW (1986) Depression of focal interictal epileptiform discharges by intracerebroventricular perfusion with the calcium channel blocker verapamil. In: Speckmann E-J, Schulze H, Walden J (eds) Epilepsy and calcium. Urban und Schwarzenberg, München, p 335

10 Hyperactivity and Semistarvation in the Rat: An Animal Model for Anorexia Nervosa

K.M. Pirke, A. Broocks, U.Schweiger

Patients with anorexia nervosa often show physical hyperactivity and in some patients hyperactivity is even the first symptom. Weight loss develops later on. Kron et al. (1978) observed hyperactivity in 25 out of 33 anorectic patients. Among physically active young women such as ballet dancers and marathon runners anorexia nervosa occurs more frequently than in sedentary, age-matched controls. Hyperactivity in anorectics is considered by many experts as just another means of losing weight. Epling and Pierce (1983) speculated on the possible causative role of hyperactivity for the development of anorexia and on its role in maintaining low body weight.

Routtenberg and Kuznesof (1967) observed that restricted availability of food

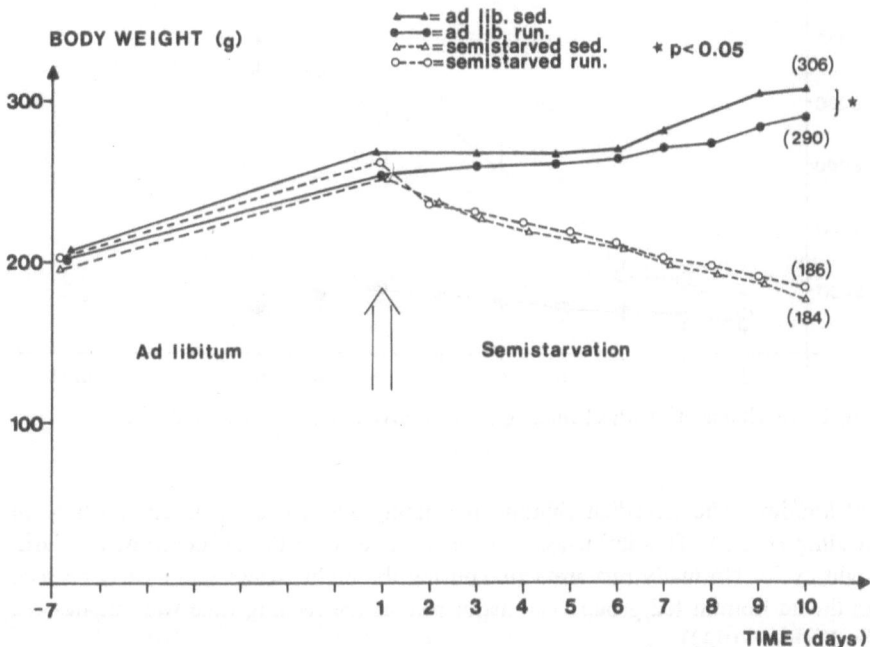

Fig.1. Body weight before and during the semistarvation experiment. All rats were kept in single cages with or without a running wheel. Numbers in parantheses show the average final weight for all experimental groups

induced hyperactivity in rats living in a running wheel. We consider this animal model as very valuable since it allows us to study the influence of semistarvation and hyperactivity on neurotransmitter activity in different parts of the brain. The mechanisms responsible for the development of hyperactivity can thus be evaluated. The hypothesis on the development of hyperactivity in semistarvation formulated on the basis of animal studies might then be evaluated later by pharmacological studies in patients with anorexia.

Figure 1 shows the development of body weight in the four groups of experimental animals: ad libitum fed sedentary controls, ad libitum fed rats living in running wheels, semistarved rats living in running wheels and semistarved rats kept in single cages without access to a running wheel. Semistarved rats were fed individually in order to achieve a constant weight loss (see Fig. 1). There was a 12-h dark-light schedule with darkness from 5 P.M. to 5 A.M.

Figure 2 shows the development of hyperactivity in semistarved rats. A maximum is achieved after about 10 days when individual rats were running up to

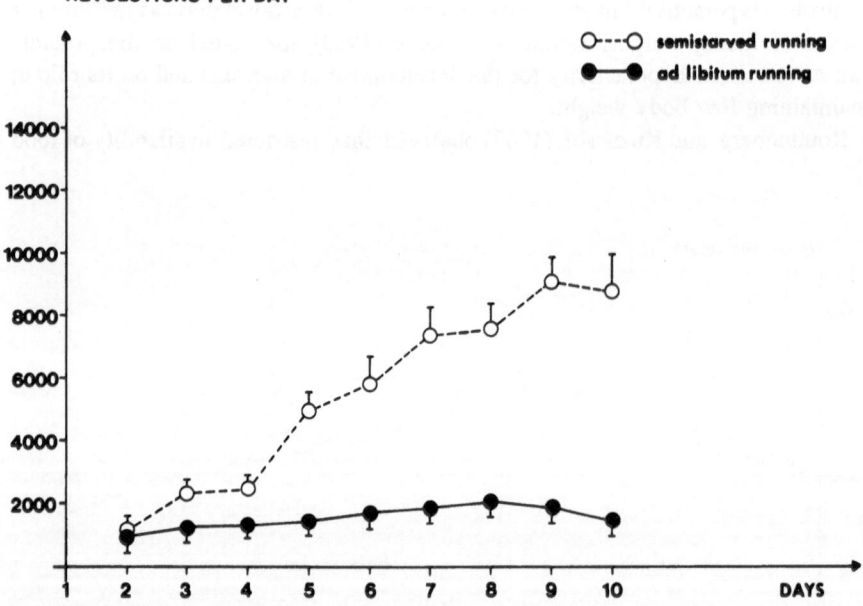

Fig.2. Development of wheel running in semistarved and ad libitum fed rats

20 km/day. The circadian rhythm of running activity depends on the time of feeding (Fig.3). This influence is much stronger than the influence of the dark-light cycle. Normally rats are active during the night, which can clearly be seen in the ad libitum fed group. The major role of the feeding time was emphasized by Richter (1922).

In order to measure the norepinephrin (NE) and serotonin (5-HT) turnover we measured NE and its main metabolite methoxyhydroxy-phenylglycol (MOPEG),

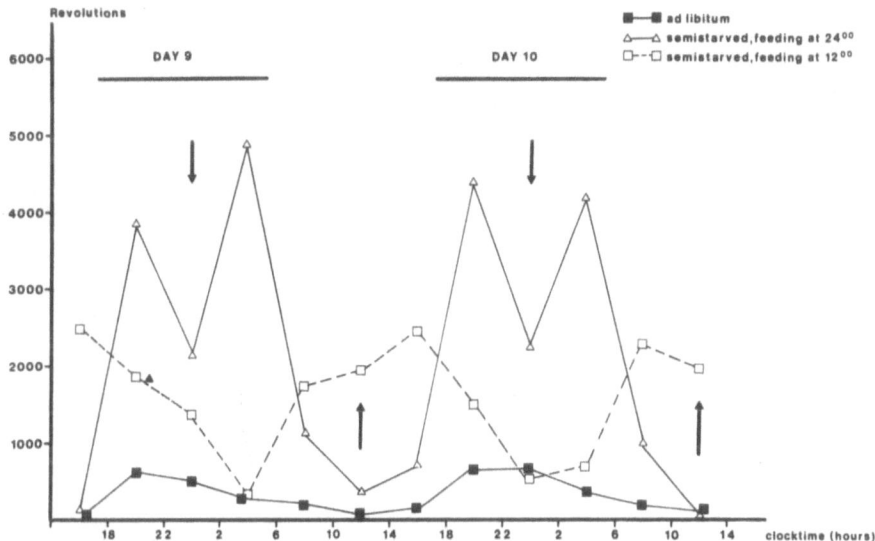

Fig.3. Circadian rhythms of running activity in semistarved and ad libitum fed animals. Black bars indicate the dark period. Arrows show the time of feeding in the semistarved groups. As can be seen, maximal activity is reached around feeding time, independent of the fact of whether it was light or dark

5-HT, and its metabolite 5-hydroxy-indole acetic acid (5-HIAA) in the medial basal hypothalamus. Although this method to measure neurotransmitter turnover has its drawbacks as with all other methods available, the concentrations of the metabolites give a fairly good estimate of the activity of serotonergic and noradrenergic neurons (Korf et al. 1973).

In earlier studies applying two different methods of turnover measurement, we observed reduced noradrenergic activity in the brain of the starved rat (Pirke and Spyra 1982, Schweiger et al. 1985). This effect of starvation is easily reversed by hyperactivity as shown in Fig.4. The rats in this experiment were fed at noon. The circadian rhythm of MOPEG concentrations parallel the running activity (see Fig.2). Activity also increased MOPEG concentrations in ad libitum fed rats. These data indicate that running wheel activity can compensate for the semistarvation-induced reduction of noradrenergic activity. Similar changes were seen in the preoptic area (data not shown here).

The mechanisms causing increased NE turnover in the brain during hyperactivity remain unclear. We have demonstrated previously that starvation causes a reduced influx of tyrosine into the brain (Schweiger et al. 1985). Tyrosine influx was calculated from the ratio tyrosine/large neutral amino acids (Tyr/LNAA) measured in peripheral plasma (Pardridge and Oldendorf 1975). According to Fernstrom and Wurtman (1973), a reduced availability of the norepinephrine precursor tyrosine may cause a reduced activity of the central norepinephrine system. During the

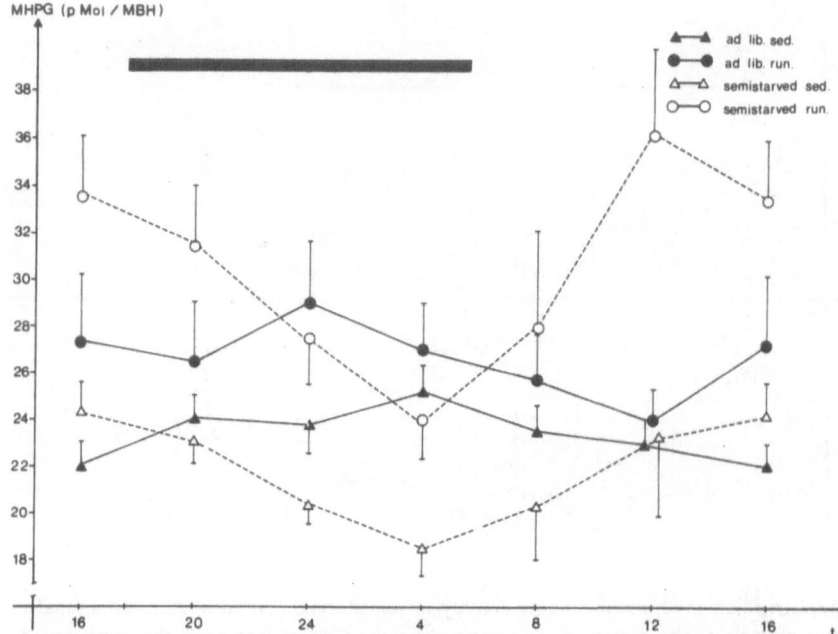

Fig.4. Circadian rhythms of the NE metabolite MHPG sulfate in the medial basal hypothalamus of semistarved and ad libitum fed rats. Hyperactivity stimulates NE turnover in both groups

state of starvation alone reduced tyrosine influx into the brain is one of the causes for reduced norepinephrine turnover (Schweiger et al. 1985). We measured Tyr/LNAA ratios also in the blood of semistarved hyperactive rats. If precursor availability plays a role in the activation of the noradrenergic activity, we should expect increased Tyr/LNAA ratios in peripheral blood. The opposite was true: Hyperactivity caused a further decrease in the Tyr/LNAA ratios as compared with semistarvation alone. Although the tyrosine influx was low, norepinephrine concentrations and norepinephrine turnover were high. These data indicate that precursor availability is not a regulatory factor for the activity of the central noradrenergic activity in semistarvation-induced hyperactivity.

The second neurotransmitter system studied was the serotonergic system. Figure 5 shows the circadian rhythm of the serotonin metabolite 5-HIAA in the medial basal hypothalamus. As can be seen, semistarvation alone increases 5-HIAA concentrations. Hyperactivity augmented 5-HIAA levels in both ad lib fed and semistarved rats. The combined effects of semistarvation and hyperactivity are a strong stimulator for hypothalamic serotonin turnover.

Based on these observations we have proposed the hypothesis that hyperactivity causes neurotransmitter changes, which may be recognized by the animal as positive and pleasant sensations. Thus the animal might learn to generate these pleasant sensations in order to overcome the negative effects of semistarvation. As a consequence the animal runs more and more. If this hypothesis is correct the application of noradrenergic or serotonergic agonists should prevent hyperactivity. In a detailed pharmacological study (Wilckens et al. in preparation) using all known centrally acting noradrenergic and serotonergic agonists (and the equivalent antagonists), we have shown that hyperactivity cannot be prevented by noradrenergic agonists but by serotonin 1c agonists. These observations suggest the important role of serotonin in the development of starvation induced hyperactivity in the rat.

These data, however, do not prove that serotonin plays a role in the development of hyperactivity in anorectic patients. They do suggest pharmacological experiments in anorectic patients to test this hypothesis. We have recently demonstrated (Pirke et al., in preparation) that hyperactivity is responsible for up to 50% of the energy expenditure in anorectic patients. Thus the development of pharmacological methods to influence hyperactivity in anorectic patients may provide a valuable treatment which could facilitate normalization of body weight in the beginning of body weight normalization.

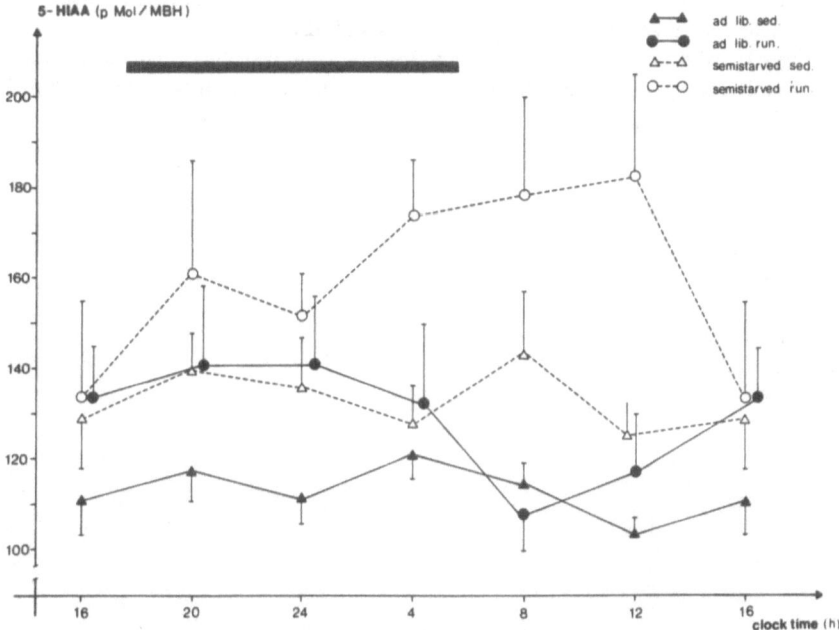

Fig. 5. Circadian rhythms of 5-HIAA, the serotonin metabolite in the medial basal hypothalamus. Semistarvation and hyperactivity stimulate serotonin turnover

References

Epling WF, Pierce WD (1983) Activity-based anorexia in rats as a function of opportunity to run on an activity wheel. Nutr Behav 2:37-49

Korf J, Aghajanian GK, Roth RH (1973) Stimulation and destruction of the locus coeruleus: opposite effects on 3-methoxy-4-hydroxyphenylglycol-sulfate levels in the rat cerebral cortex. Eur J Pharmacol 21:305-310

Kron L, Katz JL, Gorzyuski G, Weiner H (1978) Hyperactivity in anorexia nervosa: a fundamental clinical feature. Compr Psychiatry 19:433-440

Pardridge WM, Oldendorff WH (1975) Kinetic analysis of blood-rain barrier transport of amino acids. Biochim Biophys Acta 401:128-136

Pirke KM, Spyra B (1982) Catecholamine turnover in the brain and the regulation of luteinizing hormone and corticosterone in starved male rats. Acta Endocrinol (Copenh) 100:168-176

Richter CP (1922) A behavioristic study on the activity of the rat. Comp Psychol Mongr 1:1-55

Routtenberg A, Kuznesof AW (1967) Self-starvation of rats living in activity wheels on a restricted feeding schedule. J Comp Physiol 64:414-421

Schweiger U, Warnhoff M, Pirke KM (1985) Brain tyrosine availability and the depression of central nervous norepinephrine turnover in acute and chronic starvation in adult male rats. Brain Res 335:207-212

11 Effect of Starvation on Brain Morphology and Function in Anorexia Nervosa and Bulimia Nervosa

J.-C. Krieg

In the past several years there have been numerous studies on the neuroanatomical abnormalities of patients with psychiatric disorders, mainly using the method of computed tomography. This brain imaging technique enables in vivo examinations to be carried out with the aim of
- Identifying structural brain alterations such as developmental abnormalities, local or global atrophy, and changes in brain density or signal intensity as a sign of histological alterations in the cerebral tissue;
- Assessing functional abnormalities, for example, of the regional cerebral blood flow (CBF) or of the regional cerebral glucose metabolism as evidence for reduced neuronal activity.

Up to now most of the brain imaging studies in psychiatry have been performed on patients with schizophrenia and affective disorders. We have focused our interest on patients with eating disorders, i.e., anorexia nervosa and bulimia nervosa, as this group of patients provides the opportunity to study the influence of the disease process with its related neurobiological alterations on brain morphology and function.

Table 1. Clinical parameters and CT measurements of patients with anorexia nervosa and bulimia nervosa in comparison with a control group. Values are presented as mean ± SD.

	Anorexia nervosa (n = 50)	Bulimia nervosa (n = 50)	Controls (n = 50)
Age (years)	21.5 ± 3.4	22.5 ± 3.5	21.6± 3.6
Body weight (% IBW)	69 ± 6	97 ± 10	100 ± 9
Duration of the eating disorder (months)	40 ± 31	88 ± 43	—
VBR (%)	7.2 ± 3.5	4.6 ± 2.7	2.5 ± 1.1
Subjects with abnormally high VBR values (%)	70	44	0
Subjects with enlarged cortical sulci (%)	86	36	16

(%IBW, percentage of the ideal body weight; VBR, ventricle brain ratio)

In a prospective study the cranial computer tomograms (CT scans) of 50 consecutively admitted inpatients with anorexia nervosa were examined and sulcal width and ventricular brain ratio (VBR) as a measure of ventricular size were compared with the data of an age- and sex-matched control group with normal body weight (Krieg et al. 1988).

Eighty-six percent of the anorectic patients showed enlarged cortical sulci and 70% of them showed dilated ventricles (Table 1). Patients with sulcal widening were also found to have significantly higher VBR values than patients with normal-sized cortical sulci, indicating an overall enlargement of the CSF spaces in anorexia nervosa.

Figure 1 shows a magnetic resonance (MR) image of a patient with anorexia nervosa: the markedly enlarged ventricles can be clearly identified. Regarding the

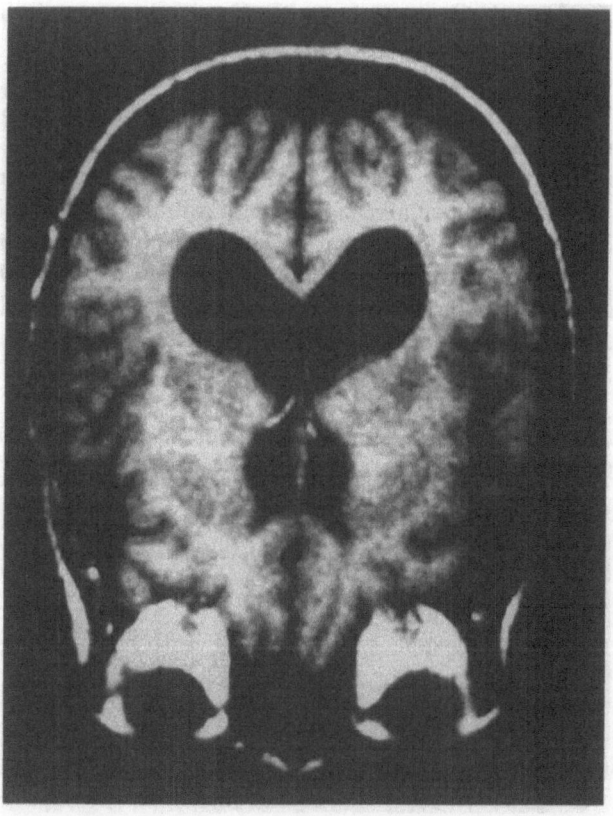

Fig. 1. Magnetic resonance image of a patient with anorexia nervosa showing enlarged ventricles

clinical parameters, there was a significant inverse relationship between the degree of the structural brain alterations and the body weight. There was, however, no association between the degree of the respective neuroradiological abnormalities and the duration of the illness, indicating that the severity and not the duration of the disorder is likely to be an important factor for the development of the structural brain abnormalities. A CT reexamination of 25 anorectic patients on discharge from hospital, which took place approximately 3 months after hospital admission and resulted in a weight gain of an average of 16% of the ideal body weight, showed a significant decrease in ventricular and sulcal size, indicating at least a partial reversibility of the neuroradiological alterations (Fig. 2).

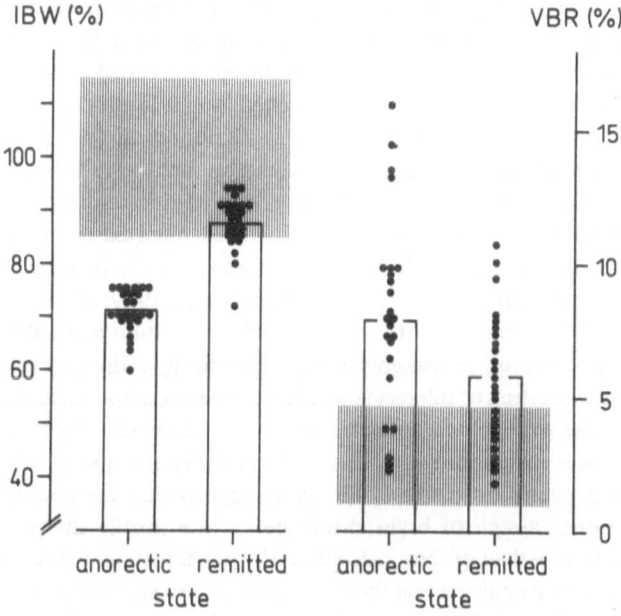

Fig. 2. Body weight (% *IBW*) and ventricular brain ratio (*VBR*) of 25 patients with anorexia nervosa in the anorexic and remitted state (*shaded areas* represent the normal range)

Surprisingly, the CT examinations, performed on 50 normal weight patients with bulimia nervosa, revealed anorexia-nervosa-like structural brain abnormalities in nearly half of the bulimic patients (Table 1). Further analysis showed that normal weight bulimic patients with a past history of anorexia nervosa did not more frequently display enlarged CSF spaces than did the bulimic patients without such a history; this finding rejects the explanation that in normal weight bulimic patients the neuromorphological alterations may be a residue of a previous anorectic state. There were no significant relationships between the neuroradiological findings and clinical parameters, such as body weight, duration of the eating disorder, and frequency of bingeing and vomiting (Krieg et al. 1989; Lauer et al. 1990). Whether the CT alterations found in bulimia nervosa are as reversible after clinical improvement as in anorexia nervosa has not yet been shown.

Provided that one and the same pathogenetic mechanism causes the structural brain abnormalities in anorexia and bulimia nervosa, being underweight per se cannot be a determining factor as the bulimic patients studied were of normal body weight. One rather has to hypothesize that the pathophysiological consequences of the disturbed eating behavior are responsible for the development of the neuro-radiological alterations, especially since it could be demonstrated that not only anorectic patients but also normal weight bulimic patients show endocrine and metabolic indices of starvation (Pirke et al. 1985). In good agreement with this assumption is the finding that in eating disorder patients (i.e., anorectic and bulimic patients) there is a close relationship between hormonal and neuroradio-logical alterations: thus the plasma cortisol levels correlated positively and the triiodotyronine serum concentrations correlated negatively with the size of the cortical sulci and the ventricles, respectively (Krieg et al. 1988; Krieg et. al. 1989). In this context it is of special interest that patients with hypercortisolemia, for example, on the basis of Cushing's disease, a corticosteroid drug treatment, an affective disorder,or alcoholism, have also been reported to exhibit enlarged CSF spaces (e.g., Momose et al. 1971; Heinz et al. 1977; Bentson et al. 1978; Okuno et al. 1980; Kellner et al. 1983; Schlegel et al. 1989; Carlen et al. 1978; Artmann et al. 1981) and furthermore ventricular dilatation and sulcal widening have also been observed in patients with a chronic hypothyroid state (Jellenik 1962). A further question of interest is whether the neuroradiological abnormalities in eating disorder patients are an expression of a real brain atrophy with loss of neural tissue. The reversibility of the structural brain alterations, observed in a great number of anorectic patients, however,suggests that the neuroradiological findings are rather a sign of brain shrinkage — presumably due to changes in water distribution — than of brain atrophy. The phenomenon of reversibility also speaks against the assumption that the CT alterations are signs of an early acquired brain lesion which makes the individual vulnerable for the development of a psychiatric disorder. Up to now systematic neuropathological examinations performed on eating disorder patients have been too rare to answer these questions convincingly.

Due to the finding of enlarged cortical sulci and dilated ventricles in eating disorder patients, the question arises of whether these structural alterations have a functional correlate. Therefore the regional cerebral blood flow (rCBF) was measured by using the xenon-133 inhalation method in 12 female anorectic patients and once again after weight gain. Although nine of the patients showed ventricular and/or sulcal widening in their CT scans, all patients except one displayed normal CBF rates in the anorectic state. Comparing the groups "anorectic versus remitted state versus controls," the mean flow rates, separately assessed at two (subcortical and cortical) levels for the right and left hemisphere, did not significantly differ among each other (Table 2). Moreover, no significant right-left differences in the flow rates could be observed in the different states (Krieg et al. 1989).

Table 2. Clinical parameters, and CT and CBF measurements of patients with anorexia nervosa at the first and second examination in comparison to a control group. Values are presented as mean ± SD.

| | Anorexia nervosa (n = 12) | | Controls (n = 12) |
	Admission	Discharge	
Age (years)	21.3 ± 3.0		31.0 ± 7.0
Body weight (% IBW)	73.3 ± 8.4	85.0 ± 7.0	107.0 ± 15.4
VBR (%)	7.0 ± 3.4	4.4 ± 3.4	—
rCBF (ml/100 g/min)			
Left HS 2	60 ± 10	62 ± 8	61 ± 8
Right HS 2	61 ± 11	62 ± 10	61 ± 7
Left HS 3	56 ± 11	59 ± 8	56 ± 7
Right HS 3	57 ± 13	58 ± 10	57 ± 7

% IBW, percentage of the ideal body weight; VBR, ventricle brain ratio; rCBF, regional cerebral blood flow; HS,half-slice 2, subcortical level; HS 3, half-slice 3, cortical level

In addition, the resting regional cerebral glucose metabolism using positron emission tomography (PET) and [^{18}F]2-fluoro-2-deoxyglucose as tracer was assessed in seven anorexic patients (72 ± 6% IBW), and once again in five of them after an average weight gain of 16% IBW. Furthermore the regional cerebral glucose metabolism was measured in nine normal weight bulimic patients. The result was that the mean global metabolic rates, assessed in the anorectic and remitted patients, in the bulimic patients and in the controls did not differ significantly among each other; again no significant left-right differences in the metabolic rates could be detected (Krieg et al. 1986, 1991; Herholz et al. 1987).

Summarizing the results of the functional-orientated computed tomography studies, one has to conclude that despite the CT findings of structural brain abnormalities, which in addition were rather pronounced in a number of cases, the measurements of the rCBF and glucose metabolism gave no evidence for a reduced functioning of certain brain areas in eating disorder patients. This result is in good agreement with other functional-orientated studies we performed on eating disorder patients: thus patients with ventricular dilatation did not perform worse in a vigilance task than patients with normally sized ventricles (Laessle et al. 1989) and EEG sleep parameters, assessed in both anorectic and bulimic patients, were within the normal range (Lauer et al. 1990).

References

Artmann H, Gall MV, Hacker H, Herrlich J (1981) Reversible enlargement of cerebral spinal fluid spaces in chronic alcoholics. Am J Neuroradiol 2:23-27

Bentson J, Reza M, Winter J, Wilson G (1978) Steroids and apparent cerebral atrophy on computed tomography scans. J Comput Assist Tomogr 2:16-23

Carlen PL, Wortzman G, Holgate RC, Wilkinson DA, Rankin JG (1978) Reversible cerebral atrophy in recently abstinent chronic alcoholics measured by computed tomography scans. Science 200:1076-1078

Heinz ER, Martinez J, Haenggeli A (1977) Reversibility of cerebral atrophy in anorexia nervosa and Cushing's syndrome. J Comput Assist Tomogr 1:415-418

Herholz K, Krieg JC, Emrich HM, Pawlik G, Beil C, Pirke KM, Pahl JJ, Wagner R, Wienhard K, Ploog D, Heiss W-D (1987) Regional cerebral glucose metabolism in anorexia nervosa measured by positron emission tomography. Biol Psychiatry 22:43-51

Jellinek EH (1962) Fits, faints, coma, and dementia in myxoedema. Lancet 3:1010-1012

Kellner CH, Rubinow DR, Gold PW, Post RM (1983) Relationship of cortisol hypersecretion to brain CT scan alterations in depressed patients. Psychiatry Res 8:191-197

Krieg J-C, Emrich HM, Backmund H, Pirke KM, Herholz K, Pawlik G, Heiss WD (1986) Brain morphology (CT) and cerebral metabolism (PET) in anorexia nervosa. In: Ferrari E, Brambilla F (eds) Disorders of eating behaviour. A psychoneuroendocrine approach. Pergamon, Oxford, p 247

Krieg J-C, Pirke K-M, Lauer C, Backmund H (1988) Endocrine, metabolic, and cranial computed tomographic findings in anorexia nervosa. Biol Psychiatry 23:377-387

Krieg J-C, Lauer C, Leinsinger G, Pahl J, Schreiber W, Pirke K-M, Moser EA (1989) Brain morphology and regional cerebral blood flow in anorexia nervosa. Biol Psychiatry 25:1041-1048

Krieg J-C, Lauer C, Pirke K-M (1989) Structural brain abnoralities in patients with bulimia nervosa. Psychiatry Res 27:39-48

Krieg J-C, Holthoff V, Schreiber W, Pirke KM, Herholz K (1991) Glucose metabolism in the caudate nuclei of patients with eating disorders, measured by PET. Eur Arch Psychiatry Clin Neurosci 240:331-333

Laessle RG, Krieg JC, Fichter MM, Pirke KM (1989) Cerebral atrophy and vigilance performance in patients with anorexia nervosa and bulimia nervosa. Neuropsychobiology 21:187-191

Lauer CJ, Lässle RG, Fichter MM, Pirke K-M, Krieg J-C (1990) Structural brain alterations and bingeing and vomiting behavior in eating disorder patients. Int J Eating Disord 9:161-166

Lauer CJ, Krieg J-C, Riemann D, Zulley J, Berger M (1990) A polysomnographic study in young psychiatric inpatients: major depression, anorexia nervosa, bulimia nervosa. J Affective Disord 18:235-245

Momose KJ, Kjellberg RN, Kliman B (1971) High incidence of cortical atrophy of the cerebral and cerebellar hemispheres in Cushing's disease. Radiology 99:341-348

Okuno T, Ito M, Konishi Y, Yoshioka M, Nakano Y (1980) Cere-bral atrophy following ACTH therapy. J Comput assist Tomogr 4:20-23

Pirke KM, Pahl J, Schweiger U, Warnhoff M (1985) Metabolic and endocrine indices of starvation in bulimia: a comparison with anorexia nervosa. Psychiatry Res 15:33-39

Schlegel S, von Bardeleben U, Wiedemann K, Frommberger U, Holsboer F (1989) Computerized brain tomography measures compared with spontaneous and suppressed plasma cortisol levels in major depression. Psychoneuroendocrinol 14:209-216

Part III: Psychiatric Aspects of Chronobiology and Sleep

12 On Self-Assessed Mood and Efficiency During Long-Term Isolation

J. Aschoff

In the 1960s, when plans were made to construct an underground isolation unit at Andechs, little was known about the effects of long-lasting isolation on mood and well-being, but sensory deprivation was a much discussed issue among psychologists (Solomon et al. 1961). I visited one of the laboratories where such experiments were done, and I was warned that to live in isolation for days and weeks would probably be harmful. It was considered essential that we should keep an eye on our subjects continuously, either via one-way windows or by closed-circuit TV. We refrained from doing so, and it turned out that nothing serious ever happened. Contrary to the expectations of psychologists, our subjects usually enjoyed staying in the unit, and many agreed to come a second time. It is partly for this reason that we have made little effort to study in detail the feelings of our subjects in the course of an experiment (Wever 1979, 1982). The present report demonstrates that various self-assessed measures of mood correlate in a systematic manner with the duration of wakefulness.

Methods

Data were available from 48 subjects (12 female, 36 male) with a mean age of 24.4 years (range 21 - 32 years). The subjects lived singly in the isolation unit (cf. Figs. 10, 11 in Wever 1979) for a mean duration of 23.3 $\pm$ 6.0 days (range 15 - 41 days) in one of three different conditions: a) constant illumination ($n = 31$); b) light-dark cycles which were not effective as an entraining zeitgeber ($n = 6$); and c) light-dark cycles complemented by regular gong signals which entrained the circadian rhythms ($n = 11$). For its main part, this report concentrates on the data from groups a and b. All subjects of these two groups developed free-running circadian rhythms with a mean period τ of 25.3 $\pm$ 2.5 h. Thirteen subjects remained internally synchronized (mean $\tau = 24.7 \pm 3.9$ h). In ten subjects internal synchronization was sometimes interrupted by a few cycles of desynchronization (mean $\tau = 25.1 \pm 0.9$ h). Fourteen subjects were more or less permanently desynchronized, either by a lengthening of the sleep-wake cycle (long desynchronization; mean $\tau = 40.7 \pm 8.1$ h) or by a shortening of the cycle (short desynchronization; mean $\tau = 21.8 \pm 1.4$ h). The characteristic features of long and short desynchronization have been described earlier (Aschoff and Wever 1976; Aschoff 1985; Aschoff et al. 1986).

The subjects were asked to fill in, at the end of each "day," a questionnaire that consisted of 20 items. Each item had to be scored on a visual analogue scale of 9 cm length, without the segmentation advocated by some authors (cf. Eastwood et al. 1984). The horizontal line was designated with " + " at its left end, and with "-" at its right end. The items were defined by catchwords such as "health," "contentment," "efficiency," or "tiredness." After completion, the questionnaire had to be stored in between the two doors of the lock which formed the entrance to the unit; hence, on the following day, the subjects could not check what scores they had given on the preceding day. As measures for the duration of sleep and wakefulness the intervals were used between two signals given by the subjects immediately after waking up and at the time of turning off their bedside reading lamp (Aschoff 1991). Further experimental details are described in Wever (1979).

Results

Much has been written about the usefulness of visual analogue scales in assessing feelings. On the one hand it has been said that "graphic rating scales are simple, self-explanatory, concrete and definite" (Hayes and Patterson 1921), and that they are preferable to the discrete-point type scale (Champney 1941). It is, on the other hand, obvious that any measurement of feelings by a visual analogue scale remains questionable: "Feelings are subjective phenomena, beyond absolute analysis; no final judgement of validity can ever be given" (Aitken 1969). In spite of these shortcomings it has been shown that scores derived from visual analogue scales correlate highly with other kinds of rating (Folstein and Luria 1973; Luria 1975). Yet, one has to keep in mind that one does not know to what extent a subject is able to make use of the scale as intended. The problem one is faced with has been described by Clarke and Spear (1964): "For such a test to express feelings reliably, the patient must be able to carry out the perceptual-motor task of putting the cross accurately where he intends it to be, but this is not enough for the test to be considered fully reliable and sensitive. The scores must be shown to remain stable when the patient reassesses his feelings unless 'something has happened' to him or within him, but to be sensitive the scores must not remain stable if his feelings have changed."

Within the whole of subjects who filled in the questionnaire there were a few who marked some of the scales, day after day, at almost exactly the same point, predominantly at its left (positive) or right (negative) end. These protocols were considered "insensitive" (according to Clarke and Spear 1964) and were not included in the analysis. In looking through the protocols of the remaining 48 subjects it became evident that some subjects needed a few days to reach a scoring which varied around a stable mean; they started making marks at the positive or negative end and moved into the scale on succeeding days. Other subjects distributed their marks around a long-term mean from the very beginning. These two types are illustrated in Fig. 1. The six diagrams present, for three items, the

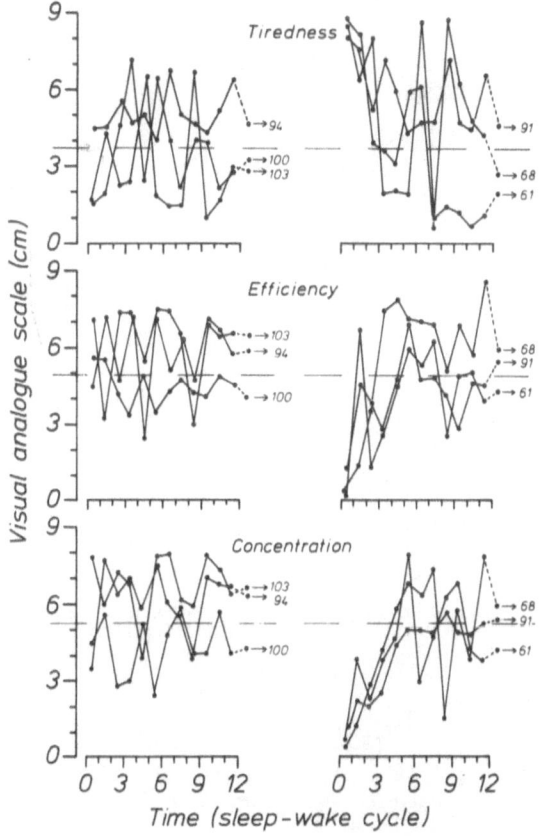

Fig. 1. Daily scores given for three items on a visual analogue scale during the first 12 days in isolation. At the ordinate, *zero* represents the negative and *nine* the positive end of the scale. *Left*, data from three subjects who did not show an initial trend in scoring. *Right*, data from three subjects with a trend during the first few days. In each curve, the last point (*at the end of the dotted line, followed by an arrow*) is drawn at the individual long-term mean of scores of the subject indicated by number. *Horizontal dashed lines* represent the overall means of scores from 48 subjects

first 12 scores as made by three subjects (left) who did not show a trend within the first few days, and those made by three subjects (right) who began scoring either at the positive or at the negative end of the scale. (To draw Fig. 1, the horizontal scale of the questionnaire has been rotated by 90°; zero represents the negative, and nine the positive end of the scale.) From the data plotted at the right half of Fig. 1 it could be assumed that these subjects, during the very first days of living in the unit, did feel extremely tired and completely deficient of efficiency and concentration. It is, however, as likely that the subjects had to get used to the task. In view of this uncertainty, the data of the first 2 or 3 days from subjects showing such a trend in scoring were discarded from the further analysis.

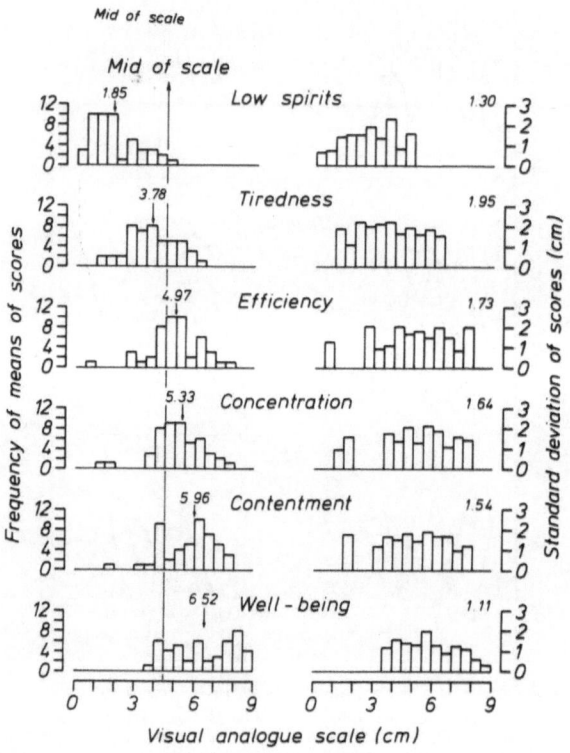

Fig. 2. Scores given for six items on a visual analogue scale, with *zero* representing the negative and *nine* the positive end of the scale. Data from 48 subjects who lived singly in isolation for a mean duration of 23.3 ± 6.0 days. *Left*, frequency of individual means of scores; numbers at histograms give the overall means (in centimeters). *Right*, standard deviation (SD) of scores, related to the individual means (averaged from several subjects in 0.5-h bins); numbers at histograms give the overall means of SD (in ± centimeters)

Ideally, the mean of scores given by a subject to a certain item could be expected to be close to the middle of the scale, i.e., close to 4.5 cm. This was found to be true for only a few of the subjects and for the minority of items. As shown in the left diagrams of Fig. 2, the individual means of scores cover large parts of the scale in each of the six items plotted. It is also noteworthy that for the item "low spirits" all but one subject had their mean score in the lower half of the scale (overall mean = 1.85 cm); that means that the subjects hardly ever felt really "low-spirited." This scoring fits to the mostly positive scores given by the subjects to "contentment" (overall mean = 5.96 cm) and "well-being" (overall mean = 6.25 cm). Closest to the "ideal" scoring comes the overall mean for the item "efficiency" (4.97 cm). Of greater interest is the intraindividual variability of scores. The right diagrams in Fig. 2 show that, intraindividually, the standard deviation (SD) of scores is more or less independent of the mean score, but varies considerably between items. The overall mean of SD is small for "low spirits" (± 1.30 cm) and "well-being" (± 1.11 cm), and reaches high values for "tiredness" (± 1.95 cm) and "efficiency" (± 1.73 cm). It is hard to say to what extent this reflects differences in the dependence of items on changing conditions within the organism or differences in the capability of the subjects to "realize" changes in their feelings. In any case, items with a relatively large variability as measured by SD are likely to indicate the day-to-day changes in feelings better than items with a low variability. Furthermore, there are large interindividual differences: some subjects have a high variability of scores in all items, other subjects a consistently low variability. This is illustrated in Fig. 3 by the data from four subjects whose SD values (except two) were above ± 2.0 cm in all six items, and from four subjects whose SD values were all below ± 2.0 cm. Finally, females exceeded

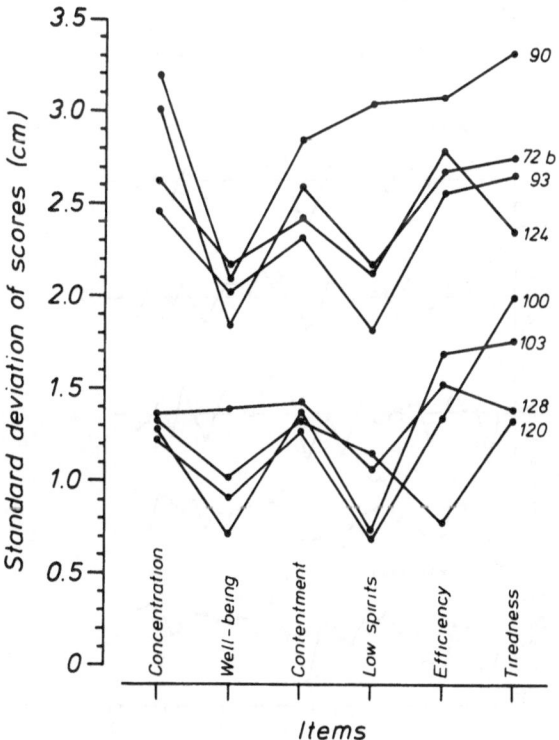

Fig. 3. Standard deviations of scores for six items, given in isolation by four subjects (*numbers at curves*) with a consistent high variability in scoring (*upper four lines*) and by four subjects with a low variability (*below*)

males in the variability of scoring: for the six items listed in Fig. 2 the SD values of the 12 females were, on average, 29.5% larger than those of the 36 males.

As a next step of the analysis, the deviations of daily scores from their mean were computed intraindividually. Furthermore, to have a similar meaning of positive (or negative) deviations in all items, the signs of the scale were reversed (i.e., minus became plus) for "low spirits," which then was labeled "mood," and for "tiredness" which was labeled "alertness." Data transformed in this way are summarized in Fig. 4 for a male subject who was temporarily short-desynchronized and went through 33 sleep-wake cycles. The curves drawn for the five items again demonstrate the differences in variability (small for "mood," large for "alertness"). They are further typical for most of the subjects insofar as they lack any long-term trend in scoring. In other words: at the end of the experiment the subjects did feel, on the average, neither worse nor better than on the day when they entered the isolation unit.

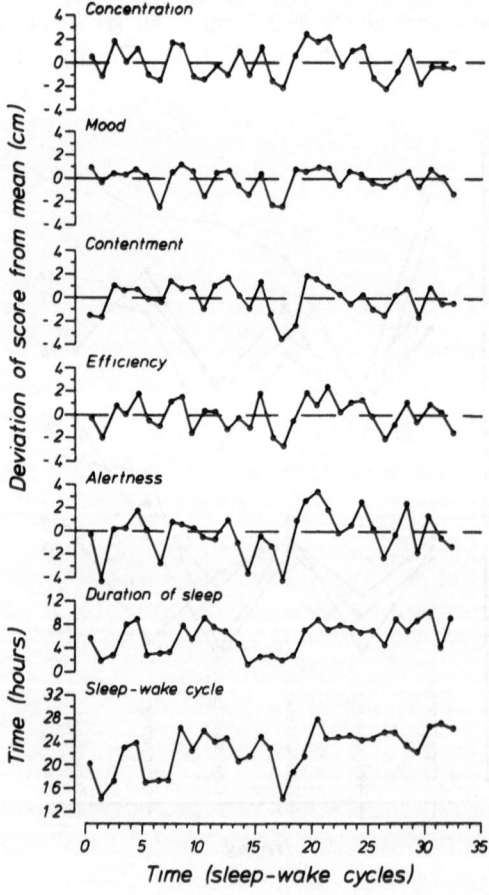

Fig. 4. Deviations of daily scores from mean, given for five items by a male subject during long-term isolation. *Bottom two rows*, duration of sleep and of the sleep-wake cycle

A closer inspection of the data presented in Fig. 4 suggests that a correlation might exist between scores and the duration of the sleep-wake cycle (cf. days 6 - 8, and day 18). To evaluate such a relationship, the daily deviations of scores from mean were plotted as a function of the sleep-wake cycle (Fig. 5). Coefficients of correlation were computed separately for all data below and above a

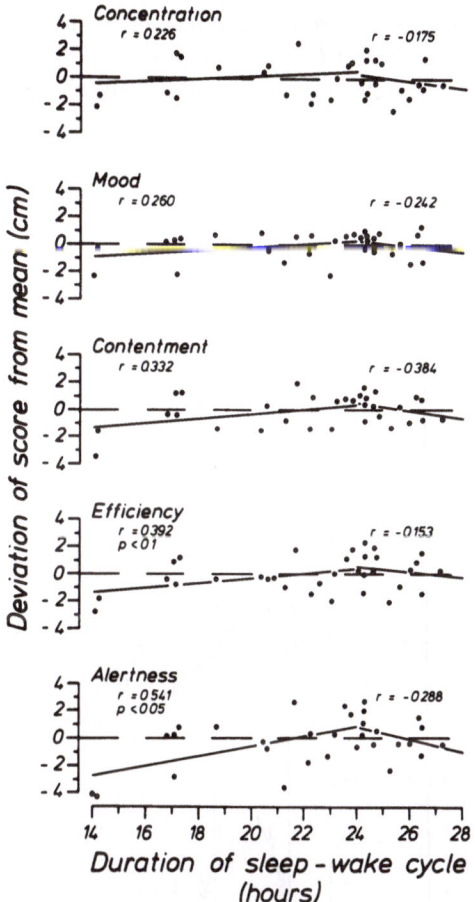

Fig. 5. Deviations of daily scores from mean, drawn as a function of the sleep-wake cycle. Data from the same subjects as in Fig. 4. *Dashed lines*, regressions through all data points below and above 24 h, respectively. *r*, coefficient of correlation

cycle duration of 24 h. The coefficients were all positive to the left of the arbitrarily chosen point of separation, and negative to the right of it. Although mostly nonsignificant, the uniformity in signs of the coefficients of correlation indicates that, in all items, the scores are above the mean when the sleep-wake cycle is close to 24 h and fall below the mean with increasing and decreasing durations of the cycle. In the next step of the analysis, scores were averaged in 1-h bins, a procedure that allowed computation of means from several subjects. The results of such computations, based on the protocols of ten subjects, are shown for three items in Fig. 6. On the average, scores remain above their mean when the sleep-wake cycle varies from 22 to 28 h; outside this range, the scores are mostly below the mean. Sleep-wake cycles of 22 and 28 h represent the limits within which free-running circadian rhythms usually remain internally synchronized. Hence, the results summarized in Fig. 6 are compatible with the hypothesis that the feelings of the subjects are relatively good as long as the rhythms remain internally synchronized and grow worse with either long or short desynchronization.

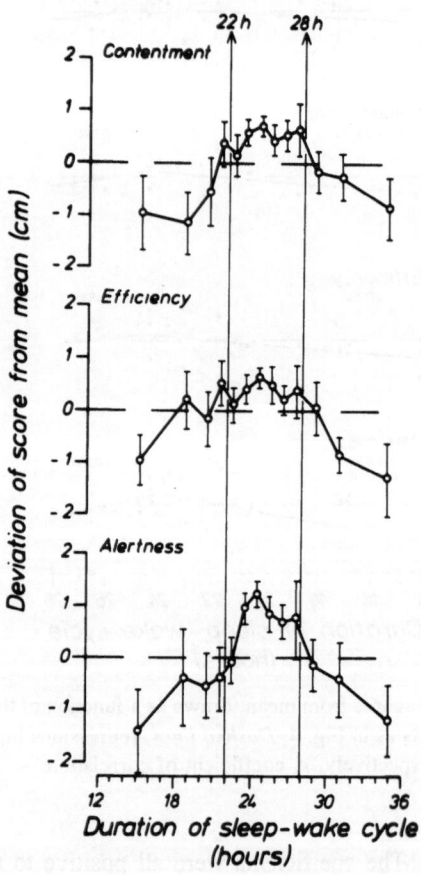

Fig. 6. Deviations of daily scores from mean, drawn for three items as a function of the sleep-wake cycle. Data averaged in 1-h bins from the protocols of ten subjects who in the course of the experiment became internally desynchronized. *Vertical lines*, standard error

When confronted with a set of data such as that shown in Fig. 4, it seems a plausible first approach to examine the correlation between scores and the period τ of the sleep-wake cycle, as in Figs. 5 and 6. However, there is the possibility that scores are related equally well or even stronger to the two constituents of τ, i.e., to the duration of wakefulness α or to the duration of sleep ρ. With this end in view, standard deviations were computed intraindividually for the 24 subjects who became internally desynchronized, and the 24 SD values of scores were then related to the proper SD values of τ, α and ρ, respectively.

Table 1. Coefficients of correlation between the standard deviation (SD) of scores for three items and the SD of the sleep-wake cycle τ, the duration of wakefulness α, and the duration of sleep ρ. Means, computed by z-transformation, from 24 subjects with temporary or permanent internal desynchronization

Items	Coefficients of correlation between SD of scores and SD of		
	τ	α	ρ
Tiredness	0.435	0.534	0.063
Concentration	0.235	0.475	-0.003
Efficiency	0.193	0.420	0.213

As shown in Table 1, in the three items tested the coefficients of correlation are strongest with α and close to zero with ρ. Hence, α was used in the following analysis the purpose of which was to find out interindividual differences. In view of the fact that, for one individual, there were often not enough data to make a fine grid with 1-h bins meaningful, the data were summed in 3-h bins and, furthermore, averaged for six items. The results computed in this way from the protocols of six subjects are presented in the lower half of Fig. 7. In each of the six curves there is a tendency for the scores to be above their mean when α is of medium duration and to fall below the mean with increasing and decreasing α-values. It is further evident that the α-values corresponding to high scores differ drastically among individuals. This difference disappears when interindividual differences in the mean duration of α are taken into account. Such normalization is used to draw the upper diagram in Fig. 7, in which the scores are plotted relative to the deviation of α from the individual mean. Now all six curves reach a maximum when α is close to its mean; the scores become negative when α is lengthened or shortened by more than 3 h.

The results summarized in Fig. 7 are again compatible with the assumption that internal desynchronization might be the cause for feelings to deteriorate. Other

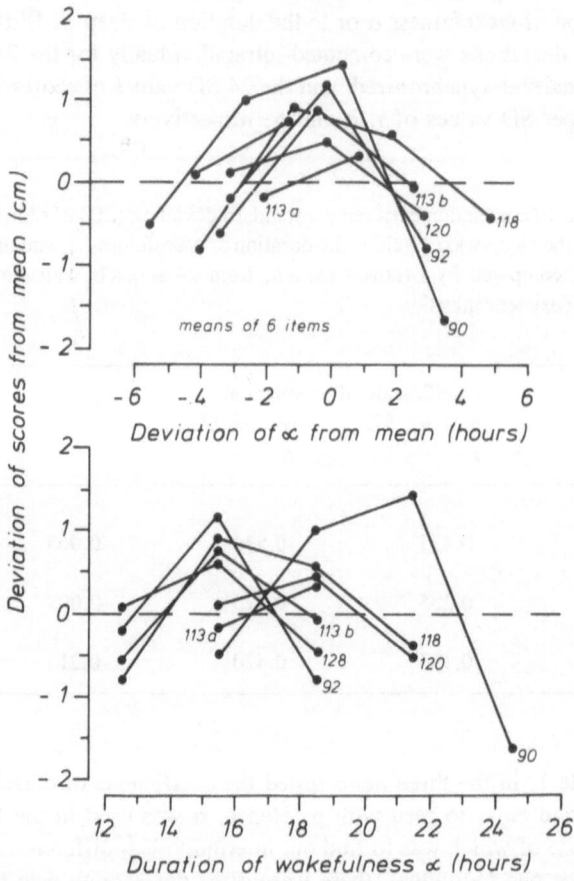

Fig. 7. Deviations of daily scores from mean, drawn as a function of wakefulness α. Data averaged in 3-h bins for six items from the protocols of six subjects (*numbers at curves*) with internal desynchronization. *Below*, original data; *above*, data normalized with regard to the individual means of α

findings contradict such a conclusion. As shown in Fig. 8, the scores of five subjects who remained internally synchronized are correlated with α in a manner similar to that found in desynchronized subjects. The scores are positive when α is close to the individual mean and become negative with increasing and decreasing α-values. It should be noted that the upper diagram in Fig. 8 differs from the upper diagram of Fig. 7 in two ways: the maximal deviations of scores from their mean are only about 20% of those shown by desynchronized subjects (cf. the differences in ordinate scales), and the α-values remain within a limit of ± 3 h of the individual mean α. In spite of the small variations in α and the relatively small changes in scoring, the uniformity of trends discernible in the five curves of Fig. 8 suggests that internal desynchronization is not needed for feelings to grow worse. The conclusion seems justified that mood and efficiency have a relationship to α which, in principle, is the same in internally synchronized as in desynchronized rhythms.

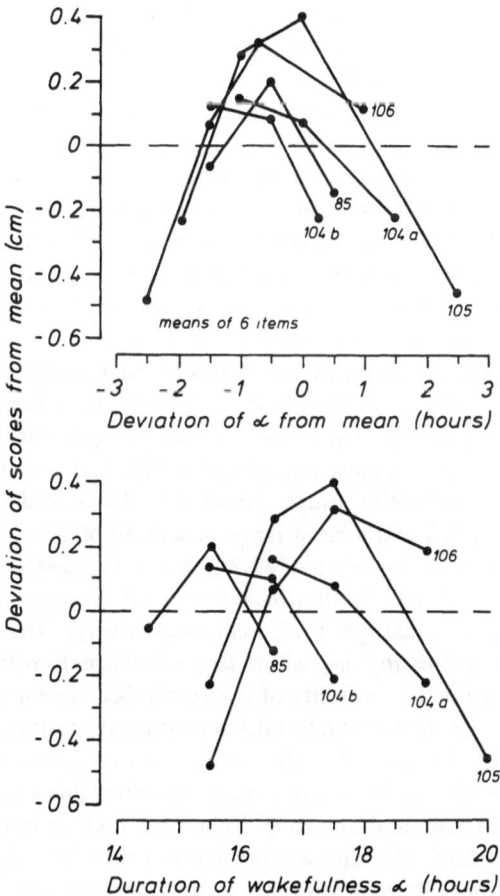

Fig. 8. Deviations of daily scores from mean, drawn as a function of wakefulness α. Data averaged in 3-h bins for six items from the protocols of five subjects (*numbers at curves*) who remained internally synchronized. *Below*, original data. *Above*, data normalized with regard to the individual means of α

Discussion

This study rests on the assumption that scores made daily once on a visual analogue scale reflect, at least to some extent, day-to-day changes in the feelings of subjects. It presupposes that the subjects can realize the direction and quantify the amount of such changes and are capable of using the scale in an appropriate manner. A second assumption is that day-to-day changes in feelings are related to changes in the physiological organization of the organism (Thayer 1989), especially as they are reflected in parameters of the circadian system. If these two assumptions are valid, a measure of variability in scores should correlate positively with the variability of the circadian parameter chosen. As mentioned earlier, such correlations were found to be strong between scores and either τ or α, but close to zero between scores and ρ (Table 1).

In evaluating the scores, three characteristics must be kept in mind: (1) The variability of scores differs among items; it is largest for "alertness" (the converse of "tiredness") and smallest for "well-being" (Fig. 2). (2) On average, females have about a 30% larger variability than males. (3) There are large interindividual differences in variability (Fig. 3). The latter observation indicates that personality factors determine either the degree to which feelings correlate with changes in the circadian system or the capability of subjects to express their feelings. An example is given by the protocols from 11 subjects whose degree of neuroticism was determined by using the questionnaire developed by Brengelmann and Brengelmann (1960), which is similar to the Maudsley Personality Inventory (Eysenck 1959). In the same subjects, the dependence of feelings on α was determined by measuring, in diagrams such as those reproduced in Fig. 7, the range between the extremes of positive and negative scores. Six of the subjects had a mean neuroticism rating of 16.8 $\pm$ 6.7 and a mean range in scoring of 1.6 $\pm$ 0.6 cm. Five subjects had a mean neuroticism rating of 29.2 $\pm$ 8.5 and a mean range in scoring of 1.0 $\pm$ 0.4 cm. Interestingly, both groups had about the same mean standard deviation of scores ($\pm$ 14.9 cm and $\pm$ 13.5 cm, respectively). These preliminary results suggest that an increasing disposition to neuroticism decreases the dependence of feelings on α (or the capability of subjects to become aware of it). This is somewhat surprising in view of the fact that a neurotic disposition increases the tendency of a subject to become internally desynchronized (Lund 1974).

It must be remembered that, in the experiments on which this analysis is based, scores were made once daily in the evening. Therefore, nothing can be said about the circadian time structure of feelings in our subjects and its interrelationship with other rhythmic functions. It is known that rhythms in mood and efficiency are partly related to the rhythm of body temperature but can become uncoupled from it during forced internal desynchronization (Wever 1982). The results of recent experiments in which isolated subjects were exposed to zeitgeber periods of either 23 or 26 h indicate that alertness is under the control of both the pacemaker, which is responsible for the rhythm in body temperature, and the sleep-wake cycle (Monk et al. 1989). In the present study, emphasis is placed on the relationship to the sleep-wake cycle and to α. Possible effects of temperature, either of its mean level or its actual value at the time of scoring, have yet to be explored.

According to the results presented in Figs. 6 and 7, the scores correlate with both τ and α in a similar manner, indicating "optimal" feelings within a medium range of τ- and α-values. Since in free-running rhythms τ and α are positively correlated with each other (Wever 1984; Aschoff et al. 1986), it is not surprising that coefficients of the same order of magnitude are found for the correlation between scores and both the circadian measures. However, the stronger correlation with α suggests that the duration of wakefulness is the crucial factor. It is tempting to speculate that indeed feelings depend on α, but the inverse relationship, i.e., a dependence of α on feelings, cannot be excluded. "In humans the decision to retire to bed is determined to a major extent by the subjective level of alertness or sleepiness that is experienced" (Monk et al. 1989). In this context it has to be mentioned that in humans whose rhythms are free-running in isolation the hourly means of locomotor activity are negatively correlated with α (Aschoff 1990). As a consequence, scores of feelings correlate with activity in a similar way as with α: subjects are in high spirits and feel well during "days" when activity is kept to a medium level, and feelings grow worse with an increase as well as with a decrease in mean hourly activity. Whatever the final answer may be to the question of cause and effect, to stay awake either too short or too long apparently is accompanied by discomfort, as was already known to Hippocrates (Jones 1967; Aphorisms II, 3): "Sleep or wakefulness, in undue measure, these are both bad symptoms."

References

Aitken RCB (1969) Measurement of feelings using visual analogue scales. Proc R Soc Med 62:989-939

Aschoff J (1985) On the perception of time during prolonged temporal isolation. Hum Neurobiol 4:41-52

Aschoff J (1990) Interdependence between locomotor activity and duration of wakefulness in humans during isolation. Experientia 46:870-871

Aschoff J (1991) Estimates on the duration of sleep and wakefulness made in isolation. Chronobiol Internat (to be published)

Aschoff J, von Goetz Ch, Wildgruber Ch, Wever RA (1986) Meal timing in man during isolation without time cues. J Biol Rhythms 1:151-162

Aschoff J, Wever R (1976) Human circadian rhythms: a multi-oscillator system. Fed Proc 35:2326-2332

Brengelmann JC, Brengelmann L (1960) Deutsche Validierung von Fragebogen der Extraversion, neurotischen Tendenz und Rigidität. Z Exp Angew Psychol 7:291-331

Champney H (1941) The measurement of parent behavior. Child Dev 12:131-166

Clarke PRF, Spear FG (1964) Reliability and sensitivity in the self-assessment of well-being. Br Bull Psychol Soc 17:18A

Eastwood MR, Whitton JL, Kramer PM (1984) A brief instrument for longitudinal monitoring of mood states. Psychiatry Res 11:119-125

Eysenck HJ (1959) Maudsley Personality Inventory. London University Press, London

Folstein MF, Luria R (1973) Reliability, validity, and clinical application of the visual analogue mood scale. Psychol Med 3:479-486

Hayes MHS, Patterson DG (1921) Experimental development of the graphic rating method. Psychol Bull 18:98

Jones WHS (1967) Hippokrates. Heinemann, London

Lund R (1974) Personality factors and desynchronization of circadian rhythms. Psychosom Med 36:224-228

Luria RE (1975) The validity and reliability of the visual analogue mood scale. J Psychiatr Res 12:51-57

Monk TH, Moline ML, Fookson JE, Peetz SM (1989) Circadian determinants of subjective alertness. J Biol Rhythms 4:393-404

Solomon P, Kubzansky PE, Leideman PH, Mendelson JH, Trumbull R, Wexler D (1961) Sensory deprivation. Harvard   University Press, Cambridge

Thayer RE (1989) The biopsychology of mood and arousal. Oxford University Press, Oxford

Wever RA (1979) The circadian system of man. Springer, Berlin Heidelberg New York

Wever RA (1982) Behavioral aspects of circadian rhythmicity. In: Brown FM, Graeber RC (eds) Rhythmic aspects of behavior. Erlbaum, London, pp 105-171

Wever RA (1984) Properties of human sleep-wake cycles: parameters of internally synchronized free-running rhythms. Sleep 7:27-51

13 Possible Relations Between Disorders in Circadian Rhythmicity and Mental Disorders

Rütger A. Wever

Introduction

The human circadian system is governed by strong principles which keep the dynamics of the rhythms within remarkably narrow limits. This is at least true for data from healthy and young subjects; consequently, in rhythms of these subjects numerous significant correlations can be observed, between different parameters of the same rhythm, between different rhythms in the same condition, and between changes in the rhythm in changing experimental conditions among different subjects. However, when rhythms of ill patients or aged subjects are analyzed, various systematic deviations from these correlations can be observed. It might be suggested, therefore, that there are realtionships between disorders in the structure of the circadian system, on the one hand, and health disorders and, in particular, mental disorders, on the other hand. It remains, however, an open question whether or not there is a causal relationship between rhythm and health disorders, and, if so, in what direction it operates.

This chapter describes examples of the characteristics of the circadian rhythm in healthy subjects and of deviations from such a normal picture in ill or old subjects. It was not possible to perform systematic experiments with ill patients in a series of long-term experiments, running continuously for more than 25 years and including more than 450 subjects. There were only a few accidental cases where subjects contracted fever (or other complaints) for a time during the course of the experiment, but they insisted on continuing the experiment; in most of these cases an infection was confirmed by a measured reaction of the immune system: the urinary excretion of neopterin and monapterin (as an indication of T-cell activity) increased up to about 5 times the original (and final) value. In several experiments where such diseases arose, a physician entered the isolation facility to examine the subjects, without the subjects becoming aware of the objective time. Moreover, 15 subjects aged between 60 and 81 years participated in the long-term isolation experiments. They were, of course, far from being senile (otherwise they could not participate in such experiments). Their rhythms, however, just as the rhythms of the temporarily ill subjects, showed systematic deviations from the rhythms of healthy and young subjects in several respects; data obtained from these subjects, therefore, may be considered as representative of data from ill and old subjects.

Under natural conditions, circadian rhythmicity is governed by a combination of endogenous and exogenous impulses. The influences of endogenous control can be evaluated separately, in experiments where subjects live under constant environmental conditions with no time cues; only in rhythms which freerun under such conditions can pure biological factors of circadian rhythmicity be investigated. Under natural conditions the rhythms are modified by external zeitgebers which synchronize the rhythms to the period of the day-night cycle; the process of synchronization does not affect only the period of the previously freerunning rhythms but also all other rhythm parameters. Under such conditions where the subjects are aware of the time of day, in addition, in particular the duration of sleep (but possibly also other rhythm parameters) is manipulated by (real, or even imagined) social constraints. This means that biological factors of circadian rhythmicity are confused to an unknown degree by external cues in experiments with natural zeitgebers. It is for this reason that rhythm disorders, which are relevant in the context of this paper, can be evaluated only in experiments with temporal isolation; these are either experiments with constant conditions with no time cues, or they are experiments using the influence of artificial zeitgebers with periods deviating from the 24-hour day.

Rhythm Disorders

The rhythm disorder which is most obvious and most easily detectable is internal desynchronization, i.e., the state in which rhythms of different variables in a subject run with different periods in the steady state. It is based on the multioscillatory structure of the circadian system, which includes several basic oscillators, or pacemakers, with different properties (Wever 1975, 1979). Mainly, the oscillatory strengths differ from each other; e.g., the oscillator dominantly controlling the rhythm of body temperature is about 12 times stronger than the oscillator dominantly controlling sleep-wake; consequently, the interindividual variabilities of the intrinsic periods are much larger, and also the ranges of entrainment under the influence of an external zeitgeber are much wider in the rhythm of sleep-wake than in that of body temperature. Moreover, the mean intrinsic periods differ slightly; e.g., it is about 1 h longer in the oscillator dominantly controlling sleep-wake than in the oscillator dominantly controlling body temperature. Due to mutual interactions between all the different oscillators, the total system normally runs in internal synchrony; it appears outwardly as if controlled by only one oscillator, or pacemaker. Internal desynchronization occurs spontaneously when the intrinsic periods of the different oscillators are out of the mutual ranges of entrainment; and this can occur under two different preconditions: (1) the different intrinsic periods are too far from each other so that they are outside a mutual range of entrainment of common size, even when the interaction between the two rhythms has a normal strength; or (2) the mutual interaction between the different oscillators is too weak to overcome a common interval between the intrinsic periods of different oscillators, i.e., the mutual range of entrainment is considerably smaller than it is normally. Consequently, the two rhythm abnormalities which are the preconditions for the occurrence of internal desynchronization may be correlated to health (mental) disorders, and in different ways; the state of internal desynchronization itself can only hint at the existence of such a rhythm disorder.

On the other hand, internal desynchronization under the influence of specific zeitgebers occurs when this zeitgeber synchronizes only a part of the rhythms (which are inside its range of entrainment) while other rhythms (which are outside the range of entrainment of this zeitgeber) freerun. Consequently, the occurrence of internal desynchronization of this type depends primarily on the experimental conditions, i.e., mainly on the strength and the period of the controlling zeitgeber. Hence, it can be forced in every subject, independent of his or her personality data (including age) and his or her health state. In other words, internal desynchronization, when forced by a zeitgeber, must not be correlated to health (mental) disorders in any way.

The state of internal desynchronization is the most obvious type of rhythm disorder; it may therefore be called rhythm disorder of the first order. For the reasons just discussed, however, this state is of minor interest in the present context, because it cannot be correlated directly to health (mental) disorders. Rather, rhythm disorders which are not very obvious but can be recognized only in sophisticated analyses have to be preferred in the search for indicators of health disorders; such disorders may be designated as second-order phenomena. The state of internal desynchronization, particularly when forced by a zeitgeber, which had been shown previously to give an insight into the dynamics of the circadian system that cannot be gained in another way, may only assist in the analysis of such more subtle disorders. In the following, correlations between rhythm disorders of the second order and health (mental) disorders will be illustrated in the light of typical examples.

Disorders in Freerunning Rhythms

In freerunning and internally synchronized rhythms, data obtained from ill or old subjects deviate from data of healthy and young subjects. Initially, there is the power of the internal rhythm stabilization which is expressed in negative serial correlations among successive cycles (i.e., any deviation of the cycle length from the individual mean is corrected, with a high probability, by opposite deviations of the lengths of the following and the following but one cycle from the mean); in particular, it is the sum of the coefficients of serial correlation of the first (correction by the next cycle) and second order (correction by the next but one cycle) which is significantly smaller in older than in younger subjects (Wever 1984).

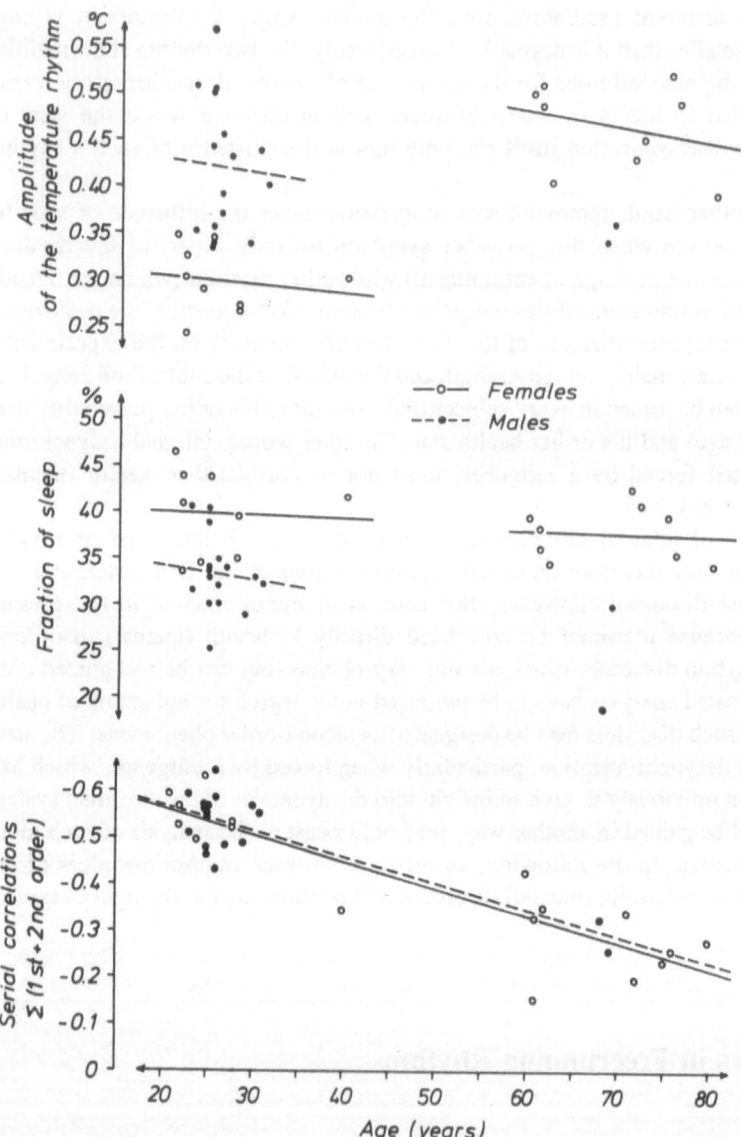

Fig.1. Three different types of sex difference and age dependence in parameters of human circadian rhythms (taken from a homogeneous sample of long-term experiments under constant conditions). *Lower*, serial correlations among successive sleep-wake cycles; no sex difference, consistent and significant age dependence. *Middle*, fraction of sleep within the sleep-wake cycle; significant sex difference, no age dependence. *Upper*, amplitude of the rhythm of body temperature; significant sex difference, but only when female subjects up to an age of about 55 years are compared with males (of any age); no sex difference when older females are compared with males (of any age). No consistent age dependence, but a threshold age in female subjects, above which the amplitude is significantly larger than below it

Figure 1, lower part, shows data from a homogenous sample of experiments, i.e., the values of this "overall stabilization power" depending on the age of the subjects and drawn separately for females and males. The figure shows that there is no sex difference in these values, in neither the older nor the younger subjects. Moreover, a very high consistency of the data can be seen in the group of the younger subjects aged below 40 years (the mean $\pm$ SD in this group of 24 subjects is -0.539 $\pm$ 0.054; the median is -0.548 with a 99% confidence interval between -0.568 and -0.505) (the coefficient of serial correlation of the first order when considered solely shows a variability which is more than three times greater, but deviates from zero at a still very high level of significance). In the group of older subjects (aged between 40 and 80 years), not only is the mean lower but also the consistency (mean $\pm$ SD in this group of 12 subjects: -0.291 $\pm$ 0.074). The difference between the "overall stabilization powers" of the two groups (0.248 $\pm$ 0.061) is highly significant: parametric ($t = 11.39$; $p < 10^{-12}$) and non-parametric (no overlap in the data; $w = 4.80$; $p < 10^{-6}$). Fig. 1 shows, in addition, that there is a high correlation between age and stabilization power when all the data are considered: parametric ($r = 0.891$; $p < 10^{-12}$) and non-parametric (Spearman's $R = 0.746$; $p \ll 10^{-3}$); the regressions are nearly identical in females and males.

These results indicate that the power of the intrinsic stabilization mechanism (which concerns the rhythm of body temperature just as that of sleep-wake) reduces with increasing age. On the other hand, the mechanism generating the rhythms is not impaired in old subjects; in females, rather, the amplitude of the body temperature rhythm is significantly larger in older than in younger subjects, with a threshold age at about 55 years (Fig. 1, top). Consequently, the efficacy of the stabilization mechanism is independent of that of the generating mechanism and, hence, the mechanism first mentioned can be disturbed independent of the second mechanism mentioned. The impairment in the stabilization power has been shown to depend on age; it must be expected, however, that such an impairment also occurs under other circumstances, e.g., in mentally ill patients. The crucial point is that disorders in the rhythm generating mechanism are easily detectable but not disorders in the rhythm stabilizing mechanism (the latter disorders can be recognized only by careful analyses of serial correlations); and this means that an obvious integrity of rhythm cannot exclude an impairment in the stability of this rhythm as an indicator for a health (mental) disorder.

It may be argued that the evaluation of long-term stability of freerunning rhythms is irrelevant for considerations of rhythm disorders in normal life; here, the rhythms are under the constant influence of a 24-hour zeitgeber which guarantees the long-term stability of the period. However, the period of a freerunning rhythm (or better: its relation to the zeitgeber period) determines the phase relationship of this rhythm under the influence of a zeitgeber to this zeitgeber. This means an instability of the period of a freerunning rhythm creates an instability of the phase relationship of this rhythm when under the influence of a zeitgeber (the period of which, by definition, is highly stable). In other words: when in old (and possibly also in ill) subjects the intrinsic stabilization mechanism in freerunning rhythms is impaired, the same subjects show a considerably less stable phase position of their rhythms within the day-night cycle than do young and healthy subjects. And this impairment in the temporal fit of the rhythmic system within the day-night cycle, in fact, is of relevance in the natural 24 h-day.

In nearly all other rhythm parameters, there is either no age dependence or an age dependence of another type. Parameters of the sleep-wake rhythm such as period or fraction of sleep are independent of the age of the subjects (but dependent on the sex); as an example, Fig. 1, middle, shows the sleep fractions in the same homogeneous sample of long-term experiments as in Fig. 1, bottom. Parameters of the body temperature rhythm, on the other hand, show — in females but not in males — a clear dependence on the age of the subjects: data from younger females (up to age about 55 years; obviously this is the age of the menopause) deviate significantly from the data of males of any age and, in addition, from data of older females; the data from older females, on the other hand, cannot be differentiated from data of males. Within each of the three samples — older females, younger females, and males — when considered separately, age dependences of the data are not recognizable. This type of parameter dependence on subject age and sex is illustrated in Fig.1, top, with regard to the amplitude of the rhythm of body temperature (taken from the same sample as Fig.1, bottom, middle).

Apart from the serial correlations as mentioned above, there are many intercorrelations between different parameters of the same rhythm, e.g., between period, amplitude, and wave shape. A summary of several of these correlations is presented in Fig. 2. Several of the correlations are valid independent of subject sex and age; they are inherent properties of the rhythm. Other correlations differ between females and males (in all these cases, the data from females older than about 55 years fit the regressions of males); the collective consideration of data from both sexes would not lead to relevant correlations. It is remarkable that all these correlations are relatively narrow when data of healthy subjects are considered; exceptions originate from ill subjects. This means that, again, disorders from the strong characteristics of human circadian rhythmicity may be related to health (mental) disorders.

Of particular interest is a correlation which has previously been discussed in detail: the correlation between amplitude of body temperature rhythm and sleep fraction (Wever 1989b). From the data of this highly significant correlation, the position of a threshold can be deduced which separates the two different stages of wake and sleep. These investigations showed that the position of this threshold is a highly stable and individual constant, which is not affected by changes in the experimental conditions (even when all other rhythm parameters are changed) but which is different in the two sexes (expressed in temperature; females, 37.08 °C ± 0.09 °C; males, 36.79 °C ± 0.08 °C; the difference is significant with $p <$ 10^{-6}); the consistency of the threshold data within both sexes, and also the (relative) difference between the threshold data of the two sexes, is higher than in any other rhythm parameter. However, again, this statement is valid only when females aged up to about 55 years are considered; threshold data from older females (36.77 °C ± 0.04 °C) cannot be differented from data of males of any age (Wever 1989b).

This means that the position of the threshold separating wake and sleep, though independent of external conditions, can be affected by hormonal changes and, hence, by changes in internal conditions. And this means that special health disorders (sleep disorders in particular) must not necessarily reflect disorders in the virtual rhythms but possibly shifts in the threshold position. To give an examp-

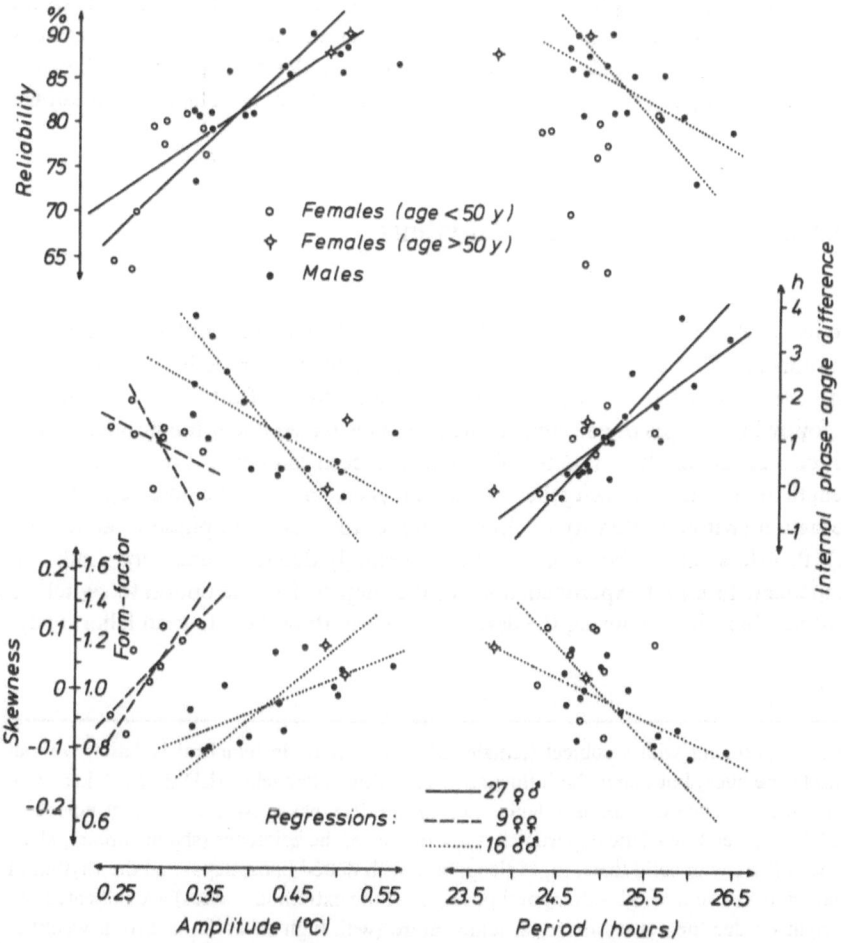

Fig.2. Intercorrelations between several parameters of human circadian rhythms (taken from a homogeneous sample of long-term experiments under constant conditions); arbitrarily, amplitude of the temperature rhythm and period are taken for reference. In some cases, significant correlations exist when all data are considered; in other cases, significant correlations exist only when data from (younger) female and male subjects are considered separately (in these cases, the data of the older females fit the regressions of the males). Only in case of significant correlations, regression lines (in both directions) are drawn

le: a young (27-year-old) female patient with heavy sleep disorders (Lund et al. 1988) showed in a study carried out with constant conditions a nearly normal rhythm of rectal temperature (amplitude, 0.237 °C; mean amplitude in healthy young females, 0.296 °C ± 0.036 °C)); her rest time fraction was unusually long (as it is often the case in sleep disturbed patients), her polygraphically determined fraction of real sleep, however, was considerably smaller [35.2 % vs. 48.7 % of the sleep-wake cycle; in healthy subjects, on the other hand, the real sleep time is commonly at most a few minutes shorter than the rest time, according to the always recorded and carefully analyzed sleep movements (Wever 1979)]. This patient showed a threshold temperature (at 36.78 °C; deduced on the basis of the real sleep time) which was considerably lower than the normal threshold in young females but which coincided with the threshold in older females or in males (see above). Such an exception in the threshold position from the respective mean has never been observed in a healthy subject.

Disorders in Synchronized Rhythms

The most relevant parameter in synchronized rhythms is the width of the range of entrainment. This range is a measure of the zeitgeber strength (relative to the oscillatory strength), and it is different for the rhythms of different variables. In the following, ranges of entrainment will be investigated under the influence of an artificial zeitgeber the strength of which had been shown to be similar to the strength of the natural zeitgeber. This zeitgeber, in fact, includes a light-dark alternation (with an intensity of illumination during the light phase of about 300 lux); its effectiveness, however, is overwhelmingly due to a behavioral (indirect) component. In a first experimental series the subjects had the option to switch on small auxiliary lamps during the dark phase, permitting them to read laboriously;

---▶

Fig.3. Experiment with a subject (female, 21 years) living in temporal isolation without natural time cues, but under the influence of an artificial zeitgeber (LD 300:0.1 lux, with the option to switch on auxiliary lamps during the dark phase) with a constant period of 25.25 h. *Left,* course of the experiment; dark phases of the zeitgeber (shaded areas), sleep episodes (bars with solid lines, night sleep; bars with dotted lines, naps) and the rhythm of rectal temperature (triangles: temporal positions of the extremum values) are indicated. At the right border the course of rectal temperature (with high fever for nearly a week) is drawn. *Middle,* periodogram analyses of several variables; night sleeps and naps are separated according to the subjective scoring. *Right,* educed cycles of the same variables as in the middle diagram, calculated with the freerunning (24.5 h) and the zeitgeber period (25.25 h) each. From the rectal temperature data the educing of the freerunning cycle had been calculated, not only by using all data (as usual) but also by using data obtained exclusively during the wake episodes and exclusively during the sleep episodes (independent of its subjective scoring).

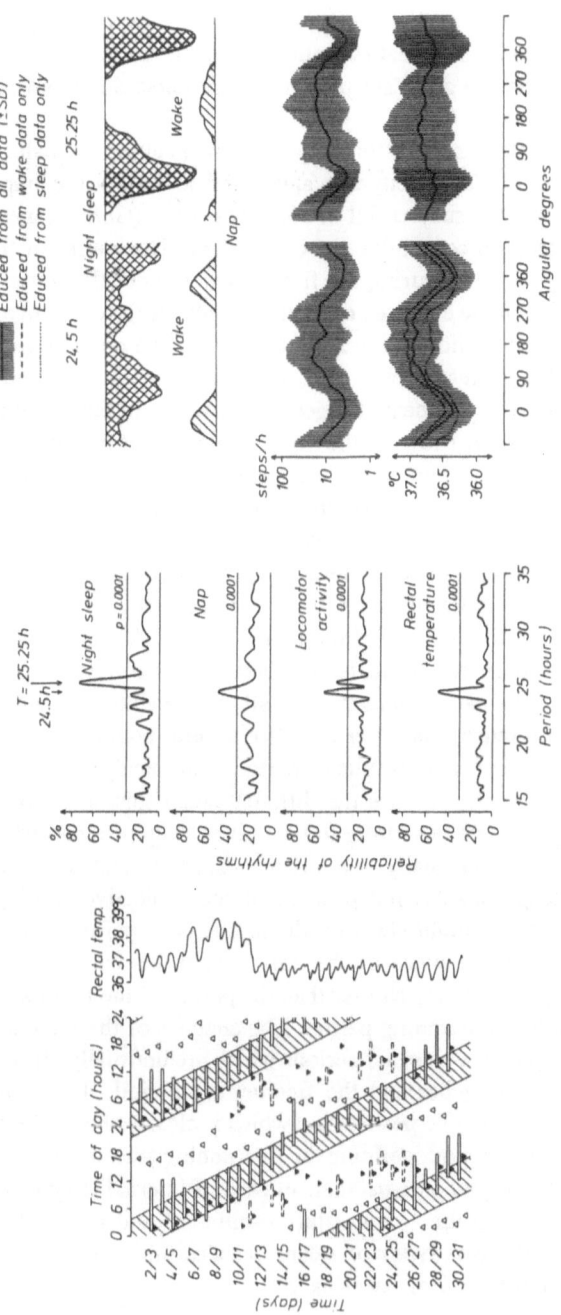

hence, they were not forced to rest with the transition from light to dark. This situation corresponds to the natural situation where the evening twilight likewise does not compel one to go to sleep but rather prompts one to switch on artificial illumination (Wever 1979).

In one of the experiments of this series, where a subject (female, 21 years old) was exposed to a 25.25-h zeitgeber and asked to follow the imposed schedule whenever possible, the subject fell ill after some days (German measles with high fever), but insisted on continuing the experiment. The course of this experiment is shown in Fig. 3, left. During the first 5 days (before the fever occurred), the experiment followed the expected course: Not only sleep-wake but also the rhythm of rectal temperature followed the zeitgeber. As shown on the right side of Fig.3, left, thereafter the subject's fever rose up to more than 39 °C, and from this day on the course of the experiment changed. Sleep-wake, in fact, continued to follow the zeitgeber as before, showing the high motivation of the subject to follow the instructions; the rhythm of rectal temperature, however, loosened from the zeitgeber and started to freerun (with a period of 24.5 h). This means, with the occurrence of the fever, the rhythms desynchronized internally; and also after the recovery from the illness after a few days, the rhythms did not resynchronize. Unlike all other experiments with forced internal desynchronization, here the difference between the periods of the two separated rhythms was not more than 45 min (i.e., not more than the difference between the common freerunning period and the period of the natural zeitgeber; in all experiments with young and healthy subjects, this difference was never less than several hours).

Fig. 3, middle, shows the results of periodogram analyses of several rhythms. For the sleep analyses, for once the different sleep episodes had been separated according to the subjective scoring to be a night sleep or a nap which was unambiguous in all cases (normally, i.e., if not expressly stated, sleep analyses are based on all sleep episodes independent of the subjective scoring). As Fig. 3 shows, the analysis of night sleep results in one peak period coinciding with the zeitgeber period; the analysis of the naps results likewise in one peak period which, however, was clearly shorter than the period of the night sleep, and which coincided with the freerunning period. The analysis of the locomotor activity of the subject results in two relevant periods which are unusually close together; they coincide with the zeitgeber and the freerunning period. The analysis of rectal temperature shows only one peak period which is clearly shorter than the zeitgeber (and the sleep-wake) period, defining the freerunning period. The comparison with the analysis of the naps confirms that, in case of internal desynchronization, the naps are controlled by the "temperature oscillator" and not by the "sleep-wake oscillator"; i.e., the two types of sleep episodes are controlled dominantly by different basic oscillators, or pacemakers.

In Fig. 3, right, educed cycles are presented, from the same rhythms as shown in Fig.3, middle, and calculated with the two resulting dominant periods, 24.5 and 25.25 h. In the sleep cycles, the more pronounced alternation (with clear phases without any sleep) is shown in the night sleep with the zeitgeber period (25.25 h) and in the naps with the freerunning period (24.5 h). With each of the other periods, there is some rhythmicity; this is due, however, to the small size of the interval between the two periods relative to the duration of the total experiment (i.e., if the experiment had been continued for 2 or 3 more weeks, the distributions with the "wrong" period each would have been considerably flattened). The educed cycles of locomotor activity are nearly equally pronounced with both relevant periods. The educed cycle of rectal temperature is clearly more pronounced with the freerunning than the zeitgeber period. Here, the educing is calculated not only from all temperature data but, in addition, also from temperature data obtained exclusively during the wake episodes and exclusively during the sleep episodes (independent of its subjective scoring). The difference between the wake and sleep temperature cycles, which run widely parallel to each other, is the "masking effect" (Wever 1985a).

In the majority of relevant experiments, the subjects did not have the option to switch on any illumination during the dark phase, and the light-dark alternation was supplemented by regular gong signals requesting the subjects for miction and the performance of several tests; during the sleep episodes the subjects were awakened by the signals. The most relevant reason to introduce the structurizing signals was to obtain performance and other psychic data regularly around the clock (body temperature had been measured continuously during wake and sleep; urine data reflect, at least, the mean over the preceding interval, independent of its length; in contrast, performance data are instantaneous values which tell us nothing about the course of performance during the preceding interval). In experiments with constant conditions, or in zeitgeber experiments without the structurizing signals (cf. Fig. 3), there is mostly a consistent night gap in the data, preventing the estimation of corresponding rhythms (a data gap of one-third of the full cycle corresponds in period analyses, independent of the number of data points obtained during the remaining part of the cycle, to an analysis using only three equidistant data points, which is, according to established rules, insufficient for the deduction of any statement about rhythmicity).

In several constant condition experiments subjects awoke occasionally from sleep and performed the tests; in these cases, however, the "night classes" of data include considerably less than 10% of the data of the "day classes", so that an equivalent consideration of night and day data would be unfair. On the other hand, these experiments by themselves allow an evaluation of the influence of the "night gap" (Wever 1982): A formal sine wave approximation is possible, of course, without consideration of the sporadic night data (as it would be inevitable in most constant condition experiments, where no night data are available); in most cases, this procedure does not lead to a significant rhythmicity at all. In a next step, a sine wave approximation had been calculated with consideration of the sporadic night data; this procedure (though unfair; see above) leads, in nearly all cases, to significant rhythmicities; in all cases, however, the parameters of such a rhythmicity (e.g., amplitude, phase, and mainly mean value) are considerably different from the parameters obtained in analyses without consideration of the night data. They are similar, rather, to rhythm parameters calculated from experiments with zeitgebers including the regular signals where night gaps in the data do not exist.

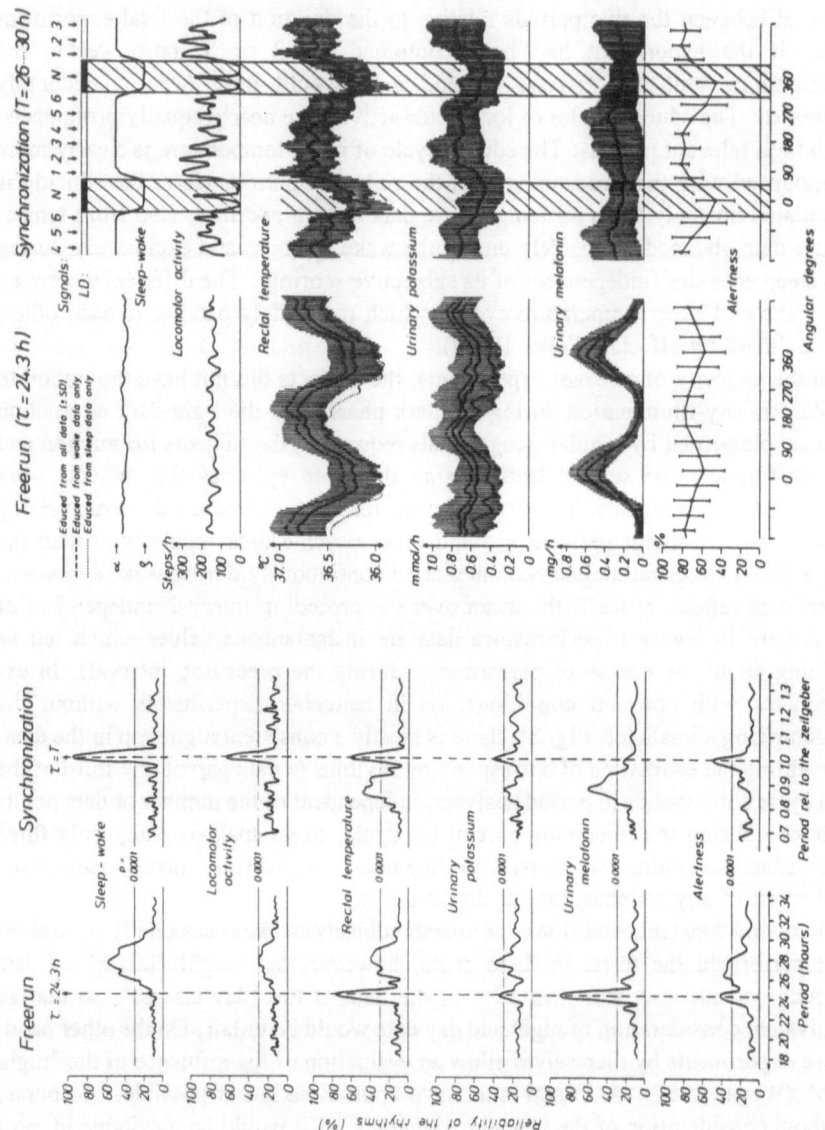

Fig. 4. Experiment with a subject (female, 81 years) living under temporal isolation without natural time cues, but under the influence of an artificial zeitgeber (LD 300:0.1 lux, and 7 signals per cycle requesting the subject for mictions and several tests) with a slowly and steadily lengthening period (starting with a period of 26 h which was maintained for 4 days; thereafter, every period was 10 min longer than the preceding one). *Left*, periodogram analyses of several variables, calculated twice each, i.e., on an absolute time base, and on a time base relative to the actual zeitgeber cycle. *Right*, educed cycles of the same variables as in *diagrams on the left*, calculated twice each, i.e., with the prominent period of the absolute analyses (24.3 h), and with the actual zeitgeber cycle as the (relative) period

Above all, without inclusion of consistent night data serious misinterpretations can occur (but, of course, must not occur necessarily in every single case) when sections of an experiment with different conditions should be compared.

In the experiments to be discussed in the following, the zeitgeber period had been altered slowly and steadily, to evaluate precisely the entrainment limits of the different rhythms ("fractional desynchronization"; Wever 1983). In a series of 19 experiments of this type, performed with young and healthy subjects, the range of entrainment of the rhythm of rectal temperature (with a range of $\pm$ 2.34 h $\pm$ 0.17 h) had been shown to be positioned nearly symmetrically around the freerunning period (24.67 h $\pm$ 0.24 h). The lengthening experiments of this series started with a zeitgeber period of 26.0 h (shorter entrainment limits are very unlikely in healthy subjects) which was maintained for four cycles (to guarantee a steady state), and every following zeitgeber cycle was 10 min longer than the preceding one; they resulted in an upper entrainment limit of 26.91 °C $\pm$ 0.24 °C (Wever 1983).

The same experimental protocol was also applied to an older female subject (81 years old), with a different result: the physiological rhythms freeran from the beginning of the experiment. This can be deduced also from Fig. 4, left, where periodogram analyses from this experiment are presented (as is common in such experiments, the analyses are computed twice, with an absolute time base, and with a time base relative to the actual zeitgeber period). Only in sleep-wake and locomotor activity is there only a rhythm running synchronously to the zeitgeber; and only in melatonin is there only a freerunning rhythm. All other variables show two rhythmicities each, a synchronized and a freerunning component. This could be interpreted as a succession of the two rhythm states, i.e., as a synchronization during a first section of the experiment and a freerun during a second section. However, sequential analyses show similar pictures with the two rhythms each from the beginning of the experiment; and the melatonin which is known to be not deformed by a masking effect (Wever 1986), shows only one rhythmicity. Hence, these analyses force one to the conclusion that the two rhythms (in proportions which change from variable to variable) coexist during the entire experiment. Consequently, a freerunning component in all physiological rhythms is present from the beginning of the experiment (a masking component is simultaneouly present in most rhythms). And this means that the upper entrainment limit in this subject was less than 26.0 h; i.e., it was so far out of the range obtained in young and healthy subjects (a deviation from the mean of more than four times the standard deviation is very unlikely) that it should not be included in the same sample.

Similar results originated from two more subjects. One of these was a 62-year-old woman suffering from different diseases (but with a special recommendation of her physician to participate in a long-term experiment); the other was a 32-year old man who contracted an infection (of unknown origin) with fever (up to 39.5 °C) a few days after the start of the experiment which disappeared after a few days (controlled by the analyses of pteridine data; see above). In spite of the small number of relevant experiments (but with additional consideration of the experiment on which Fig.3 is based), the impression is given that the range of entrainment is considerably reduced in ill and old subjects. The result of the experiment on which Fig. 3 is based even shows that, in such cases, a zeitgeber of normal strength may be too weak to synchronize the physiological rhythms to the 24-h day, but is still able to synchronize the sleep-wake rhythm.

The experiments discussed above simultaneously open up another approach to the correlation between rhythm abnormalities and health (mental) disorders. In the rhythm state of internal desynchronization, it is possible to determine the masking effect quantitatively (Wever 1985a). The corresponding procedure was also applied to the rhythms of patients the range of entrainment of whom had been shown to be abnormally small (see above): Educed cycles had been calculated, not only by using all data, but also by using data which had been obtained exclusively during the wake episodes or exclusively during the sleep episodes. In Fig.4, right, educed cycles from the 81-year old lady are presented, each calculated with the two relevant periods (the — absolute — dominant period of the physiological rhythms and the — relative — dominant period of sleep-wake); in all (freerunning) physiological rhythms and in the alertness rhythm, in addition, the mentioned separation into a wake and a sleep cycle has been performed. The result on the whole is that the "educed wake cycle" of every variable shows higher values than the corresponding "educed sleep cycle"; this statement is valid also with regard to melatonin (measured in the urine as aMT6s) where a masking effect is usually not detectable.

In freerunning rhythms, the mean masking effect in the rhythm of rectal temperature had been estimated to be 0.28 °C ± 0.06 °C (Wever 1985a); this value is relatively high, evidently because spontaneous internal desynchronization (which is a precondition for the detection of the masking effect in this way) occurs significantly more often in (younger) subjects with high neurotic scores or in old subjects than in young and healthy subjects (Wever 1979). In these experiments, the masking effect is clearly greater than normal in subjects who are under behavioral stress than in others, so it can be utilized as a predictor for stress. Under the influence of a zeitgeber where internal desynchronization can occur in every subject, it is distinctly smaller (about 0.22 °C; Wever 1985a). In the experiment on which Fig. 4 based, however, the masking effect of the temperature rhythm is distinctly greater (0.39 °C). When considered with the zeitgeber period (diagrams most on the right), the pattern of masking with the overshoots at the onsets of wake and of sleep is more obviously pronounced than in other experiments; even the timing of the 7 requesting signals per cycle is reflected, not only (as usual) in locomotor activity but also (uniquely) in the course of rectal temperature. Moreover, a masking effect is detectable even in melatonin (when in the course of the internal desynchronization the melatonin peak was positioned in a wake episode and, hence, the light-phase, it was just twice as high as when it was positioned in a sleep episode and, hence, the dark-phase; Wever 1989c). In other experiments, a difference between melatonin wake and sleep cycles had been observed only under constant bright illumination, where the wake cycle (from data obtained with open eyes under the bright light which is known to suppress melatonin; Lewy et al. 1980) is distinctly lower than the sleep cycle (from data with closed eyes where the bright light cannot be effective; Wever 1986). The experiment on which Fig. 4 is based, consequently, supports the earlier suggestion that the masking effect is larger in older and in stressed (and possibly in ill) subjects than it is in young and healthy subjects.

The lowermost diagrams in Fig. 4 show remarkably high values of alertness. This is due not only to the general sense of well-being of this subject (it was her third long-term experiment), but also to the particular experimental conditions: It is a general experience that subjectively scored well-being and objectively measured performance are increased under forced internal desynchronization. Particularly in experiments where the subject's rhythms run internally synchronized in one or more sections and internally desynchronized in other sections, subjective feeling and objective performance are significantly better, without exception in more than 50 experiments with various changes in the temporal sequence of the sections compared, under internal desynchronization than under synchronization (Wever 1982); this apparently paradoxical result was also found by other authors who performed similar experiments (Folkard et al. 1985). This result can indeed be confirmed, on principle, only in zeitgeber experiments; in experiments under constant conditions where evaluations of psychic rhythms are not very meaningful on principle (see above), consistent differences in sections with internal synchronization and desynchronization have not been found in psychic rhythms. Hence, also the question for differences in spontaneously (under constant conditions) or forcedly (under a zeitgeber) occurring internal desynchronization with regard to psychic variables cannot be answered (considering only data from wake episodes which are present equally in both types of desynchronization, and that in experimental sections with equal periods, systematic differences cannot be observed).

Practical Implications

In all cases where rhythm disorders lead to health (mental) disorders, an enlargement in the amplitude or the strength of the controlling zeitgeber can improve the situation (Wever 1988). In humans, the most relevant zeitgeber is of behavioral origin; it is social contact with the environment. Its relevance is based on the fact that it is, though it is not the strongest possible zeitgeber, ubiquitous. Indeed, particularly in old and ill patients, where rhythm disorders have been observed most frequently, the effective zeitgeber may be not strong enough to synchronize all rhythms of the patients to 24 h. Such an external desynchronization is easy to recognize when it concerns all rhythms including sleep-wake. As the example of Fig.3 shows, however, a missing synchronization of only the physiological rhythms (which is much more probable because of their much smaller ranges of entrainment) is much harder to realize. In such cases the overall zeitgeber strength can be intensified by the utilization of the "bright-light zeitgeber." This zeitgeber, although of minor relevance under normal conditions, had been shown to be the strongest zeitgeber and, moreover, to be able to be superimposed on the social zeitgeber nearly additively (Wever 1989a).

In applying the bright-light zeitgeber, one is confronted with an apparent contradiction: Although the bright-light zeitgeber is considerably stronger than the normal-light zeitgeber, it leads to an amplitude of the circadian temperature rhythm which is clearly smaller than under the influence of a normal-light zeitgeber (on average, by about 25%). A reduction of the temperature amplitude with the transition to bright light has been shown under a 24-h zeitgeber, and that in phase shift experiments which show simultaneously the considerable strenghtening of the zeitgeber (by halving the duration of reentrainment of the rhythm to the shifted zeitgeber; Wever 1985b); and it has been shown in other experiments under a 25-h zeitgeber, which has been selected to avoid additional indirect effects on the amplitude due to changes in the phase relationship between rhythm and zeitgeber (which are unavoidable after changes of the zeitgeber strength when the zeitgeber period deviates from the intrinsic period of the rhythm). Finally these results of zeitgeber experiments agree with results of experiments in constant conditions where the amplitude of the temperature rhythm is clearly smaller under constant bright light than under constant light of normal intensity (Wever 1986). The solution of the apparent paradoxon, a reduction of the amplitude of the temperature rhythm with strengthening the zeitgeber, is based on the observation that the relation between amplitude and zeitgeber strength is ambiguous: under a zeitgeber of medium strength (e.g., the normal-light or the information zeitgeber), in fact, the amplitude is larger than in freerunning rhymths (Wever 1979); with further increase of the zeitgeber strength, however, the amplitude passes a maximum value, and it becomes smaller eventually (due to an "overmodulation" of the system). Possibly, the reduction of the amplitude with increasing light intensity has another aspect: the same reduction should occur in patients with an increased sensitiveness to light (e.g., in depressives) already under illumination of normal intensity. This would mean that the observed reduction of the amplitude in depressives may be due, at least in part, to the increased sensitiveness of the circadian system to light which is known in such patients.

To constitute an affective bright-light zeitgeber, the intensity of illumination during the light phase must be more than 2500 lux; this value can be reached indoors only by an expensive technical equipment. In most of the hitherto discussed zeitgeber experiments, the bright light was in operation during the full light phase, i.e., for at least 16 h/day. Hence, it is still an open question how long humans must be exposed to the bright light to take advantage of the high zeitgeber strength; preliminary studies showed that, at least, several hours of exposure are necessary (necessary means the constitution of a zeitgeber with a range of entrainment of, at least, 1 h either side, to overcome the interval between the normal period of freerunning rhythms and the 24-h day). And this means that in our industrial society only a negligible number of people are able to make use of the bright-light zeitgeber; particularly old and ill patients who suffer from a lack of social contacts (and, hence, may suffer from insufficient synchronization of their physiological rhythms) are mostly unable to stay outdoors for many hours. Here, the installation of artificial bright light devices should be considered, despite the high technical cost. A precondition for the application of therapy applying the bright-light zeitgeber, however, is the knowledge of how many hours per day the patients have to be exposed to the bright light.

Two experimental series have been performed to test the sufficiency of a bright-light zeitgeber with 6 h of bright light/cycle.In a first series the pure effect of light was tested, without participation of a behavioral component. To test the concept, healthy subjects were exposed to alternations of light und dark where the ratio between the light intensities during the light and dark phases was only 10:1, so that the subjects could also perform all the activities during the dark phases ("relative LD").

Fig.5 shows the outcomes of three typical experiments where subjects were exposed to such light-dark alternations with coinciding temporal protocols, each starting with a period of 24.0 h and continuing with a steady shortening of the period of 10 min/cycle. In Fig.5, left, the light intensities werde 300:30 lux, with a temporal ratio of 75 %:25 %; the result was a clear freerun of all rhythms from the beginning of the experiment. In Fig.5, right, the light intensities were 10 times higher (i.e., 3000:300 lux) with the same temporal ratio (the subjects experienced an even smaller contrast in the light intensities than with the lower light intensities); the result was clear synchronization within a wide range, i.e., down to about 20.5 h. In Fig.5, middle, the light intensities were the same as in Fig.5, right, but the temporal ratio was reversed (i.e., it was 25 %:75 %); as a result, the rhythms were synchronized (with maintaining internal synchronization) only within small ranges, i.e., down to about 23 h. In summary, while normal artificial illumination (Fig.5, left) exerts no zeitgeber effect and bright light for the full light phase (Fig.5, right) exerts strong zeitgeber effects, 6 h bright light/cycle (Fig.5, middle) shows a zeitgeber effectiveness which is just sufficient to synchronize human circadian rhythms to the 24-h day. Similar results have also been obtained in corresponding experiments with a steady lengthening of the zeitgeber period.

In the other experimental series the intensity of illumination during the dark phase was close to zero, so that the subjects were forced to rest during the dark phase ("absolute LD"); consequently, sleep-wake was synchronized to the zeitgeber within a wide range (in these experiments this meaans, during the entire experiments), and only the range of entrainment of the physiological rhythms could be considered. In other words, the zeitgeber included a behavioral component, constituted by the requests to rest which were transmitted by the light-dark transitions. It is known that such a behavioral component when given solely (e.g., by acoustic signals under constant illumination or darkness) exerts a zeitgeber with a range of entrainment of about 2 h either side of the freerunning period. And it is also known that, under a light-dark alternation with intensities of common artificial illumination, the range of entrainment is at most the same (in a large sample, the upper entrainment limit was 26.91 h $\pm$ 0.27 h; see above); the additional direct effect of light, hence, is negligible.

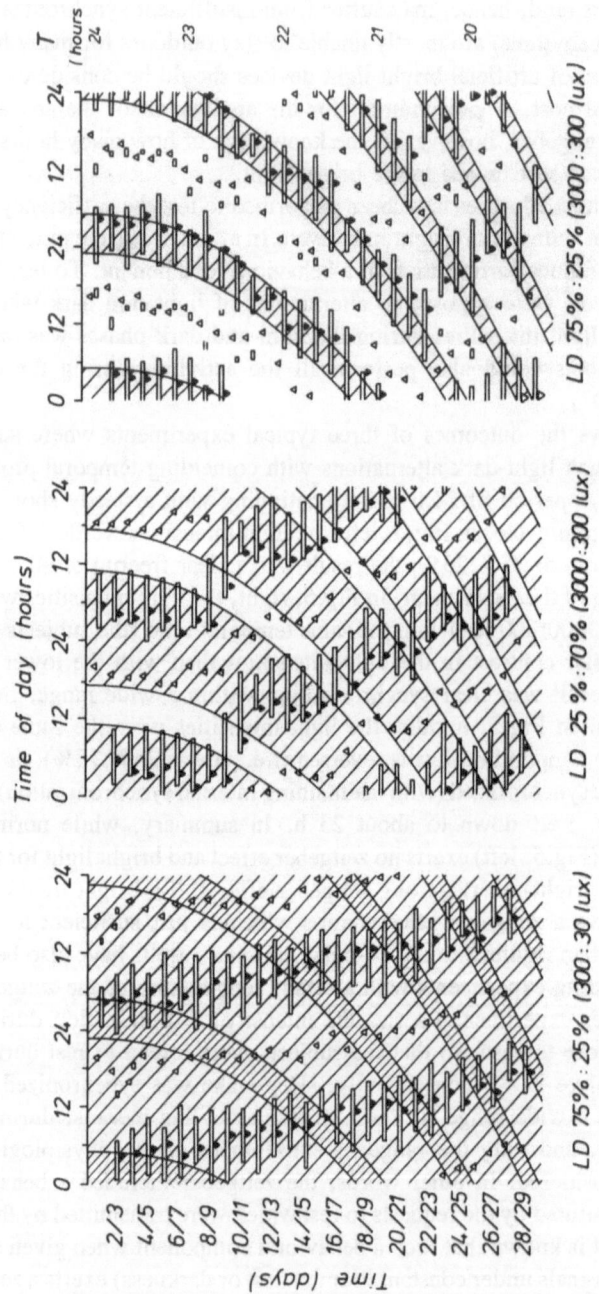

Fig.6 shows 4 typical examples from this series. Fig.6, left, shows the course of an experiment as discussed earlier, with an intensity of illumination of about 300 lux during the light phase; this results in an upper entrainment limit of the temperature rhythm of about 27 h (which was due only to the behavioral zeitgeber component; see above). In the exemplary experiment on which Fig.6, right, is based, the intensity of illumination during the full light phase was more than 3000 lux; as a result, not only sleep-wake but also the rhythm of body temperature was synchronized to the zeitgeber up to the end of the experiment, i.e., the entrainment limits were higher than about 30 h. In Fig.6, middle, courses of 2 experiments are shown where the bright light was in operation only during a third of the light phase, i.e., for 6 h in the initial 26-h day, while in the remaining two thirds the light intensity was about 300 lux; also in these experiments, the behavioral component was based on the full light phase, as it was in the other experiments. In these experiments the entrainment limits of the temperature rhythm was clearly higher than in the experiment with normal illumination throughout, on average for about 1 h; on the other hand, they were considerably lower than in the experiment with bright illumination throughout. A closer inspection shows that it is relevant to the entrainment limit whether the bright light section is positioned at the beginning or the end of the light phase; according to the phase response curve applicable in this case (Wever 1989a), the upper entrainment limit is extended more when the bright light is in the last third of the light phase (at about 28 h) than when it is in the first third (at about 27.5 h). These experiments, therefore, show an extension of the range of entrainment by the supplementation of the behavioral zeitgeber by 6 h of bright light for about 1 h. Similar results have also been obtained in corresponding experiments with a steady shortening of the zeitgeber period (here, the lower entrainment limit is extended more when the bright light is in the first third of the light phase than when it is in the last third). In summary, the results of the experiments which include a behavioral component fully agree with the results of the experiments which do not include such a component.

◄───

Fig.5. Courses of three exemplary experiments where subjects lived in temporal isolation without natural time cues, but under the influence of artificial zeitgebers (LD with a ratio of light intensities of only 10:1) with slowly and steadily shortening periods (starting with a period of 24 h, every period was 10 min shorter than the preceding one); the actual zeitgeber periods are indicated *at the right border*. Due to the applied zeitgeber ("relative LD"; i.e., without participation of a behavioral component), the rhythms were internally synchronized, in all experiments, until the end of the experiment. *Left*, LD (300:30 lux) with a temporal ratio of 75%:25%; no external synchronization at all. *Right*, LD with 10 times higher light intensities as in the left diagram (i.e., 3000:300 lux) but identical temporal ratios (75%:25%); external synchronization down to about 20.5 h. *Middle*, LD with the same light intensities as in the right diagram (3000:300 lux), but in reversed temporal ratio (i.e., 25%:75%); external synchronization only down to about 23 h

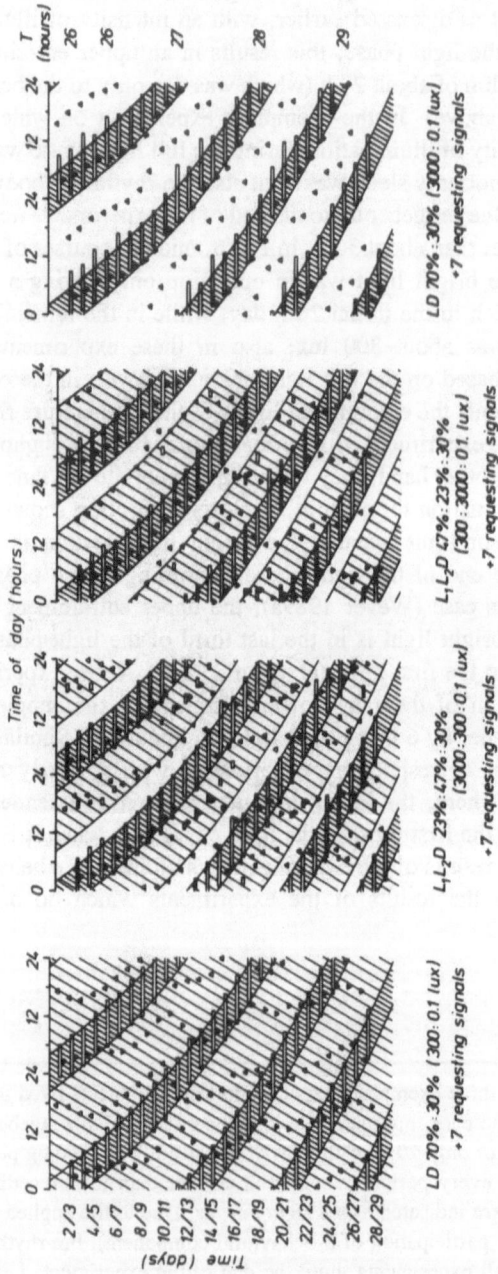

In the experiments discussed here the period of the zeitgeber was changed slowly and steadily. It would be possible to obtain the desired results also in other ways, for instance, by holding the zeitgeber period constant (at a value guaranteeing a sufficient range of entrainment; e.g., at 23.5 h) but by changing the temporal L:D ratio slowly and steadily. The method used here, however, has a special advantage, which is to enable the phase and amplitude response curves to be determined simultaneously (Wever 1989a). The knowledge of such curves makes it possible to predict the effects of bright-light pulses (or of sections with social contacts, respectively) on phase and amplitude of the rhythm depending on the phase of the rhythm hit by the stimulus; i.e., to predict the most effective time of day for a light pulse or a social contact, when a specific change in the rhythm is demanded.

In summary, the bright light experiments have shown that a sufficient zeitgeber effectiveness demands at least 6 h of bright light/day, with an intensity of more than 2500 lux. Such a zeitgeber is able to synchronize human circadian rhythms to the 24-h day, independent of the behavioral zeitgeber. When supplementing an — when given solely — insufficient behavioral zeitgeber, even a shorter bright light pulse would be able to make an overall zeitgeber sufficient. A therapy utilizing the bright-light zeitgeber has already been proposed (Wever 1985b, 1986, 1988) on the basis of more preliminary results. Apparently, the first applications of such a therapy in old patients have shown positive results (Dietzel et al. 1989). Moreover, it may be possible that the bright-light therapy which is helpful in special types of depression (seasonal affective disorder) is based on a strengthening of the effective zeitgeber. Now, more quantitative data about the effectiveness of bright-light zeitgebers are available, so that there should be an even better chance to make use of a therapy applying the bright-light zeitgeber.

◄──

Fig. 6. Courses of 4 exemplary experiments where subjects lived under temporal isolation without natural time cues, but under the influence of artificial zeitgebers (LD with basis intensities of 300:0.1 lux and a temporal ratio of 70%:30%, and 7 signals/cycle requesting the subjects for miction and several tests), with slowly and steadily lengthening periods (starting with a period of 26 h maintained for 4 days; thereafter, every period was 10 min longer than the preceding one); the actual zeitgeber periods are indicated *at the right border*. Due to the applied zeitgeber ("absolute LD"; i.e., with participation of a behavioral component), sleep wake was synchronized, in all experiments, until the end of the experiment; consequently, after the external desynchronization of the physiological rhythms, internal desynchronization also occurred. *Left*, LD with light intensities of 300:0.1 lux; synchronization of the physiological rhythms up to about 27 h. *Right*, LD with light intensities of 3000:0.1 lux (i.e., with bright light during the entire light phase); synchronization of the physiological rhythms up the end of the experiment, i.e., up to at least 30 h. *Middle diagrams*, with bright light (3000 lux) during a third of the light-phase, *in the middle left diagram* during the first third and *in the middle right diagram* during the last third of the light phase; synchronization of the physiological rhythms up to about 27.5 h when the bright light was in the first and up to about 28 h when the bright light was in the last third of the light-phase

References

Dietzel M, Saletu B (1989) Der Einfluss von intensivem Licht auf Schlafdauer und Schlafar-chitektur geriatrischer Patienten. In: Saletu B (ed) Biologische Psychiatrie. Thieme, Stuttgart, pp 388-391

Folkard S, Hume KI, Minors DS, Waterhouse JM, Watson FL (1985) Independence of the circadian rhythm in alertness from the sleep/wake cycle. Nature 313: 678-679

Lewy, AJ, Wehr TA, Goodwin FK, Newsome DA, Markey SP (1980) Light suppresses melatonin secretion in humans. Science 210: 1267-1269

Lund R, Rüther E, Wever R (1987) Untersuchungen an schlafgestörten Patienten und gesunden Kontrollpersonen unter zeitgeberfreien Bedingungen. In: Hippius H, Rüther E, Schmauss M (eds) Schlaf-Wach-Funktionen. Springer, Berlin Heidelberg New York, pp 11-25

Wever R (1975) The circadian multi-oscillator system of man. Int J Chronobiol 3: 19-55

Wever RA (1979) The circadian system of man. Springer, Berlin Heidelberg New York

Wever RA (1982) Behavioral aspects of circadian rhythmicity. In: Brown FM, Graeber RC (eds) Rhythmic aspects of behavior. Erlbaum, Hillsdale, pp 105-171

Wever RA (1983) Fractional desynchronization of human circadian rhythms: a method for evaluating entrainment limits and functional interdependences. Pflügers Arch 396: 128-137

Wever RA (1984) Properties of human sleep-wake cycles: parameters of internally synchro-nized freerunning rhythms. Sleep 7: 27-51

Wever RA (1985a) Internal interactions within the human circadian system: masking effects. Experientia 4: 332-342

Wever RA (1985b) Use of light to treat jet lag: differential effects of normal and bright artificial light on human circadian rhythms. In: Medical and biological effects of light. Ann N Y Acad Sci 453: 282-304

Wever RA (1986) Characteristics of circadian rhythms in human functions. J Neural Transm Suppl 21: 323-373

Wever RA (1988) Order and disorder in human circadian rhythmicity: possible relations to mental disorders. In: Kupfer DJ, Monk TH, Barchas JD (eds) Biological rhythms and mental disorders. Guilford, New York, pp 253-347

Wever RA (1989a) Light effects on human circadian rhythms: a review of recent Andechs experiments. J Biol Rhythms 4: 161-185

Wever RA (1989b) Geschlechtsunterschiede von Schlafparametern. In: Saletu B (ed) Biologische Psychiatrie. Thieme, Stuttgart New York, 375-379

Wever RA (1989c) Schlaf und Melatonin. In: Saletu B (ed) Biologische Psychiatrie. Thieme, Stuttgart, 397-401

14 Periodic Phenomena in Affective Illness with Special Reference to Annual Cycles

D. von Zerssen, H.M. Emrich, G. Dirlich

Introduction

Periodic phenomena, i.e., rhythms consisting of regular cycles, can be observed in nature at various frequencies, from the atomic to the cosmic level. Such phenomena in living organisms form the objects of chronobiology (Aschoff 1981a; Hekkens et al. 1988) which, in romantic medicine, was consequently labeled as "periodology" (Baumgarten Crusius 1836). Chronomedicine, a branch of chronobiology, deals with regular, or almost regular, cycles of pathological processes and of the organism's reactivity to noxious or therapeutic agents (Reinberg and Smolensky 1983). In psychiatry, periodic phenomena in affective illness constitute the focal point of this kind of research (Wehr and Goodwin 1981, 1983). Recurrent forms of the disorder were formerly described as "periodic psychoses" (periodic mania, periodic melancholia, and periodic cyclic psychosis or circular insanity with alternations of mania and depression) by some authors (e.g., Kirn 1878; Kraepelin 1883), although, in the majority of cases subsumed under this term, the period, i.e., the length of the cycles (time elapsed from the onset of one episode to the next), varied considerably (see Slater 1938; Eastwood and Peter 1989). The term was later on extended to include psychoses which did not belong to the group of affective illness (e.g., Pilcz 1901; Hatotani and Nomura 1983), above all the so-called periodic catatonias (Müller 1900; Gjessing and Gjessing 1961; Gjessing 1974); yet still recurrent forms of mania, depression, and their combinations were regarded as the core disorders of this type of insanity. It is beyond any doubt that, indeed, periodic phenomena in the sense of (almost) regular cycles can be observed in affective illness much more frequently than in any other form of mental disorder (see Menninger-Lerchenthal 1960; Richter 1965).

Despite the long history of clinical observations reported in the literature, there are still divergences at the descriptive level concerning the delineation of periodic phenomena in affective illness and, as a consequence, also with respect to the frequency of their occurrence and the nosological status of the disorders displaying such periodicity. Are these disorders distinct nosological entities (e.g., Hitzig 1898) or variants of a recurrent disorder that usually takes a less regular course (Kraepelin 1899)? Above all, the explanation of periodicity in terms of chronobiologically defined mechanisms remains a matter of debate. Four groups of mechanism (see Aschoff 1981a) have to be considered in this context:

1. A disturbance of "internal clocks" generating endogenous rhythms within the organism, such as the pacemaker(s) for circadian rhythmicity. One of the following three is true:
   - The physiological pacemaker(s) is/are deficient, e.g., generate(s) rhythms of abnormal period or phase (e.g., Halberg 1968; Wehr and Goodwin 1981).
   - The rhythm of a set of hypothetical pacemakers, which, under normal circumstances, generate a cycling of the same period but at different phases, has become synchronized so that the usually concealed rhythm becomes evident (Richter 1960).
   - The disease process in the brain underlying the formation of affective symptomatology has established a new, unphysiological pacemaker, e.g., in the case of 48-h cycles (see below).
2. Induction of periodicity by periodic changes in the environment, e.g., seasonal changes in sunshine or ambient temperature (see Aschoff 1981b; Roenneberg and Aschoff 1990).
3. Modification of a primarily aperiodic pathological process by periodic influences from the environment or by overt rhythms within the organism (e.g., by the circadian rhythm of sleep or motor activity) (von Zerssen 1983, 1987) — influences not mediated by the internal clock(s).
4. Coupling of the disease process in the brain to physiological clock mechanisms (Dirlich et al. 1981; von Zerssen et al. 1985, 1987).

It should be noted that only the mechanisms under 1. imply a disturbance within the time-keeping system of the organism, whereas the three others are perceived as essentially similar to the mechanisms that are at work in generating normal rhythmicity of biological functions. The concepts according to which the periodicity of affective symptomatology is caused by physiological mechanisms (von Zerssen 1983, 1987; Healy and Waterhouse 1990) and not by dysfunctions of the rhythm-generating system are not very popular in the current psychiatric literature (see Wehr and Goodwin 1983; Halaris 1987; Pflug 1987). However, they have the advantage of not postulating an otherwise unknown pathology.

In the following, we will review the evidence for and against the different kinds of hypothetical mechanisms in the causation of periodic phenomena in affective illness. The review is based on the literature, with special reference to our own observations and data analyses, also including material that has not yet been published in detail. Only three kinds of periods, namely annual rhythms, bidian (48-h) rhythms, and diurnal variation in symptomatology, are considered here, these being most thoroughly documented in the literature and covered by research of our own. In earlier reports, we have extensively discussed problems of 48-h cycles (Doerr et al. 1979; Emrich et al. 1979; Dirlich et al. 1981; von Zerssen et al. 1979, 1983) and of diurnal variation in depression (von Zerssen et al. 1985, 1987; von Zerssen 1988). Therefore, in this paper we will focus on annual cycles.

Annual Cycles

Description

Annual rhythms are widespread in the plant and animal kingdoms, depending largely on climatic changes during the course of the year and thus increasing with geographic distance from the equator up to 40° latitude (see Aschoff 1981b). In several species, an endogenous component of circannual rhythms has been demonstrated, e.g., for seasonal migration in birds, and for seasonal coat changes and hibernation in mammals (see Gwinner 1986). In humans, several physiological functions display seasonal variations (see Lacoste and Wirz-Justice 1989). However, nothing is known about an "internal clock" generating an endogenous circannual rhythm in man in the absence of seasonal changes in the environment. The overt rhythms may well be entirely induced by changes in climate, food, and other circumstances of living (see Aschoff 1981b; Roenneberg and Aschoff 1990).

With respect to annual rhythms in affective illness, one can find clear descriptions of the phenomenon as far back as the medical literature of the eighteenth century: "Once every year in December, Helwig noted in a man the recurrence of melancholy, which was heralded by sleeplessness and terminated by a headache. During the episode, he was mute, destroyed, like a child, things that were lying around, and had a hearty appetite" (translated from Medicus 1764, pp. 43f.). The same book mentions a nobleman from Graubünden (Switzerland) who was melancholic during the winter but manic during the summer (idem, p. 44). In the early nineteenth century, annual cycles of a bipolar II disorder (see Dunner et al. 1970) were described in detail as "a periodic melancholia" (Wolff 1821).

Toward the end of the nineteenth century, however, Kraepelin (1899) abandoned the concept of periodic psychoses as separate nosological entities and subsumed periodic mania, periodic melancholia and circular insanity under the heading of "manic-depressive insanity": "First of all, one can speak of a truly strict periodic recurrence of episodes only in a proportionally rather small number of observations. From here, there is a vast range of gradual transitions to the forms displaying a quite irregular course" (translated; p. 403). He estimated the portion of cases exhibiting regular changes during their lives at 4%-5%. "Repeatedly, I saw the moodiness set in in fall and pass over to excitement in spring 'when the sap shoots into the trees', in a certain sense corresponding to mood changes which even overcome healthy individuals during seasonal changes. As a rule, they seem to represent forms taking a very mild course, i.e. hypomania and simple retardation" (p.410f.; see also Georgi 1947). In the past decade, such seasonally recurring disturbances of mood were extensively described as "seasonal affective disorder" (SAD: Rosenthal et al. 1984; see Rosenthal and Blehar 1989; Thompson and Silverstone 1989).

The most frequent form of the disorder is the combination of a mild to moderate atypical depression (see Liebowitz et al. 1984) in the winter season (called "winter depression") with hypomania in spring/summer (Rosenthal et al. 1984; Thompson and Isaacs 1988). The depression is characterized by sadness, often accompanied by an admixture of anxiety and irritability, reduced activity, increased appetite, with carbohydrate craving and subsequent weight gain, and by hypersomnia. Yet also unipolar depression, severe depression accompanied by weight loss and hyposomnia, and bipolar I disorder (see Dunner et al. 1970) may exhibit a similar seasonal course. A reverse course, with "summer depression" and (hypo)mania in fall/winter, can also be observed, though far less frequently (Wehr et al. 1987). The symptom picture of "summer depression" is often characterized by loss of appetite and hyposomnia (Boyce and Parker 1988) and is thus more typical of depressions in general (Wehr and Rosenthal 1989). There are, however, exceptions to this rule (see, e.g., Zaudig et al., submitted for publication).

In accordance with Kraepelin's above description, less pronounced seasonal mood cycles have been revealed in a large proportion of the general population (Thompson et al. 1988; Kasper et al. 1989b, and others). The prevalence figures vary considerably around one-fourth in adults, depending on latitude and the methods of case finding and case definition. The majority of subjects afflicted with this so-called "subsyndromal SAD" (Kasper et al. 1989a) report a decrease in well-being to occur during the winter season; a minority feel worse during the summer. Spring and fall are rarely mentioned as the most critical seasons.

In the revised version of the third edition of the *Diagnostic and Statistical Manual of the American Psychiatric Association*, DSM-III-R (American Psychiatric Association 1987), SAD was incorporated into the section on Mood Disorder (another term for "Affective Disorder" as used in DSM-III: American Psychiatric Association 1980); however, it was not defined as a nosological subtype but rather as a special form of the course that different subtypes ("Major Depression, Recurrent," "Bipolar Disorder" and the mixed group of "Affective Disorder, Not Otherwise Specified") may take. DSM-III-R criteria for the diagnosis of SAD are:

- Regular temporal relationship of the onset of an episode of depression and/or (hypo)mania to a particular 60-day period of the year, e.g., the occurrence of a depressive episode between the beginning of October and the end of November, independent of regularly recurring psychosocial stressors like unemployment during the winter season
- Complete remission or transition from depression to (hypo)mania, also within a specified 60-day period of the year
- At least three episodes of this kind, of which two should occur in subsequent years
- A ratio of seasonal to nonseasonal epsiodes of at least 3:1

The last two criteria indicate that even irregular cycles of an affective illness are included in the definition of SAD if there is a statistical linkage of the onset and offset of episodes to a certain time of the year. It should be noted, too, that only three episodes are sufficient for the diagnosis. Hence, SAD, in general, cannot be regarded as a periodic disorder in the strict sense, as this would demand regular cycles over so many years that a temporal random distribution of episodes becomes highly improbable (see Mrosovsky 1989). This has to be kept in mind when estimating the frequency of periodic phenomena in affective illness and discussing the underlying causes.

Although the existence of variants of an affective illness meeting the criteria for SAD, with a large preponderance of winter depression over summer depression,

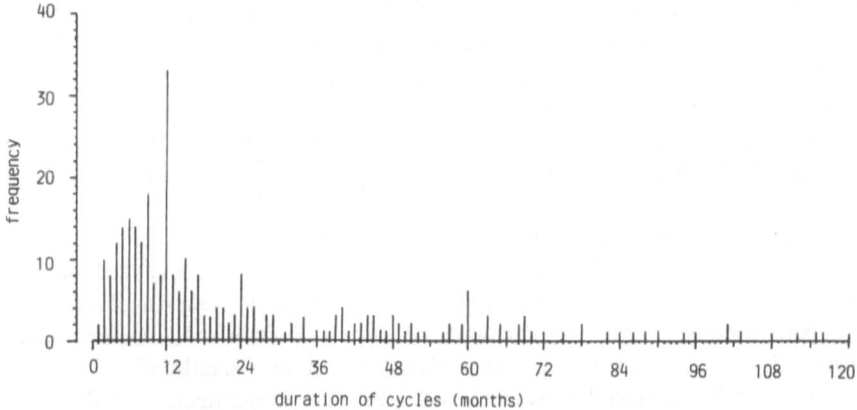

Fig.1 Frequency distribution of the duration of retrospectively assessed cycles in the subsample from Glostrup, Denmark

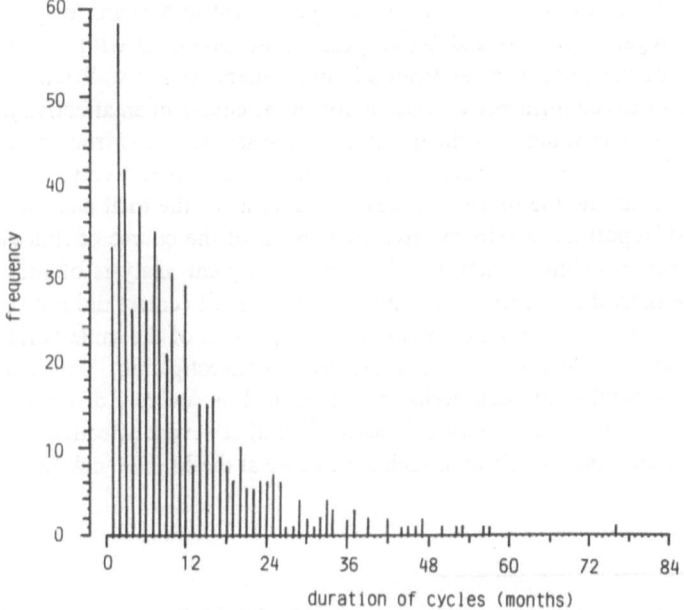

Fig.2 Frequency distribution of the duration of prospectively assessed cycles in the subsample from Glostrup, Denmark

seems fairly well established, these variants constitute only a very small proportion of clinical cases. Otherwise it could hardly be explained that, in agreement with the incidence of suicides in the general population (see Aschoff 1981b), hospital admissions for depression tend to occur most often in spring; autumn is another season with an increased admission rate for depression, but usually not the predominant one (see Faust and Sarreither 1975; Eastwood and Stiasny 1978, Thompson 1989a). The same trend toward a comparatively high incidence of depressive episodes in spring and not only in fall or winter is revealed by the retrospective assessment of the onset of episodes (Mitchell 1897; Slater 1938; Angst et al. 1969). It has to be mentioned, though, that a British study of the seasonal variation of depression in general practice did in fact show a winter peak for the onset of major depression (Blacker and Clare 1988). This fits in with the description of winter depression as an atypical form of depression rarely deman-ding hospital treatment.

In order to estimate the frequency of regular cycles of all frequencies in affec-tive and schizoaffective disorders in need of inpatient care, we analyzed data on cycle lengths in patients investigated within a multicenter study involving four European centers (Prague, Czechoslovakia; Zurich, Switzerland; Landeck, Ger-many; Glostrup, Denmark) and one Canadian center (Hamilton)[*]. The total sample comprised almost 2000 subjects with altogether approximately 7000 cycles. The majority of patients suffered from severe unipolar depression or bipolar disorder with a preponderence of depression over (hypo)mania. Figure 1 presents, as an example, the frequency distribution of cycle lengths assessed retrospectively at Glostrup. Three peaks are clearly discernible, the highest one at 1 year (annual cycles), the other two at 2 years (biannual cycles) and at 5 years, respectively. The finding regarding the 1- and 2-year peaks is in agreement with the result of the analysis of the total data set from all five centers. It fits well with the as-sumption of a marked influence of seasonality on the course of an affective illness. However, when analyzing only the prospectively assessed cycles from the Danish subsample (Fig.2), the three peaks at 1, 2, and 5 years, respectively, disappear. It can be inferred that the result obtained on the basis of the total data set is due to the bias of reporting in retrospective assessment of the course of illness. It is in concordance with this conclusion that our subsequent analysis of individual cycles in the most thoroughly documented cases from all centers did not reveal a single case exhibiting a periodic course with a repetition of the same duration of cycles over the whole time span covered by the investigation. This does not exclude the possibility of such periodic courses in less severely disturbed cases (see Kinkelin 1954) or in exceptional cases of a rather severe affective disorder. We had the opportunity to observe such a rare case at the Max Planck Institute of Psychiatry.

---

[*] We are indebted to the authors of that study, Drs. Paul Grof (Prague, Landeck, Hamil-ton), Jules Angst (Zurich), and Christian Baastrup (Glostrup) for providing us with the respective data.

The 60-year-old female patient had several first- or second-degree family members who had suffered from depression and/or attempted or committed suicide. The patient's report on her own previous history of SAD was confirmed by her husband. There was little doubt that she had suffered from regular annual cycles of major depression in winter followed by hypomania in spring/summer for the previous 15 years (see Fig.3). The cycles had not responded clearly to

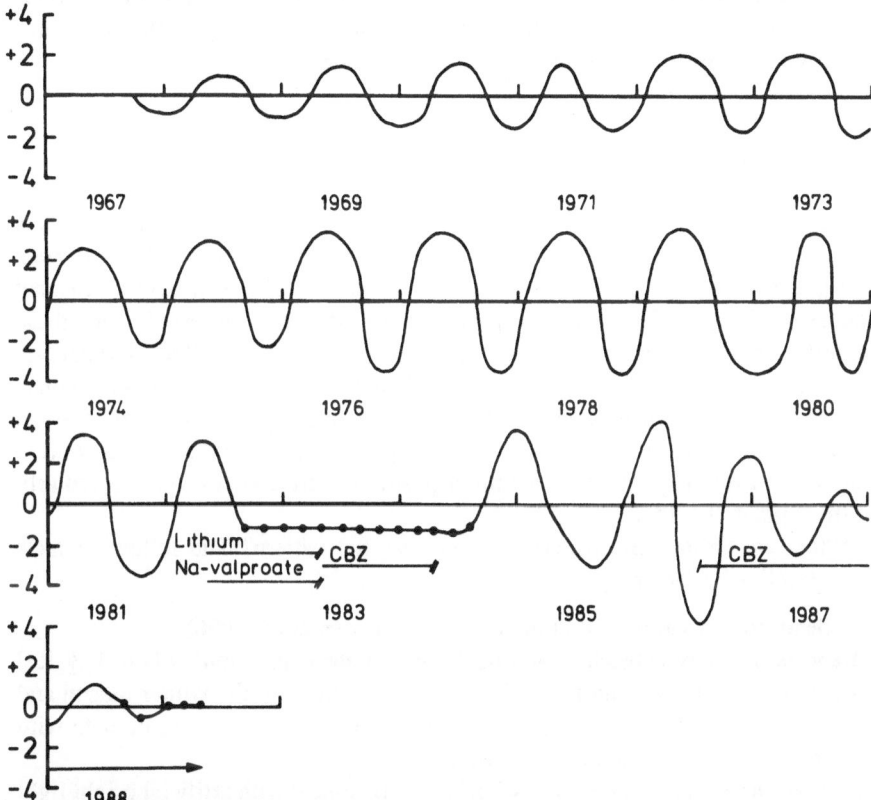

Fig.3 Global rating of the course of a bipolar II disorder with seasonal cycles. Nine-point scale for retrospective assessment until 1982, from that time onwards for prospective assessment: 0, euthymia; +, (hypo)mania; -, Depression; *CBZ*, carbamazepine

antidepressants and tranquilizers. This was also true of the subsequent treatment by one of the authors (H.M.E.). Therefore, only the application of lithium and anticonvulsants (see Emrich et al. 1985) is documented in Fig. 3. It can be seen that the patient received a combination of lithium and sodiumvalproate for almost 1 year. Owing to weight gain, this medication was then replaced by carbamazepine for another year. Under this drug regime the patient was constantly subdepressive. However, after she had stopped taking carbamazepine, the annual cycling reappeared, yet, compared with the preceding years, with a complete phase reversal, i.e., hypomania in the winter season and depression during summertime. After two such cycles, the patient agreed to take carbamazepine again. She then experienced two further cycles of decreasing intensity, with partial recurrence of the original pattern, i.e., hypomania in spring/summer and depression in fall.

A phase shift of episodes has also been observed in other cases of SAD (e.g., Rosenthal et al. 1983, 1984). This indicates that neither depression nor hypomania as such are induced by environmental changes during the seasons of the year; rather, endogenous cycles are triggered or modulated by climatic influences. This point will be considered in the following subsection.

Causal Interpretations

Among the factors causing SAD, heredity seems to play an important role, as is indicated by the high prevalence of affective disorders in the families of index cases; but only a minority of afflicted family members also display a seasonal course of the disorder (see Thompson 1989b). It can be inferred from these findings that SAD is genetically closely linked to nonseasonal affective disorders and does not represent a distinct nosological subtype of affective illness. Rather, the periodicity of course is caused by a kind of trigger mechanism of seasonal influences in some of the individuals — predominantly young women (see Thompson 1989b) — who bear the predisposition to affective illness, particularly of the bipolar II subtype.

Which are the specific triggers for the seasonal pattern? The following facts point to climatic factors:

- Dependence on latitude (Potkin et al. 1986; Rosen et al. 1990)
- Reports of many subjects suffering from "winter depression" when they feel bothered by the cold and particularly by the darkness of the winter season and that their depression may decrease or even disappear in a warmer climate with more sunshine (Rosenthal et al. 1984)
- Responsiveness of "winter depression" to the treatment with artificial bright light (> 2000 lux) for at least 1 - 2 h on several consecutive days (Lewy et al. 1982; Rosenthal et al. 1984; Dietzel et al. 1986; Wirz-Justice et al. 1986; Terman 1988; Lam et al. 1989; Dietzel 1990). Although a placebo effect cannot definitely be ruled out, this procedure seems to be more effective than dim light and more effective in "winter depression" than in nonseasonal forms of depression. A lengthening of the photoperiod or a time shifting of the melatonin rhythm, originally assumed to be of major importance (see Lewy et al. 1988), are apparently not involved in the action mechanism of phototherapy; rather, the total amount of light seems to be the crucial factor (Wehr et al. 1986; Jacobsen et al. 1987; Issacs et al. 1988; Rosenthal et al. 1988; Arendt et al. 1989; Checkley et al. 1989)
- The temporal relationship of the incidence of manic episodes to the amount of sunshine (not to ambient temperature: Carney et al. 1988)

- Reports of subjects suffering from "summer depression" asserting that they cannot bear a high ambient temperature (Wehr and Rosenthal 1989)
- Responsiveness of the aforementioned disorder to therapeutic exposure to cold (Wehr at al. 1987)

Conclusions

Regular annual cycles of affective states are apparently a rather widespread phenomenon. Severe forms of SAD with a periodic course over so many years that a random distribution of cycles becomes extremely improbable are, however, very rare. The question arises whether these rare cases are, indeed, variants of the same general phenomenon of seasonal fluctuations of well-being, the mildest form of which is represented by the so-called subsyndromal SAD. This assumption would imply that severe forms of an affective illness displaying regular annual cycles represent the extreme of environmentally induced periodic disturbances of well-being and are thus etiologically basically different from aperiodic forms of an affective disorder. This is, however, very unlikely because of:

- The symptomatic similarity between periodic and aperiodic forms
- The changes of an aperiodic to a periodic course and vice versa in the same individual
- The family loading with mainly aperiodic forms of an affective disorder

For these reasons, it seems more probable that periodic annual cycles of an affective illness represent a special form of the course of such disorders under the influence of seasonal changes in the environment as implied in the DSM-III-R definition of SAD (see above). It is still unexplained why milder forms of bipolar II disorders are particularly prone to such a modification of their courses. Possibly, bipolar disorder in general tends toward a more regular course than unipolar forms of depression, and bipolar I disorder is so severe that the endogenous cycles are less easily modified by external influences such as light and heat.

Subsyndromal forms of SAD are probably unrelated to the specific etiology of bipolar affective disorders; rather they are entirely induced by seasonal influences on variations in well-being within the normal range, whereas in clinically relevant cases of SAD a morbid predisposition — indicated by the high hereditary load with (usually nonseasonal) affective disorders — becomes activated by these influences. This situation is comparable with that of postpartum psychoses, namely disorders originally regarded as constituting a distinct nosological group of exogenous psychoses; more recent epidemiological, family history, and follow-up investigations, however, point to a hereditary predisposition to an endogenous psychosis of the affective or schizoaffective type, with an increased vulnerability to the puerperal stage as a trigger of a psychotic episode (e.g., Whalley et al. 1982; Davidson and Robertson 1985; Kendell et al. 1987) — at least in the vast majority of cases (Schoepf et al. 1984, 1985). In SAD, a vulnerability to certain seasonal influences seems to exist as an additional risk factor for the manifestation of an episode of an affective disorder. Family studies in subsyndromal SAD cases within the general population should be performed using strictly defined diagnostic criteria in order to clarify the etiological relationship of annual cycles in well-being to the morbid forms of affective disturbances (major depression and bipolar disorders).

Bidian Cycles

Description

Regular bidian (48-h) cycles have not yet been observed in nature except for rare occasions, e.g., malaria or experimental isolation from external time cues in humans. Even in such isolation experiments, a 48-h rhythm does not occur regularly, and it is restricted to the sleep-wake cycle and its masking effects on other rhythms which remain near 24-h (usually around 25-h); i.e., a circabidian component is superimposed upon a circadian rhythm, for example that of core body temperature (see Wever 1979). It is therefore remarkable that clear bidian rhythms have repeatedly been observed in mental disorders, particularly depressions of the unipolar and bipolar II variants. Usually one "bad day" of depressed mood is followed by a "good day" of euthymia or by a day of hyperactivity and elated mood, despite an ongoing 24-h sleep-wake cycle.

More than 70 such cases have been described in the psychiatric literature since the eighteenth century (von Zerssen et al. 1983). "Reimann observed a melancholy appearing every other day in a 60-year-old man who became despaired of God's mercy and intended to commit suicide but, at the same time, was timid like a child. During the intervals, he was considerate and cried about his weakness, and Teichmann thought of an adolescent who became anxious and sad in the morning every other day" (translated from Medicus, 1764 p.42f). Since the last century (Ziegler 1864; Schaefer 1896), several physiological and biochemical concomitants of these abnormal cycles in mood and behavior have been recorded, e.g., regarding urinary excretion of water and electrolytes and of body temperature. During the past few decades, hypercortisolism was among the bodily variables found to coincide with days of depression; it was absent the next day when the patient was manic or euthymic (Bunney et al. 1965; Doerr et al. 1979). The 48-h mood cycles may commence as such in hitherto healthy subjects (often after child birth, head injury, or a hemorrhage) or as a secondary phenomenon in a preexisting affective disorder of a primarily irregular course. In any case, they are rather enduring and may persist with little variation over years and even decades. As far as familiy history data are available, a slightly increased morbidity rate of affective disorders in relatives becomes apparent, but a similar periodic course in secondary cases seems to be the exception rather than the rule. More often there is a hint of brain damage in the patients themselves (see von Zerssen et al. 1979). However, an organic basis for the abnormal cycling cannot be demonstrated in many other cases.

One typical feature of 48-h cycles is that the switch into depression and, usually, also the shift from depression into (hypo)mania or euthymia occurs during night sleep (see Sitaram et al. 1978; notable exception: Paschalis et al. 1980). Three such patients were studied for 8-14 days in an environment devoid of time cues, one of them together with his attending psychiatrist (Jenner et al. 1968). In this case the time routine was condensed to a 22-h period — a change not noticed by either the patient or his attendant. Both their sleep-wake cycles adapted to this routine, whereas the biological rhythms exhibited a 22-h and a 24-h component in both of them and additional 44-h and 48-h components in the patient. The time course of his psychopathology clearly followed the sleep-wake cycle, with a change from one state to the other (i.e., from depression to hypomania and vice versa) still occurring during the major sleep episodes every 22 h.

In another case observed in the freerun of rhythms during a 2-week period (Dirlich et al. 1981), internal desynchronization (see Wever 1979) occurred due to a fragmentation of the sleep-wake cycle, which resulted in a reduction of the average cycle length to approximately 19 h in the presence of a near 24-h rhythm of biological functions. The changes from a euthymic to a depressed state still took place only during sleep, whereas a normalization of mood gradually developed during the subsequent wake time. This was similar to the situation under a 24-h routine on a psychiatric ward or the patient's time routine at home (von Zerssen et al. 1983). In spite of the obvious coupling of the patient's psychopathology to the sleep-wake cycle, he still exhibited, on average, a 48-h period of changes in affectivity, thus compensating for the irregularity and shortness of his free-running sleep-wake cycle. This points to an involvement of the circadian system in addition to the states of sleep and wake in inducing the cycles of psychopathology. The dependency of the 48-h cycles on signals from the circadian system is also documented by the fact that, during a night of total sleep deprivation on the ward after a "good day," a rather sudden change from euthymia to depression occurred in the early morning hours around 5 A.M. (von Zerssen et al. 1983). Thus, the sleep state as such was only a promoting but unnecessary condition for the switch to depression.

The third case (Welsh et al. 1986) concerns a very mild bipolar II disorder with 48-h cycles which had emerged more than 2 years previously. During 8 days in a time-cue free environment, the rest-activity cycle became rather irregular; the first four cycles were, on average, longer than previously; the next four cycles, however, were clearly shorter. Unfortunately, this finding is difficult to interpret because lithium was administered from the fourth cycle onwards. It is therefore not clear whether — in contrast to the finding in plants and animals (e.g. Engelmann 1973; Kripke and Wyborney 1980; Welsh and Moore-Ede 1990) — lithium had lengthened the period of the "internal clock" for circadian rhythmicity or whether the changes in cycle length were the expression of a random distribution during freerun (see Dirlich 1984; Wehr et al. 1985; von Zerssen et al. 1989), which was not markedly influenced by lithium.

In all three cases described above, occasional phase jumps of the cycles of psychopathology were recorded; sometimes, but not always, they occurred when the time schedule had been changed. Drug treatment proved more (lithium) or less effective (antidepressants, carbamazepine) in these (Hanna et al. 1972; von Zerssen et al. 1983; Welsh et al. 1986) and other cases (Delay et al. 1961; Gelenberg and Klerman 1978; King et al. 1979; Dinner 1980; Paschalis et al. 1980; Berger et al. 1990). The range of bidian oscillation of mood and activity was usually only attenuated by antidepressants and by carbamazepine; however, the cycling disappeared in most patients who were treated with lithium. In one of the two patients described above in more detail, antidepressants caused a marked irregularity of cycles with a concomitant reduction of "bad days" compared with "good days." The course then resembled the one observed before the onset of the 48-h rhythm more than 13 years ago (von Zerssen et al. 1983). This points to a close relationship of bidian cycles to irregular cycles of short duration.

Causal Interpretations

Obviously, bidian cycles represent an extremely short and precise form of "rapid cycling" (Dunner and Fieve 1974) in affective illness, at least at a phenomenological level. Three hypotheses (see "Introduction") which could explain this kind of rapid cycling have been formulated. They have been discussed extensively in earlier publications (von Zerssen et al. 1979, 1983) and will therefore not be described in detail here. They are:

- "Shock-phase" hypothesis (Richter 1960)
- Desynchronization hypothesis (Halberg 1968)
- Entrainment model (Dirlich et al. 1981)

The possibility that a localized lesion (e.g., by trauma) may induce an abnormal pacemaker in certain, e.g., hypothalamic (see Beringer 1942), brain regions or change the properties of the circadian clock also has to be taken into account. Such a hypothesis may be applicable, not only to bidian cycles (see Arndt 1930; Frank and Harrer 1980), but also to cycles of longer duration (see Aiginger and Neumayer 1949). We will, however, not elaborate this issue here because we are not aware of any publications dealing with it specifically. Thus, in the following, only the three aforementioned hypotheses will be referred to.

Richter's hypothesis could explain the sudden occurrence of 48-h cycles after a stressful event (head injury, hemorrhage etc.). It is, however, not in accord with the adaptability of cycles to experimental changes in the time routine as in Jenner's case (Jenner et al. 1968).

Halberg's hypothesis would predict a marked change in the period of the abnormal rhythm of affectivity to occur in a 22-h routine, as in Jenner's case (namely from 48 h to 88 h), forthe ups and downs of mood and activity are conceived of as a "beat phenomenon" resulting from an interaction between a (hypothetical) free-running rhythm and the rhythm of those biological functions that remain entrained to the (usually 24 h) routine of daily life (see also Kripke et al. 1978). It is apparently not in line with the data.

The entrainment model, however, is consonant with the findings under all three time schedules: 24-h routine (in all cases reported in the literature), 22-h routine (Jenner et al. 1968), and freerun (Dirlich et. al 1981; Welsh et al. 1986). The basic assumption of the model is an intrinsic cycling of psychopathology that varies within the range of 1 - 2 days and becomes coupled to the circadian system by a gating mechanism. This mechanism would allow switches from one state to the other, i.e., from depression to euthymia or (hypo)mania, only during restricted time intervals of circadian rhythms. Computer simulations based on the entrainment model are characterized by a rather regular 48-h rhythm with occasional phase jumps similar to those in fact observed in the most thoroughly studied cases of bidian cycles in affective psychopathology (see above).

The irregular cycles which preceded the 48-h rhythms in several cases indicate that the nature of the cycling process is, in accord with the model, basically of a stochastic nature and becomes regular only by a coupling to the circadian rhythmicity if the frequency of cycling has increased to nearly one cycle/day. According to this interpretation, the 48-h variant of periodic psychoses is a borderline phenomenon in a random distribution of cycle lengths in affective illness; this phenomenon tends to occur at the end of the distribution with extremely short cycles, described by Angst et al. (1990) as "recurrent brief depression." It can be assumed that cycles of a year or so (see chapter on annual cycles) but also short cycles with comparatively little variation mainly occur in bipolar II disorders. Otherwise, the relatively high prevalence of the bipolar II type among the 48-h cyclers could hardly be explained.

Conclusions

Whereas relatively short and relatively regular cycles of an affective disorder may become coupled to the endogenous rhythm of the circadian system, resulting in 48-h cycles of psychopathology, much longer cycles in the order of 1 year (counted from the onset of one episode to that of the next one) may be prone to influences of seasonal rhythms in the environment. In both instances, the strict periodicity would not underly the psychopathological process but rather be imposed on its fluctuations if these happen to approach the cycle length of a profound internal (circadian) or external (annual) rhythm. Thus, the most striking examples of periodic psychoses can well be explained as variants of a usually aperiodic illness, as originally suggested by Kraepelin (1899).

Diurnal Variation

Description

Diurnal variations constitute a universal phenomenon in nature. They are inherent in all organisms in the form of an intrinsic circadian (i.e., circa 24-h) rhythm independent of external time cues (see Aschoff 1981a). Proof of this fact has also been procured in humans under conditions devoid of external time cues (Wever 1979). Findings of animal experiments have shown that such endogenous circadian rhythms are generated in that vital processes are modulated by a kind of "internal clock." It is assumed that, in mammals, this "clock" or so-called pacemaker is located in the suprachiasmatic nuclei of the anterior hypothalamus (see Moore-Ede 1982; Schwartz and Reppert 1985; Moore-Ede 1986; Earnest and Sladek 1986). Yet, not all 24-h rhythms in living creatures — including man — can be related primarily to an "internal clock" for circadian rhythmicity; in part, they depend more on other overt rhythms in the organism itself (internal masking) or on environmental rhythms (external masking), e.g., by rhythmic changes in ambient temperature. Examples of internal masking are influences of sleep and wakefulness on bodily functions.

Pathological processes may also depend on the time of day, e.g., bronchial obstructions in asthmatics reach a peak in the second half of the night (see Reinberg and Smolensky 1983). In the field of mental disorders, several investigations have been concerned with diurnal variation (DV) of the intensity of symptomatology in melancholic patients. Krafft-Ebing (1874) was probably the first to mention this phenomenon in the psychiatric literature. Typically, such cases are characterized by a maximum intensity of depression in the early morning hours, with a gradual improvement taking place during the course of the day. Conversely, there is the less common form of DV referred to as the "inverse type" which is characterized by an increasing intensity of depression during the daytime. Furthermore, one can observe switches from one type to the other and from rhythmic to arrhythmic courses, and vice versa, within a depressive episode; moreover, there may be changes from one episode to the next. DV of the intensity of symptoms in affective illness obviously bears no relationship to the normal daily fluctuations of mood and activity in healthy individuals, as in the case of the so-called morning type or evening type. Even the morning type, who normally displays a maximum of activity during morning hours, will, during a depressive episode, most often exhibit the typical form of DV with a morning low of mood. When the depressive episode has subsided, most patients will return to their habitual rhythm or a lack of rhythmicity as before the onset of the episode (Middelhoff 1967).

In earlier studies, the frequency of DV in depression was estimated as being very high (up to 80% of the bipolar cases: Waldmann 1972) and considered a specific feature of endogenous forms of the disorder. More recent studies based on continuous observations point out, however, that DV occurs in only about 50% (see Mellerup and Rafaelsen 1979) of melancholics, or even less frequently (Tölle and Goetze 1987), and in these cases on only 40% of the days observed (Stallone et al. 1973; Reinink et al. 1990a). Hence, in the majority of cases DV does not constitute a strictly periodical phenomenon; nor is it specific for melancholia (von Knorring et al. 1977; Fähndrich and Haug 1988), although it seems to be most prevalent in severe forms of depression (von Knorring et al. 1977). However, it often disappears when the intensity of depression is reaching its maximum and then reappears with clinical improvement (Waldmann 1972). Accordingly, cross-sectional investigations have not revealed a correlation between the severity of depression and the degree of DV (Carpenter et al. 1986; Haug and Fähndrich 1990). It should be mentioned in this context that, in contrast to the findings in depression, anxiety disorders were found to show a maximum of symptom severity most often in the afternoon and/or evening, and not in the morning (Cameron et al. 1986).

Causal Interpretations

Basically, two essentially different mechanisms are used to explain DV in depression, with one not necessarily excluding the other.

On the one hand, masking effects caused by the influence of the sleep-wake rhythm on the mood state seem to play a role. Considering that, in patients with a 48-h cycle, switches into depression were found to occur almost always during night sleep and, in the case examined by the authors, the condition improved only gradually during the waking hours of the next day, it seems feasible that sleep may promote and being awake suppress depressive symptoms. This interpretation is supported by the observation that in our patient the switch to depression also occurred during sleep under free-running conditions, when his sleep-wake cycle had to a large extent been uncoupled from the rhythms of other vital functions (Doerr et al 1979; Dirlich et al. 1981) — that is, when the patient was in a state of internal desynchronization (see Wever 1979).

The assumption of a depressiogenic effect of sleep is also in line with the short-term therapeutic effect of total sleep deprivation (TSD) during 1 night in more than 50% of the cases of severe depression and the deterioration of the pathological condition in the majority of TSD responders during the "recovery" night (see Gillin et al. 1984; Kuhs and Tölle 1986). Moreover, this view, according to which the influence of sleep and wake on depression is relatively independent of the time of day, is supported by the fact that a short daytime nap (but not too short, i.e., not less than ¼ - ½ h: Gillin et al. 1988) following sleep deprivation often leads to a worsening of TSD responders' mental state (Wiegand et al. 1987a,b). Furthermore, a single case study, in which sleep and wake times were distributed irregularly, revealed that the therapeutic effect of manipulating the sleep-wake cycle was dependent only on the length of waking time, and not the time of day (Knowles et al. 1979).

Worthy of note in this context is the fact that the therapeutic effect of TSD is observed mainly in patients exhibiting typical DV, whereas it is usually missing for the "inverse type" of DV, characterized by a worsening of mood during the course of the day. In these cases, even an augmentation of depression has been observed on the day following TSD (Reinink et al. 1990b).

On the other hand, the effects of sleep deprivation do not seem to be totally independent of the time of day; for partial sleep deprivation in the second half of the night is reported to be nearly as effective as TSD (Schilgen and Tölle 1980), whereas partial sleep deprivation in the first half has proven to be largely ineffective (Goetze and Tölle 1981; see also Sack et al. 1988). Conversely, a nap in the morning or the middle of the day quite regularly leads to a reversal of the therapeutic effect of TSD during the course of the day, while an afternoon nap at around 3 P.M. does not (Wiegand et al. 1989). In this case, the lack of a depressiogenic effect of napping in TSD responders may be due to the length of the total previous wake period (= 1 day + 1 night + 3/4 day). However, this observation is also consonant with the assumption of an additional circadian factor causing varying intensities of depression at different times of day. The existence of such an influence on the course of depression is also indicated by the fact that, in our patient with a 48-h cycle, the switch to depression occurred at about 5 A.M. during TSD in the night following a "good" day (see above). This is the time of day when partial sleep deprivation generally seems to be more effective than in the first half of the night; moreover, the "switchover" point is close to the time of day when a nap tends to reverse the therapeutic effect of TSD (i.e. morning or noon) and farther away from the time when a nap usually no longer leads to such a reversal (see above).

The early morning hours during which many depressives suffer from substantial sleep disturbances — even beyond the end of the depressive episode (see von Zerssen 1987) — seem to be a particularly critical time of day for the emergence or deterioration of depression. This is the time when cortisol secretion reaches its maximum. For this reason, it had already been hypothesized in the 1960s that DV in depression could be linked with the cortisol rhythm (McClure 1966). We were in fact able to verify such an association in a chronobiological study of drug-free depressives (von Zerssen et al. 1985, 1987). Nine out of 16 cases with a definite clinical and RDC (Spitzer et al. 1978) diagnosis of endogenous depression (melancholia) exhibited significant DV. The time of day when their depressed mood reached a maximum correlated significantly with the time when the maximum of their circadian cortisol rhythm occurred. It is as yet undecided whether a direct — unilateral or mutual — influence of the cortisol rhythm and DV of depression is the case here or whether both the hormonal and the mood rhythms depend on a third factor, such as the activity rhythms of certain neurotransmitters in the brain under the control of the "circadian clock." The respective brain regions, i.e., the hypothalamus (see Carlsson et al. 1980) and parts of the limbic system (see Krieger and Krieger 1966), may be responsible for the rhythms in hormone secretion as well as in the depressive state. The complex interrelations between neurotransmitter actions, hormonal secretion, and mood pathology have to be clarified in subsequent studies, which should also shed light on the emergence of an "inverse" type of DV in depression and of changes from one type to the other.

In any case, it is not necessary to postulate a dysfunction of the "inner clock(s)" as a basis for the occurrence of periodic variation in the intensity of mood pathology during a depressive episode; it is sufficient to assume (von Zerssen et al. 1987) that the intensity of depression is modulated in a way similar to the circadian rhythm of physiological functions, such as the secretion of corticotropin-releasing hormone (CRF) - adrenocortiotropic hormone (ACTH) corticosteroids (see Sadow 1979; Keller-Wood and Dallman 1984).

Conclusions

Diurnal variation in depression is no doubt the most frequent periodic phenomenon in affective illness; it is, however, less frequent and nosologically less specific than formerly assumed. A strictly periodic course in the sense of regular variation of the severity of depression over a longer period is obviously less frequent than irregular changes of intensity. They include phase shifts (from "typical" DV with a morning low to the "inverse" type with a deterioration during the day and vice versa) and the occasional lack of any rhythmicity.

The most appropriate interpretation of DV in depression is that of a circadian modulation of the course of the disorder. Probably, there is little or no connection to the "normal" variation of mood and activity in healthy subjects or patients during their symptom-free intervals. On the one hand, the modulation may be caused by the sleep-wake rhythm in the form of a depressiogenic effect of sleep and an antidepressive effect of being awake, which can be used therapeutically. On the other hand, signals from the circadian system which are responsible for the emergence of the cortisol rhythm are likely to be involved in the modulation of the depressed state.

Concluding Remarks

The fact that periodic phenomena are apparently rare in affective illness, but nonetheless more frequent than in other mental disorders, may be a hint to the pathogenesis of this kind of disorder: the pathological processes responsible for the generation of symptoms may well take place in those parts of the brain which are also relevant for the generation of other types of periodic processes (see Ewald 1924; Beringer 1942; Krieger and Krieger 1966 and others). The emergence of an annual cycling of affective illness in the form of SAD might well be caused by processes similar to those responsible for seasonal variation in the mental states of healthy persons, the so-called subsyndromal SAD. Forty-eight-hour rhythms, however, seem to be created by the coupling of pathological processes to signals from the circadian system. In this case, sleep apparently has an additional gating function.

In SAD, as well as in a 48-h rhythm of an affective disorder, a basically aperiodic course of the disorder becomes coupled to a periodic exogenous or endogenous rhythm. In the authors' opinion, this coupling may be established when the spontaneous cycles of the disorder happen to reach a range similar to that of the endogenous or exogenous rhythms, respectively. Due to the distribution of frequencies in the duration of cycles in affective illness, this is more often the case in the range of annual rhythms than in the range of days. Bipolar II forms of an affective disorder seem to tend toward a course fulfilling these requirements. The autonomous dynamics of bipolar I disorders may be too severe to facilitate a coupling of the course of the illness to an exogenous or endogenous rhythm. Unipolar depression might, in general, tend to a less regular course than bipolar disorders, with the result that, in relation to the total frequency of all subtypes, unipolar depression less frequently displays a periodic course than the other subtypes.

Shorter spontaneous cycles of the illness than those evoking a bidian rhythm seem to be so rare that diurnal cycles in a strict sense, as in a case described by Waldmann (1969), are extreme exceptions among periodic phenomena in affective disorders. During such a cycle, depression not only ameliorates or switches to (hypo)mania in the course of the day, but even totally disappears and returns the next day, and so forth. DV in depression is basically different from such dian as well as from bidian and annual cycles of an affective illness since they are not complete cycles of the disorder, but rather changes of the intensity of symptomatology within a depressive episode. The fact that these changes occur mainly in depression and not in mania or hypomania might be due to the stronger influence of sleeping and waking on the intensity of depression than on a state of elation.

The above interpretation of periodic phenomena in affective illness is in basic agreement with Kraepelin's (1899) view outlined above in "Annual Cycles, Description". Research in the mechanism underlying the modulations of the course of an affective illness by rhythmic changes in the organism or the environment may prove quite fruitful for elucidating the pathogenesis of this kind of mental disorder.

References

Aiginger J, Neumayer E (1949) Ueber periodische, paroxysmale, pseudoneurasthenische Zustandsbilder bei Postencephalitikern. Wien Klin Wochenschr 61:314-318

American Psychiatric Association (1980) Diagnostic and statistical manual of mental disorders, 3rd edn (DSM-III). American Psychiatric Association, Washington

American Psychiatric Association (1987) Diagnostic and statistical manual of mental disorders, 3rd edn, revised (DSM-III-R). American Psychiatric Association, Washington

Angst J, Grof P, Hippius H, Pöldinger W, Varga E, Weis P, Wyss F (1969) Verlaufs-gesetzlichkeiten depressiver Syndrome. In: Hippius H, Selbach H (eds) Das depressive Syndrom. Schwarzenberg, Munich, pp 93-100

Angst J, Merikangas K, Scheidegger P, Wicki W (1990) Recurrent brief depression: a new subtype of affective disorder. J Affective Disord 19:87-98

Arendt J, Broadway S, Folkard S, Marks M (1989) The effects of light on mood and melatonin in normal subjects. In: Thompson C, Silverstone T (eds) Seasonal affective disorder. CNS, London, pp 133-143

Arndt M (1930) Über täglichen (24stündigen) Wechsel psychischer Krankheitszustände. Allg Z Psychiatrie 92:128-150

Aschoff J (1981a) Biological rhythms. Handbook of behavioral neurobiology, vol 4. Plenum, New York

Aschoff J (1981b) Annual rhythms in man. In: Aschoff J (ed) Handbook of behavioral neurobiology, vol 4. Plenum, New York, pp 475-487

Baumgarten Crusius AM (1836) Periodologie, oder die Lehre von den periodischen Veränderungen im Leben des gesunden und kranken Menschen. Schwetschke, Halle

Berger M, Fleckenstein P, Riemann D, Müller WE (1990) Experimental approaches for testing the cholinergic/noradrenergic imbalance hypothesis of affective disorders. In: Bunney WE, Hippius H, Laakmann G, Schmauss M (eds) Neuropsychopharmacology. Springer, Berlin Heidelberg New York, pp 208-220

Beringer K (1942) Rhythmischer Wechsel von Enthemmtheit und Gehemmtheit als diencephale Antriebsstörung. Nervenarzt 15:225-239

Blacker CVR, Clare AW (1988) The prevalence and treatment of depression in general practice. Psychopharmacology 95[Suppl]:S14-S17

Boyce P, Parker G (1988) Seasonal affective disorder in the southern hemisphere. Am J Psychiatry 145:96-99

Bunney WE Jr, Hartmann EL, Mason JW (1965) Study of a patient with 48-hour manic-depressive cycles. Part II. Arch Gen Psychiatry 12:619-625

Cameron OG, Lee MA, Kotun J, McPhee KM (1986) Circadian symptom fluctuations in people with anxiety disorders. J Affective Disord 11:213-218

Carlsson A, Svennerholm L, Winblad B (1980) Seasonal and circadian monoamine variations in human brains examined post mortem. Acta Psychiatr Scand 61[Suppl 280]:75-83

Carney PA, FitzGerald CT, Monaghan CE (1988) Influence of climate on the prevalence of mania. Br J Psychiatry 152:820- 823

Carpenter LL, Kupfer DJ, Frank E (1986) Is diurnal variation a meaningful symptom in unipolar depression? J Affective Disord 11:255-264

Checkley SA, Franey C, Winton F, Corn T, Arendt J (1989) A neuroendocrine study of the mechanism of action of phototherapy in seasonal affective disorder. In: Thompson C, Silverstone T (eds) Seasonal affective disorder. CNS, London, pp 223-231

Davidson J, Robertson E (1985) A follow-up study of post partum illness, 1946-1978. Acta Psychiatr Scand 71:451-457

Delay J, Pichot P, Deniker P, Jousselin D (1961) Psychose cyclique avec inversions quotidiennes de l'humeur. Ann Med Psychol (Paris) 119/2:125-129

Dietzel M (1990) Die Lichttherapie der endogenen Depression. Springer, Berlin, Heidelberg, New York

Dietzel M, Saletu B, Lesch OM, Sieghart W, Schjerve M (1986) Light treatment in depressive illness. Polysomnographic, psychometric and neuroendocrinological findings. Eur Neurol 25[Suppl 2]:93-103

Dinner PE (1980) Ein Fall von bipolarer Affektpsychose mit 48-Stunden-Rhythmus. Medical dissertation, University of Zurich

Dirlich G (1984) Looking at human circadian phenomena from a framework of simple stochastic models. In: Moore-Ede MC, Czeisler CA (eds) Mathematical models of the circadian sleep-wake cycle. Raven, New York, pp 159-185

Dirlich G, Kammerloher A, Schulz H, Lund R, Doerr P, von Zerssen D (1981) Temporal coordination of rest-activity cycle, body temperature, urinary free cortisol, and mood in a patient with 48-hour unipolar-depressive cycles in clinical and time-cue-free environments. Biol Psychiatry 16:163-179

Doerr P, von Zerssen D, Fischler M, Schulz H (1979) Relationship between mood changes and adrenal cortical activity in a patient with 48-hour unipolar-depressive cycles. J Affective Disord 1:93-104

Dunner DL, Fieve RR (1974) Clinical factors in lithium carbonate prophylaxis failure. Arch Gen Psychiatry 30:229-233

Dunner DL, Gershon ES, Goodwin FK (1970) Heritable factors in the severity of affective illness. Sci Proc Am Psychiatric Assoc 123:187-188

Earnest DJ, Sladek CD (1986) Circadian rhythms of vasopressin release from individual rat suprachiasmatic explants in vitro. Brain Res 382:129-133

Eastwood MR, Peter AM (1989) Prospective studies: infradian mood rhythms and seasonal affective disorder. In: Thompson C, Silverstone T (eds) Seasonal affective disorder. CNS, London, pp 29-36

Eastwood MR, Stiasny S (1978) Psychiatric disorder, hospital admission, and season. Arch Gen Psychiatry 35:769-771

Emrich HM, Lund R, von Zerssen D (1979) Vegetative Funktionen und körperliche Aktivität in der endogenen Depression. Verlaufsuntersuchungen von Speichelsekretion, Temperatur und Motorik bei einem Patienten mit 48-Stunden-Zyklus. Arch Psychiatr Nervenkr 227:227-240

Emrich HM, Dose M, von Zerssen D (1985) The use of sodium valproate, carbamazepine and oxcarbazepine in patients with affective disorders. J Affective Disord 8:243-250

Engelmann W (1973) A slowing down of circadian rhythms by lithium ions. Z Naturforsch 28:733-736

Ewald G (1924) Temperament und Charakter. Springer, Berlin

Fähndrich E, Haug H-J (1988) Diurnal variations of mood in psychiatric patients of different nosological groups. Neuropsychobiology 20:141-144

Faust V, Sarreither P (1975) Jahreszeit und psychische Krankheit. Med Klin 70:467-473

Frank C, Harrer G (1980) Zyklothymie mit persistierender 48-Stunden-Periodik. Chrono-pathologische Aspekte. Wien Med Wochenschr 130:45-48

Gelenberg AJ, Klerman GL (1978) The effects of amitriptyline and lithium on a patient with 48-hour recurrent depressions. J Nerv Ment Dis 166:365-368

Georgi F (1947) Psychophysische Korrelationen: III. Psychiatrische Probleme im Lichte der Rhythmusforschung. Schweiz Med Wochenschr 49:1276-1280

Gillin JC, Sitaram N, Wehr T, Duncan W, Post R, Murphy DL, Mendelson WB, Wyatt RJ, Bunney WE (1984) Sleep and affective illness. In: Post RM, Ballenger JC (eds) Neurobiology of mood disorders. Williams & Wilkens, Baltimore, pp 157-189

Gillin JC, Kripke DF, Janowsky DS, Risch SC (1988) Effects of brief naps on mood and sleep in sleep-deprived depressed patients. Psychiatry Res 27:253-265

Gjessing LR (1974) A review of periodic catatonia. Biol Psychiatry 8:23-45

Gjessing R, Gjessing L (1961) Some main trends in the clinical aspects of periodic catatonia. Acta Psychiatr Scand 37:1-13

Goetze U, Tölle R (1981) Antidepressive Wirkung des partiellen Schlafentzugs während der 1. Hälfte der Nacht. Psychiatr Clin 14:129-149

Gwinner E (1986) Circannual rhythms. Springer, Berlin, Heidelberg, New York

Halaris A (1987) Chronobiology and psychiatric disorders. Elsevier, New York

Halberg F (1968) Physiologic considerations underlying rhythmometry, with special reference to emotional illness. In: de Ajuriaguerra J (ed) Cycles biologique et psychiatrie. Masson, Paris, pp 73-126

Hanna SM, Jenner FA, Pearson IB, Sampson GA, Thompson EA (1972) The therapeutic effect of lithium carbonate on a patient with a forty-eight hour periodic psychosis. Br J Psychiatry 121:271-280

Hatotani N, Nomura J (1983) Neurobiology of periodic psychoses. Igaku-Shoin, Tokyo

Haug H-J, Fähndrich E (1990) Diurnal variations of mood in depressed patients in relation to severity of depression. J Affective Disord 19:37-41

Healy D, Waterhouse JM (1990) The circadian system and affective disorders: clocks or rhythms? Chronobiol Int 7:5-10

Hekkens WThJM, Kerkhof GA, Rietveld WJ (1988) Trends in chronobiology. Pergamon, Oxford

Hitzig E (1898) Über die nosologische Auffassung und über die Therapie der periodischen Geistesstörungen. Berl Klin Wochenschr 35:1-4, 34-39, 53-56

Isaacs G, Stainer DS, Sensky TE, Moor S, Thompson C (1988) Phototherapy and its mechanisms of action in seasonal affective disorder. J Affective Disord 14:13-19

Jacobsen FM, Wehr TA, Skwerer RA, Sack DA, Rosenthal NE (1987) Morning versus midday phototherapy of seasonal affective disorder. Am J Psychiatry 144:1301-1305

Jenner FA, Goodwin JC, Sheridan M, Tauber IJ, Lobban MC (1968) The effect of an altered time regime on biological rhythms in a 48-hour periodic psychosis. Br J Psychiatry 114:215-224

Kasper S, Rogers SLB, Yancey A, Schulz PM, Skwerer RG, Rosenthal NE (1989a) Phototherapy in individuals with and without subsyndromal seasonal affective disorder. Arch Gen Psychiatry 46:837-844

Kasper S, Wehr TA, Bartko JJ, Gaist PA, Rosenthal NE (1989b) Epidemiological findings of seasonal changes in mood and behavior. Ach Gen Psychiatry 46:823-833

Keller-Wood M, Dallman MF (1984) Corticosteroid inhibition of ACTH secretion. Endocr Rev 5:1-24

Kendell RE, Chalmers JC, Platz C (1987) Epidemiology of puerperal psychoses. Br J Psychiatry 150:662-673

King DJ, Salem SAM, Meimary NS (1979) A 48-hour periodic manic-depressive illness presenting in late life. Br J Psychiatry 135:190-191

Kinkelin M (1954) Verlauf und Prognose des Manisch-depressiven Irreseins. Schweiz Arch Neurol Psychiatr 73:100-146

Kirn L (1878) Die periodischen Psychosen. Enke, Stuttgart

Knorring von L, Perris C, Strandman E (1977) Diurnal variations in intensity of symptoms in patients of different diagnostic groups. Arch Psychiatr Nervenkr 224:295-312

Knowles JB, Southmayd SE, Delva N, MacLean AW, Cairns J, Letemendia FJ (1979) Five variations of sleep deprivation in a depressed woman. Br J Psychiatry 135:403-410

Kraepelin E (1883) Compendium der Psychiatrie. Abel, Leipzig

Kraepelin E (1899) Psychiatrie, 6th edn. Barth, Leipzig

Krafft-Ebing R von (1874) Die Melancholie. Eine klinische Studie. Enke, Erlangen

Krieger DT, Krieger HP (1966) Circadian variation of the plasma 17-hydroxycorticosteroids in central nervous system disease. J Clin Endocrinol 26:929-940

Kripke DF, Wyborney VG (1980) Lithium slows rat circadian activity rhythms. Life Sci 26:1319-1321

Kripke DF, Mullaney DJ, Atkinson M, Wolf S (1978) Circadian rhythm disorders in manic-depressives. Biol Psychiatry 13:335-351

Kuhs H, Tölle R (1986) Schlafentzug (Wachtherapie) als Antidepressivum. Fortschr Neurol Psychiatr 54:341-355

Lacoste V, Wirz-Justice A (1989) Seasonal variation in normal subjects: an update of variables current in depression research. In: Rosenthal NE, Blehar MC (eds) Seasonal affective disorders and phototherapy. Guilford, New York, pp 167-229

Lam RW, Kripke DF, Gillin JC (1989) Phototherapy for depressive disorders: a review. Can J Psychiatry 34:140-146

Lewy AJ, Kern HE, Rosenthal NE, Wehr TA (1982) Bright artificial light treatment of a manic-depressive patient with a seasonal mood cycle. Am J Psychiatry 139:1496-1498

Lewy AJ, Sack RL, Singer CM, White DM, Hoban TM (1988) Winter depression and the phase-shift hypothesis for bright light's therapeutic effects: history, theory, and experimental evidence. J Biol Rhythms 3:121-134

Liebowitz MR, Quitkin FM, Stewart JW, McGrath PJ, Harrison W, Rabkin J, Tricamo E, Markowitz JS, Klein DF (1984) Phenelzine versus imipramine in atypical depression. A preliminary report. Arch Gen Psychiatry 41:669-677

McClure DJ (1966) The effects of antidepressant medication on the diurnal plasma cortisol levels in depressed patients. J Psychosom Res 10:197-202

Medicus FC (1764) Geschichte periodischer Krankheiten. Macklot, Karlsruhe

Mellerup ET, Rafaelsen OJ (1979) Circadian rhythms in manic melancholic disorders. In: Essmann WB, Valzelli L (eds) Current developments in psychopharmacology, vol 5. Spectrum, New York, pp 51-66

Menninger-Lerchenthal E (1960), Periodizität in der Psychopathologie. Maudrich, Wien

Middelhoff HD (1967) Tagesrhythmische Schwankungen bei endogen Depressiven im symptomfreien Intervall und während der Phase. Arch Psychiatr Nervenkr 209:315-339

Mitchell SW (1897) An analysis of 3000 cases of melancholia. Trans Assoc Am Physicians 12:480-487

Moore-Ede MC (1982) The clocks that time us. Harvard University Press, Cambridge

Moore-Ede MC (1986) Physiology of the circadian timing system: predictive versus reactive homeostasis. Am J Physiol 250:R735-R752

Mrosovsky (1989) Seasonal affective disorder, hibernation, and annual cycles in animals: chipmunks in the sky. In: Rosenthal NE, Blehar MC (eds) Seasonal affective disorders and phototherapy. Guilford, New York London, pp 127-148

Müller A (1900) Periodische Katatonien. Med dissertation, University of Zürich

Paschalis C, Pavlou A, Papadimitriou A (1980) A stepped forty-eight hour manic-depressive cycle. Br J Psychiatry 137:332- 336

Pflug B (1987) Rhythmusfragen bei affektiven Psychosen. In: Kisker KP, Lauter H, Meyer J-E, Müller C, Strömgren E, (eds) Psychiatrie der Gegenwart, vol 5: Affektive Psychosen, 3rd edn. Springer, Berlin, Heidelberg, New York, pp 241-270

Pilcz A (1901) Die periodischen Geistesstörungen. Fischer, Jena

Potkin SG, Zetin M, Stamenkovic V, Kripke D, Bunney WE Jr (1986) Seasonal affective disorder: prevalence varies with latitude and climate. Clin Neuropharmacol 9[Suppl 4]:181-183

Reinberg A, Smolensky MH (1983) Biological rhythms and medicine. Springer, New York, Berlin, Heidelberg

Reinink E, Bouhuys N, Wirz-Justice A, Hoofdakker R van den (1990a) Prediction of the antidepressant response to total sleep deprivation by diurnal variation of mood. Psychiatry Res 32:113-124

Reinink E, Bouhuys N, Gordijn M, Hoofdakker R van den, Beersma D (1990b) Total sleep deprivation and diurnal variation in depression. In: Psychiatry: A world perspective, vol 1. Excerpta Medica, Amsterdam, pp 494-499

Richter CP (1960) Biological clocks in medicine and psychiatry: shockphase hypothesis. Proc Natl Acad Sci USA 46:1506-1530

Richter CP (1965) Biological clocks in medicine and psychiatry. Thomas, Springfield

Roenneberg T, Aschoff J (1990) Annual rhythm of human reproduction: II. Environmental correlations. J Biol Rhythms 5:217-240

Rosen LN, Targum SD, Terman M, Bryant MJ, Hoffman H, Kasper SF, Hamovit JR, Docherty JP, Welch B, Rosenthal NE (1990) Prevalence of seasonal affective disorder at four latitudes. Psychiatry Res 31:131-144

Rosenthal NE, Blehar MC (1989) Seasonal affective disorders and phototherapy. Guilford, New York

Rosenthal NE, Lewy AJ, Wehr TA, Kern HE, Goodwin FK (1983) Seasonal cycling in a bipolar patient. Psychiatr Res 8:25-31

Rosenthal NE, Sack DA, Gillin JC, Lewy AJ, Goodwin FK, Davenport Y, Mueller PS, Newsome DA, Wehr TA (1984) Seasonal affective disorder. A description of the syndrome and preliminary findings with light therapy. Arch Gen Psychiatry 41:72-80

Rosenthal NE, Jacobsen FM, Sack DA, Arendt J, James SP, Parry BL, Wehr TA (1988) Atenolol in seasonal affective disorder: a test of the melatonin hypothesis. Am J Psychiatry 145:52-56

Sack DA, Duncan W, Rosenthal NE, Mendelson WE, Wehr TA (1988) The timing and duration of sleep in partial sleep deprivation therapy of depression. Acta Psychiatr Scand 77:219-224

Sadow J (1979) The diurnal rhythmicity of brain, pituitary and adrenocortical hormones. In: Jones MT, Dallman MF, Gillham B, Chattopadhyay S (eds) Interaction within the brain-pituitary-adrenocortical system. Academic, London, pp 221-227

Schaefer A (1896) Stoffwechselerscheinungen bei einem eigenartigen Falle von circulärem Irresein. Neurol Centrbl 15:1067-1072

Schilgen B, Tölle (1980) Partial sleep deprivation as therapy for depression. Arch Gen Psychiatry 37:267-271

Schöpf J, Bryois C, Jonquière M, Le PK (1984) On the nosology of severe psychiatric postpartum disorders. Results of a catamnestic investigation. Eur Arch Psychiatry Neurol Sci 234:54-63

Schöpf J, Bryois C, Jonquière M, Scharfetter C (1985) A family hereditary study of postpartum "psychoses". Eur Arch Psychiatry Neurol Sci 235:164-170

Schwartz WJ, Reppert SM (1985) Neural regulation of the circadian vasopressin rhythm on cerebrospinal fluid: a pre- eminent role for the suprachiasmatic nuclei. J Neurosci 5:2771-2778

Sitaram N, Gillin JC, Bunney WE Jr (1978) Circadian variation in the time of "switch" of a patient with 48-hour manic- depressive cycles. Biol Psychiatry 13:567-574

Slater E (1938) Zur Periodik des manisch-depressiven Irreseins. Z Gesamte Neurol Psychiatr 162:794-801

Spitzer RL, Endicott J, Robins E (1978) Research diagnostic criteria. Arch Gen Psychiatry 35:773-782

Stallone F, Huba GJ, Lawlor WG, Fieve RR (1973) Longitudinal studies of diurnal variations in depression: a sample of 643 patient days. Br J Psychiatry 123:311-318

Terman M (1988) On the question of mechanism in phototherapy for seasonal affective disorder: considerations of clinical efficacy end epidemiology. J Biol Rhythms 3:155-172

Thompson C (1989) Seasonality of depression. In: Thompson C, Silverstone T (eds) Seasonal affective disorder. CNS, London, pp 1-17

Thompson C (1989b) The syndrome of seasonal affective disorder. In: Thompson C, Silverstone T (eds) Seasonal affective disorder. CNS, London, pp 37-57

Thompson C, Isaacs G (1988) Seasonal affective disorder — a British sample. Symptomatology in relation to mode of referral and diagnostic subtype. J Affective Disord 14:1-11

Thompson C, Silverstone T (1989) Seasonal affective disorder. CNS, London

Thompson C, Stinson D, Fernandez M, Fine J, Isaacs G (1988) A comparison of normal, bipolar and seasonal affective disorder subjects using the Seasonal Pattern Assessment Questionnaire. J Affective Disord 14:257-264

Tölle R, Goetze U (1987) On the daily rhythm of depression symptomatology. Psychopathology 20:237-249

Waldmann H (1969) Zirkadianer Phasenwechsel bei der manisch-depressiven Krankheit. Fortschr Neurol Psychiatr 37:83-104

Waldmann H (1972) Tagesschwankung in der Depression als rhythmisches Phänomen. Fortschr Neurol Psychiatr 40:83-104

Wehr TA, Goodwin FK (1981) Biological rhythms and psychiatry. In: Arieti S, Brodie HKH (eds) American handbook of psychiatry, vol 7, 2nd edn. Advances and new directions. Basic Books, New York, pp 46-74

Wehr TA, Goodwin FK (1983) Circadian rhythms in psychiatry, vol 2. Boxwood, Pacific Grove

Wehr TA, Rosenthal NE (1989) Seasonality and affective illness. Am J Psychiatry 146:829--839

Wehr TA, Sack DA, Duncan WC, Mendelson WB, Rosenthal NE, Gillin JC, Goodwin FK (1985) Sleep and circadian rhythms in affective patients isolated from external time cues. Psychiatry Res 15:327-339

Wehr TA, Jacobsen FM, Sack DA, Arendt J, Tamarkin L, Rosenthal NE (1986) Phototherapy of seasonal affective disorder: time of day and suppression of melatonin are not critical for antidepressant effects. Arch Gen Psychiatry 43:870-875

Wehr TA, Sack DA, Rosenthal NE (1987) Seasonal affective disorder with summer depression and winter hypomania. Am J Psychiatry 144:1602-1603

Welsh DK, Moore-Ede MC (1990) Lithium lengthens circadian period in a diurnal primate, Saimiri sciureus. Biol Psychiatry 28:117-126

Welsh DK, Nino-Murcia G, Gander PH, Keenan S, Dement WC (1986) Regular 48-hour cycling of sleep duration and mood in a 35-year-old woman: use of lithium in time isolation. Biol Psychiatry 21:527-537

Wever RA (1979) The circadian system of man. Springer, New York Heidelberg Berlin

Whalley LJ, Roberts DF, Wentzel J, Wright AF (1982) Genetic factors in puerperal affective psychoses. Acta Psychiatr Scand 65:180-193

Wiegand M, Berger M, Zulley J, Lauer Ch, Riemann D, von Zerssen D (1987a) The effect of daytime naps subsequent to sleep deprivation on the course of mood in depressives. In: Chase MH, McGinty DJ, O'Conner C (eds) Sleep research, vol 16. Brain Information Service/Brain Research Institute, University of California, Los Angeles, p 542

Wiegand M, Berger M, Zulley J, Lauer C, Zerssen D von (1987b) The influence of daytime naps on the therapeutic effect of sleep deprivation. Biol Psychiatry 22:389-392

Wiegand M, Riemann D, Zulley J, Lauer Ch, Schreiber W, Elsenga S, Berger M (1989) Effect of morning and afternoon naps on mood after sleep deprivation in depressives. In: Horne J (ed) Sleep '88. Fischer, Stuttgart, pp 227-229

Wirz-Justice A, Bucheli B, Graw P, Kielholz P, Fisch H-U, Woggon B (1986) Light treatment of seasonal affective disorder in Switzerland. Acta Psychiatr Scand 74:193-204

Wolff H (1821) Eine periodische Melancholie. Z psych Aerzte 4:124-134

Zaudig M, von Bose M, Dirlich G, Knopf H, Zulley J, Schreiber W, Pirke KM, Mombour W (submitted for publication) A possible relationship of climatic variables upon seasonal affective disorder with summer depression and winter hypomania: preliminary results of a prospective pilot-study. Am J Psychiatry

Zerssen D von (1983) Chronobiology of depression. In: Angst J (ed) The origins of depression: current concepts and approaches. Dahlem Konferenzen. Springer, Berlin, Heidelberg, New York, pp 253-271

Zerssen D von (1987) What is wrong with circadian clocks in depression? In: Halaris A (ed) Chronobiology and psychiatric disorders. Elsevier, New York, pp 159-179

Zerssen D von (1988) Circadian phenomena in depression: theoretical concepts and empirical findings. In: Hekkens WThJM, Kerkhof GA, Rietveld WJ (eds) Trends in chronobiology. Pergamon, Oxford, pp 357-366

Zerssen D von, Lund R, Doerr P, Fischler M, Emrich HM, Ploog D (1979) 48-hour-cycles of depression and their biological concomitants with and without "Zeitgebers". A case report. In: Saletu B, Berner P, Hollister L (eds) Neuro-Psychopharmacology. Pergamon, Oxford, pp 233-245

Zerssen D von, Dirlich G, Fischler M (1983) Influence of an abnormal time routine and therapeutic measures on 48-hour cycles of affective disorders: chronobiological considerations. In: Wehr TA, Goodwin FK (eds) Circadian rhythms in psychiatry, vol 2. Boxwood, Pacific Grove, pp 109- 127

Zerssen D von, Barthelmes H, Dirlich G, Doerr P, Emrich HM, von Lindern L, Lund R, Pirke KM (1985) Circadian rhythms in endogenous depression. Psychiatry Res 16:51-63

Zerssen D von, Doerr P, Emrich HM, Lund R, Pirke KM (1987) Diurnal variation of mood and the cortisol rhythm in depression and normal states of mind. Eur Arch Psychiatry Neurol Sci 237:36-45

Zerssen D von, Dirlich G, Zulley J (1989) Circadian rhythm disturbances in affective disorders: facts and fictions. In: Lerer B, Gershon S (eds) New directions in affective disorders. Springer, New York, Berlin, Heidelberg, pp 243-250

Ziegler K (1864) Über die Eigenwärme in einem Fall von Geistesstörung mit eigenthümlichen intermittirenden Erscheinungen. Ein Beitrag zu Untersuchungen über die Eigenwärme in Geistesstörungen. Allg Z Psychiatrie 21:184-194

15 Reversal of Antidepressant Sleep Deprivation Effects by Daytime Naps

M. Wiegand, D. Riemann, W. Schreiber, C. Lauer, M. Berger

Introduction

Total sleep deprivation (TSD) is an effective treatment of major depression, with a response rate of about 50% - 60%. In contrast to other antidepressant treatments, the therapeutic effect develops rapidly, but a relapse into depression virtually always occurs after the following nocturnal sleep (Gerner et al. 1979; Gillin 1983; Kuhs and Tölle 1986).

Despite its limited clinical usefulness, sleep deprivation has become an important paradigm in research on affective disorders. In order to elucidate its mechanism of action, previous studies have aimed to identify predictors of response to TSD (Roy-Byrne et al. 1984). In the present paper, a different experimental approach is presented. It is based on the clinical observation that a daytime nap after successful sleep deprivation can provoke a mood setback or even a severe relapse into depression. This phenomenon was first mentioned in an early report on the beneficial effects of TSD in depressed patients by Pflug and Tölle (1971). In a single case study, Knowles et al. (1979) described a relapse into depression provoked by a short nap of 15 min duration, and Roy-Byrne et al. (1984) observed a severe mood worsening subsequent to as little as 90 s polysomnographically recorded sleep. Southmayd et al. (1987) described a deterioration of mood in a TSD responder after several very short episodes of sleep revealed by continuous EEG monitoring. In a systematic study, Gillin et al. (1988), however, did not observe such relapses following brief (10 min) naps. In a study with patients treated with antidepressants, Giedke (1988) observed no consistent effect of daytime naps on mood.

The antidepressant effect of sleep deprivation and its reversal by sleep (daytime naps as well as nocturnal sleep) support the hypothesis that sleep can promote depressive symptomatology in depressed patients. This assumption is further supported by the frequent clinical phenomenon of positive diurnal variation of mood with a maximum of depressed mood in the morning and a gradual improvement during the course of the day.

Several hypotheses have been raised to explain the antidepressant effect of sleep deprivation and, conversely, the "depressiogenic" properties of sleep in depression. Among these, the following are presently most discussed (van den Hoofdakker and Beersma 1988):

1) Under a chronobiological perspective, major depression can be characterized by alterations of "internal clocks", e.g. desynchronization or phase shifts. Sleep deprivation is supposed to exert its antidepressant action by either resynchronizing disturbed rhythms, or by preventing sleep during a so-called "critical phase" in the early morning hours (Wehr and Wirz-Justice 1980; Kripke 1984; these aspects are discussed in more detail in the paper by von Zerssen et al., in this volume, pp 181-205). In light of these theories, the timing of a daytime nap following sleep deprivation can be expected to be crucial for its effect on mood.

2) The "two-process model" of sleep (Borbély 1987; Borbély and Wirz-Justice 1982) postulates a deficiency of a homeostatic "process S" (associated with EEG slow wave activity) in depression which may account for the impairment of mood. Sleep deprivation is supposed to increase the level of "process S" by lengthening the duration of wakefulness and thus leading to a mood improvement. This model allows the prediction that the relapse caused by a nap is related to the degree of "process S" reduction. Correspondingly, both the EEG slow wave activity during a nap (associated with nap length) and the duration of prior wakefulness can be expected to be essential for the nap-induced deterioration of mood. A model with similar implications has been proposed by Wu and Bunney (1990) who postulate a depressiogenic substance which is released by even small amounts of sleep.

3) Regarding the antidepressant effect of selective REM sleep deprivation observed by Vogel et al. (1980), it has been hypothesized that REM sleep suppression is essential for the beneficial effects of several antidepressant treatment modalities, including sleep deprivation (Berger 1987). This view is in line with the cholinergic-adrenergic imbalance model of depression (Janowsky et al. 1972) and the reciprocal interaction model of REM sleep regulation (McCarley 1982). In light of this approach, the occurrence of REM sleep during a daytime nap, as a correlate of elevated cholinergic neuronal activity, should be accompanied by a greater propensity of relapse into depression.

The induction of depressive symptomatology by short sleep episodes is a crucial experiment to test these hypotheses. The series of studies presented in this paper were designed to examine this phenomenon systematically in order to elucidate the nature of the depressiogenic properties of sleep in depression.

Methods

In the present paper, data are compiled from four studies on therapeutic sleep deprivation and daytime naps which are described in more detail in Table 1. Inpatients suffering from major depression according to DSM-III-R (296.2x, 296.3x, 296.5x) were included in the studies. The drug washout period was at least 7 days. TSDs were preceded by 2 nights in the sleep laboratory, with

Table 1. Synopsis of Studies. *MPI*, Max Planck Institute of Psychiatry, Munich, Germany; *ZI*, Central Institute of Mental Health, Mannheim, Germany; *TSD*, total sleep deprivation

	Study 1	Study 2	Study 3	Study 4	Total
Institution	MPI	MPI	MPI/ZI	MPI/ZI	
N of patients	12	3	30[*]	26[*]	50
male/female	4/ 8	0/ 3	10/20	8/18	14/36
age (mean ± SD)	40.7 ± 14.2	50.0 ± 6.1	48.7 ± 11.5	48.5 ± 13.1	46.2 ± 13.2
HAMD-21					
(mean ± SD)	26.5 ± 6.8	28.3 ± 4.0	26.9 ± 5.3	27.8 ± 4.9	27.4 ± 5.5
No. of TSDs	23	6	30	26	85
with response	12	3	20	16	51
No. of naps	22	6	28	24	80
At 0900 hours	0	6	13	24	43
At 1300 hours	22	0	0	0	22
At 1500 hours	0	0	15	0	15

[*] Patients in part identical in studies 3 and 4 (see text)

polysomnographic recordings being performed during the 2nd night. Daytime naps took place on the day subsequent to TSD and were recorded in the sleep laboratory. All sleep recordings were scored visually according to standard criteria (Rechtschaffen and Kales 1968). Mood changes during sleep deprivation and nap were scored by means of the six-item version of the Hamilton Depression Scale (HAMD-6, Bech et al., 1975). In addition, self-ratings were performed using the Adjective Mood Scale (AMS, von Zerssen, 1986). Ratings took place in the mornings before and after sleep deprivations, as well as immediately before and about 30 minutes after the termination of daytime naps. "Response" to total sleep deprivation was defined as a reduction of at least 30% in the HAMD-6 score.

Study 1: This study was designed to test the hypothesis that mood worsenings following a daytime nap after successful therapeutic sleep deprivation are associated with the occurrence of REM sleep. The study aimed at comparing naps containing REM sleep ("REM naps") with naps without REM sleep ("non-REM naps"). Naps took place at 1300 hours after sleep deprivation and were terminated either by an awakening after the first REM episode ("REM nap") or by waking the patient up immediately at the very onset of a REM episode ("non-REM nap"); patients were assigned randomly to one of both waking conditions. Those patients who awoke spontaneously without having exhibited an REM episode were included in the latter group. In patients who consented, TSD and nap were repeated one week later, with reversed waking conditions. Methodology and part of the results of this study were published by Wiegand et al. (1987a, 1987b).

Study 2: This study was designed to assess the effects of shorter (50 min) versus longer (100 min) naps at 0900 hours; naps were terminated by awakenings. TSD and nap were repeated one week later, with reversed waking conditions.

Study 3: The objective of this study was to determine the influence of the timing of a daytime nap (morning versus afternoon) on mood changes. Patients were randomly assigned to the morning nap (0900 hours) or afternoon nap (1500 hours) condition. Naps were terminated by spontanous awakenings. This study has partly been published by Wiegand et al. (1989).

Study 4: This study (partly published by Riemann et al. 1989) aimed to examine the effect of the occurrence of REM sleep on mood changes after morning naps (0900 hours), controlling for the impact of sleep length by comparing pairs of patients with REM naps and non-REM naps with nearly identical sleep lengths. Naps were terminated by experimental awakenings either 2 minutes after the termination of an REM period (REM nap) or after a non-REM sleep period equalling a previous REM nap in length (non-REM nap). Naps terminated by spontaneous awakenings before the occurrence of the first REM period were classified as non-REM naps and matched, if possible, with a REM nap with comparable duration.

Of the patients included in study 3, ten participated in study 4 about one week later. Analogously, eleven patients of study 4 later took part in study 3.

Present Analysis of the Data

The present analysis concentrates on the changes in observer-rated depression scores before versus after naps following sleep deprivation (Delta HAMD-6). It focuses on their relationship with some crucial variables regarding the major hypotheses outlined above:

- 1) Timing of the nap (0900 vs. 1300 vs. 1500 hours)
- 2) Nap sleep duration
- 3) Occurrence of REM sleep during the nap

In a first step of the analysis, the data from all studies were pooled, including the repetitions of TSDs. This resulted in a total of 85 sleep deprivations with 80 subsequent daytime naps, observed in 50 patients (in 5 cases, patients did not fall asleep at the scheduled nap time). This sample will be referred to as *"total samp-le"* and is characterized in more detail in Table 1. As the data are partly inter-dependent (30 of the 80 naps being repetitions), statistical tests cannot be per-formed on this data set, and only descriptive data will be given.

Since the main interest of the present analysis was the effects of daytime naps after *successful* TSD, a second step of data analysis concentrated on the subsample of responders to TSD. To avoid the problem of interdependent data and to allow for statistical tests, repetitions of TSD and nap were not included in this sample, each patient thus being represented only once. If a patient had responded twice, only the data from his first TSD and nap were included in the analysis. The resulting sample is referred to as the *"responders' sample"*, consisting of 33 patients (10 male / 23 female, mean age 46.6 ± 13.0 years, mean HAMD-6 score

28.6 ± 4.8), with 14 naps at 0900 hours, 8 naps at 1300 hours, and 11 naps at 1500 hours.

For the descriptive presentation of the total sample data (Fig. 1), the effects of naps on mood were classified according to the difference in HAMD-6 scores (Delta HAMD-6) before versus after the naps (severely worse = worsening of more than 3 points; slightly worse = worsening of 1 to 3 points; no change; improved). In the statistical analysis of the responders' sample (Tables 2 - 4), the effects were dichotomized (severe worsening = worsening of more than 3 points; no severe worsening = slightly worse, no change, or improved). Statistical analysis in Tables 2 and 4 is based on chi-square tests. For the comparison of nap durations at different times (Table 3), Mann-Whitney U-tests were carried out. The level of significance was set at 5% (two-tailed).

Results

Effect of Nap Timing

Figure 1 summarizes the effects of TSDs and daytime naps on mood at different times in the total sample. It is evident that in responders to TSD there was a

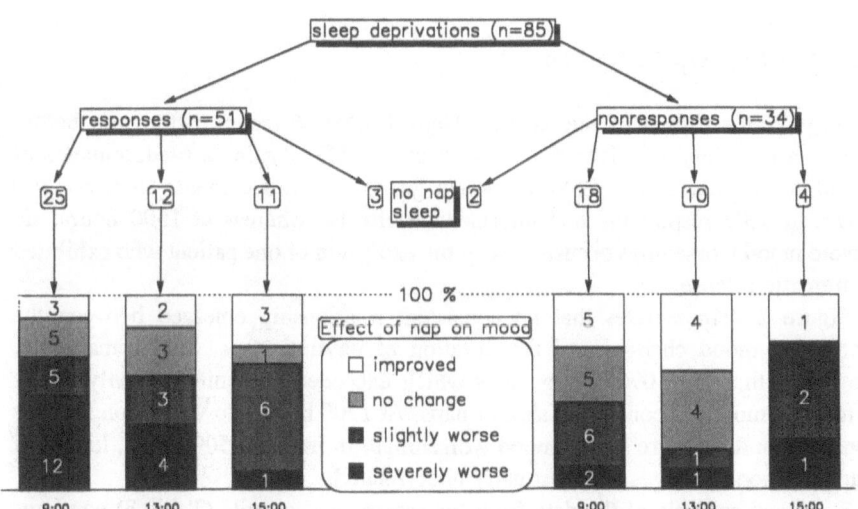

Fig. 1. Effects of sleep deprivations and daytime naps on mood in the total sample. The sections of the columns represent the percentages of patients who exhibited the respective response to a daytime nap. *Total column* = 100%; *slightly worse* = worsening of 1 to 3 points in the HAMD-6; *severely worse* = worsening of more than 3 points

relatively large number of severe mood worsenings in the 0900 hours group, compared with naps at 1500 hours, the rate of severe worsenings at 1300 hours being in-between. Improvements of mood rarely occurred, even at 1500 hours slight worsenings predominated. In contrast, after nonresponses to TSD, the majority of daytime naps at 0900 hours and 1300 hours were followed by improvement or no mood change [for naps at 1500 hours following nonresponse, the sample (n=4) appears too small for interpretation]. Severe mood worsenings were rare in nonresponders to TSD.

A statistical analysis performed in the responders' sample confirms these impressions (Table 2): severe worsenings of mood were significantly more frequent following a 0900 hours nap, compared with naps at 1300 and 1500 hours.

Table 2. Influence of nap timing on mood changes (responders' sample)

	Severe worsening (Delta HAMD-6 > 3)	No severe worsening
Nap at 0900 hours	9	5
Nap at 1300 hours	2	6
Nap at 1500 hours	1	10

Chi-square = 8.70, df = 2, p < 0.02

Effect of Nap Sleep Duration

In Fig. 2, the effects of the naps on Delta HAMD-6 (score differences before versus after naps) are given for responders to TSD. Again, a predominance of mood worsenings in the 0900 hours nap group becomes evident. Naps at 1300 hours in TSD responders had intermediate effects, whereas at 1500 hours, no severe mood worsenings occurred, with the exception of one patient who exhibited a dramatic relapse.

Figure 2 demonstrates that no consistent relationship emerged between the degree of mood changes and the duration of daytime naps. It is remarkable, however, that both 0900 hours naps which exceeded 120 min had only minor effects on mood, in contrast to shorter naps. At 1300 hours, however, longer naps tended to induce more severe mood worsenings. In naps at 1500 hours, length of nap and mood changes were virtually uncorrelated.

Statistical analysis of the data from the responders' sample (Table 3) confirms that at neither time of the day did naps leading to severe worsenings differ significantly in length from naps without this effect. For naps at 0900 hours, there was a tendency toward a negative association of mood impairment and nap length, whereas an opposite trend was present for naps at 1300 hours.

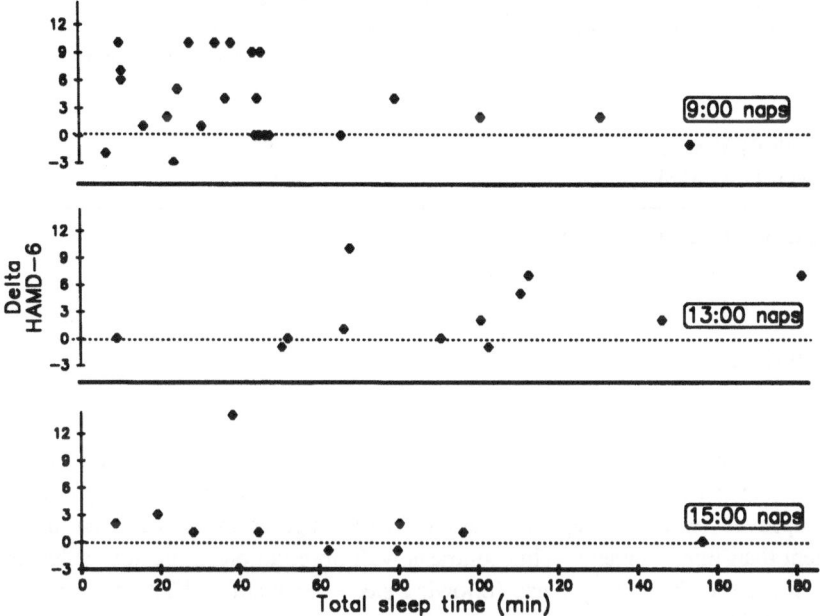

Fig. 2. Duration and mood effects of naps following response to TSD

Table 3. Influence of nap sleep duration on mood changes (responders' sample)

	Severe worsening	No severe worsening	Total	
Nap at 0900 hours duration (min)	37.2 ± 20.8	71.7 ± 65.9	49.5 ± 43.5	NS
Nap at 1300 hours duration (min)	90.0 ± 31.8	67.5 ± 36.9	73.1 ± 35.0	NS
Nap at 1500 hours duration (min)	38.0 (n=1)	61.3 ± 43.8	59.2 ± 42.2	NS
Total	46.1 ± 28.8	65.5 ± 45.7	58.5 ± 41.0	NS

NS, nonsignificant

Effect of the Occurrence of REM Sleep

The statistical analysis of data from the responders' sample (Table 4) demonstrates that the occurrence of REM sleep was not associated with severe worsenings of mood. The ratio of naps with versus without REM sleep did not vary significantly between different times of the day (not represented in Table 4).

Table 4. Influence of the occurrence of REM sleep (responders' sample)

	Severe worsening (Delta HAMD-6 > 3)	No severe worsening
Naps with REM sleep	3	9
Naps without REM sleep	9	12

Chi-square = 0.42, df = 1, NS

Discussion

The studies analyzed in the present paper confirm former observations that a daytime nap can re-induce depressive symptomatology in depressed patients who had improved by total sleep deprivation. Worsenings of mood were far more frequent than improvements. This contrasts with observations in healthy subjects who, in general, benefit by a nap following sleep deprivation (Taub et al. 1976; Naitoh 1981).

Our data show that, in depressed patients who had not responded to TSD, daytime naps had, in general, more beneficial effects than in responders. Although the present analysis (like most research in the field) focuses on the impact of nap sleep on mood in *responders* to TSD, effects observed in nonresponders should not be neglected and merit special consideration.

It might be objected that our results mirror "sleep inertia" effects occurring immediately after awakening (Naitoh 1981). However, ratings were performed about ½ h after waking up; after such a delay, sleep inertia effects are expected to be marginal (Webb and Agnew 1974). Particularly the severe relapses we observed exceed the range of slight temporary discomfort which might be the expression of sleep inertia.

Of the three variables analyzed, the timing of a nap appeared to be most important for its effect on depressive symptomatology. There was a gradient from morning naps at 0900 hours, which clearly had the most detrimental impact in responders to TSD, via naps at 1300 hours with intermediate effects, to afternoon (1500 hours) naps, which were far better tolerated. The crucial role of nap timing seems to support chronobiological hypotheses, suggesting that there may be a circadian variation of propensity to relapse into depression. In analogy to the "internal coincidence model" (Wehr and Wirz-Justice 1983), it may be speculated that a nap at 0900 hours in the morning coincides with a "vulnerable phase", during which the occurrence of sleep can provoke a relapse. The importance of chronobiological processes for the effects of sleep deprivation is further underscored by the observation that the presence of a positive diurnal variation of mood is among the few predictors of response to TSD which have as yet been identified (Reinink et al. 1990; Riemann et al. 1990).

On the other hand, in the present analyses, timing of naps is confounded with the duration of prior wakefulness, since the sleep deprivation periods began constantly at 0700 hours on the preceding day. Thus, the more detrimental impact of morning naps can alternatively be explained by the S-deficiency hypothesis: following this model, the deficient "process S" has already passed a hypothetical threshold of depressive mood in the morning after successful sleep deprivation, but can easily be diminished below this level even by small amounts of sleep. In the afternoon, process S has reached a higher level, and even long naps are not sufficient to decrease this level below the hypothetical threshold. Thus, our finding that nap timing is crucial for its effect on mood does not necessarily favor circadian models but can also point to a homeostatic process.

However, the S-deficiency hypothesis would predict that independent of nap timing, relapses into depression are more likely following longer naps, since these will contain a higher amount of EEG slow wave activity and thus lead to a higher reduction of "process S" than shorter naps. Except for a nonsignificant trend in this direction in naps at 1300 hours, our data do not support this hypothesis; after naps at 0900 hours, there was even an opposite tendency with shorter naps being more detrimental. The result by Gillin et al. (1988) that naps of 10 min maximum duration do not cause worsenings is compatible with our data since none of the naps shorter than 10 min caused a relapse. However, the observation by Roy-Byrne (1984) of an ultrashort (90 s) nap followed by a severe relapse refutes the assumption that there may be a minimum of several minutes of sleep required for severe worsenings of mood.

The data do not really contradict the S-deficiency model since EEG power spectra would be required for any critical test of this hypothesis which are not available here. However, as EEG delta power can be expected to correlate with nap sleep duration, some degree of relationship between nap length and mood worsening should be present which is clearly not supported by our data.

The occurrence of REM sleep did not turn out to be of significance for relapses into depression. This does not necessarily refute the hypothesis derived from the cholinergic-aminergic imbalance model of depression that cholinergic overactivity may be involved in relapses into depression caused by a daytime nap. Our data rather qualify the role of REM sleep as a reliable indicator of the cholinergic tone. A circadian variation of cholinergic functioning may be involved in the different pathogenic impact of naps at different times of the day, without necessarily being mirrored in variations of REM propensity in short naps.

To summarize, our main findings are basically compatible with all major hypotheses raised to explain the depressiogenic impact of sleep in depression, and do not clearly refute one of them. Further analyses will have to consider more variables with respect to their impact on mood, including nap sleep structure. Future studies in this field should attempt to separate the confounded variables "nap timing" and "duration of prior wakefulness" since this will be decisive for the differentiation between circadian and homeostatic processes with regard to the unfavorable impact of sleep on mood in depression.

References

Bech P, Gram LF, Dein E, Jacobsen O, Vitger J, Bolwig TG (1975) Quantitative rating of depressive states. Acta Psychiatr Scand 51:161-170

Berger M (1987) REM-Schlaf und cholinerges System bei depressiven Erkrankungen. In: Hippius H, Rüther E, Schmauß M (eds) Schlaf-Wach-Funktionen. Springer, Berlin Heidelberg New York London Paris Tokyo, pp 181-189

Borbély AA (1987) The S-deficiency hypothesis of depression and the two-process model of sleep regulation. Pharmacopsychiatry 20:23-29

Borbély AA, Wirz-Justice A (1982) Sleep, sleep deprivation and depression. A hypothesis derived from a model of sleep regulation. Hum Neurobiol 1:205-210

Gerner RH, Post RM, Gillin JC, Bunney WE (1979) Biological and behavioral effects of one night's sleep deprivation in depressed patients and normals. J Psychiatr Res 15:21-40

Giedke H (1988) The effect of afternoon naps on mood in depressive patients after therapeutic sleep deprivation. In: Koella WP, Obál F, Schulz H, Visser P (eds) Sleep '86. Fischer, Stuttgart, pp 451-453

Gillin JC (1983) The sleep therapies of depression. Prog Neuro-psychopharmacol Biol Psychiatry 7:351-364

Gillin JC, Kripke DF, Janowsky DS, Risch SC (1988) Effects of brief naps on mood and sleep in sleep-deprived depressed patients. Psychiatry Res 27:253-265

Hoofdakker RH van den, Beersma DGM (1988) On the contribution of sleep wake physiology to the explanation and the treatment of depression. Acta Scand[Suppl]341(77):53-71

Janowsky DS, Davis JM, El-Yousef MK, Sekerke HJ (1972) A cholinergic-adrenergic hypothesis of mania and depression. Lancet ii:632

Knowles JB, Southmayd SE, Delva N, MacLean AW, Cairns J, Letemendia FJ (1979) Five variations of sleep deprivation in a depressed woman. Br J Psychiatry 135:403-410

Kripke DF (1984) Critical interval hypothesis for depression. Chronobiol Int 1:73-80

Kuhs H, Tölle R (1986) Schlafentzug (Wachtherapie) als Antidepressivum. Fortschr Neurol Psychiat 54:341-355

McCarley RW (1982) REM sleep and depression: common neurobiological control mechanisms. Am J Psychiatry 139:565-570

Naitoh P (1981) Circadian cycles and restorative power of naps. In: Johnson LC, Tepas DI, Colquhoun WP, Colligan MP (eds) Biological rhythms, sleep and shift work. Spectrum, New York, pp 553-580

Pflug B, Tölle R (1979) Therapie endogener Depressionen durch Schlafentzug. Nervenarzt 42:117-124

Rechtschaffen A, Kales A (1968) A manual of standardized terminology, techniques and scoring system for sleep stages of human subjects. Public Health Service, Washington

Reinink E, Bouhuys N, Wirz-Justice A, Hoofdakker R van den (1990) Prediction of the antidepressant response to total sleep deprivation by diurnal variation of mood. Psychiatry Res 32:113-124

Riemann D, Wiegand M, Berger M (1990) Are there predictors for sleep deprivation response in depressed patients? Biol Psychiatry 29:707-710

Riemann D, Wiegand M, Zulley J, Lauer Ch, Schreiber W, Berger M (1989) The effect of the occurrence of REM sleep during morning naps on mood after sleep deprivation in patients with major depressive disorder. In: Horne JA (ed) Sleep '88. Fischer, Stuttgart, pp 230-232

Roy-Byrne PR, Uhde TW, Post RM (1984) Antidepressant effects of one night's sleep deprivation: clinical and theoretical implications. In: Post RM, Ballenger JC (eds) Neurobiology of mood disorders. Clin Neurosci, vol 1. Williams and Wilkins, Baltimore, pp 817- 835

Southmayd SE, Cairns J, Brunet DG (1987) Antidepressant response to sleep deprivation in relation to psychophysiologically defined wakefulness. Sleep Res 16:538

Taub JM, Tanguay PE, Clarkson D (1976) Effects of daytime naps on performance and mood in a college student population. J Abnorm Psychol 85:210-217

Vogel GW, Vogel F, McAbee RS, Turmond J (1980) Improvement of depression by REM sleep deprivation. New findings and a theory. Arch Gen Psychiatry 37:247-253

Webb WB, Agnew H (1974) The effects of a chronic limitation of sleep length. Psychophysiology 11:265-274

Wehr TA, Wirz-Justice A (1981) Internal coincidence model for sleep deprivation and depression. In: Koella WP (ed) Sleep 1980. Karger, Basel, pp 26-33

Wiegand M, Berger M, Zulley J, Lauer C, Riemann D, von Zerssen D (1987a) The effect of daytime naps subsequent to sleep deprivation on the course of mood in depressives. Sleep Research 16:542

Wiegand M, Berger M, Zulley J, Lauer C, Zerssen D von (1987b) The influence of daytime naps on the therapeutic effect of sleep deprivation. Biol Psychiatry 22:389-392

Wiegand M, Riemann D, Zulley J, Lauer C, Schreiber W, Elsenga S, Berger M (1989) Effect of morning and afternoon naps on mood after sleep deprivation in depressives. In: Horne JA (ed) Sleep '88. Fischer, Stuttgart, pp 227-229

Wu JC, Bunney WE (1990) The biological basis of an antidepressant response to sleep deprivation and relapse: review and hypothesis. Am J Psychiatry 147:14-21

Zerssen D von (1986) Clinical self-rating scales (CSRS) of the Munich Psychiatric Information System (PSYCHIS München). In: Sartorius N, Ban TA (eds) Assessment of depression. Springer, Berlin Heidelberg New York, pp 270-303

Part IV: Diagnostic and Therapeutic Aspects

16 The New Classification Systems in Psychiatry: Overview, Problems, and Consequences

W. Mombour

In psychiatry, diagnoses and classifications are used at three different levels: symptom, syndrome, and nosological group. As in the rest of medicine there are many possible reasons for the use of diagnostics and classification, of which I only want to mention four:

1. To bring some order to the confusing diversity of single phenomena
2. To choose the best therapy from the many alternatives
3. To make a prognosis, which may be important in planning the future needs of the patient
4. To facilitate the exchange of information and communication between physicians, in teaching, in publications, in correspondence, etc., by using an abbreviated diagnostic term instead of giving all the information available.

Everyone working in or writing about psychiatry uses diagnostic terms from at least one of these three levels (symptom, syndrome, nosology). Even those people who think of themselves as"antidiagnostically minded" (e.g., psychoanalysts, antipsychiatrists, behavioral therapists, and sometimes even biological psychiatrists) use diagnostic terms at least on a purely descriptive level of symptoms and syndromes. Often they are merely critical of the presently used nosological classifications and of the theoretical concepts underlying theses classifications.

Until the middle of the 1960s psychiatric diagnostics were dominated by many local schools of thought, conceptualized mostly by an important and dominating psychiatrist and professor of the local university.

Therefore psychiatric diagnoses were not comparable between countries and sometimes even not within the same country. In order to address the noncomparability of psychiatric diagnostics many scientific projects have been undertaken in the past 2 decades, aiming at a better understanding of the diagnostic process and of the reasons for diagnostic discrepancies; great efforts have been made to establish a worldwide standardization of psychiatric diagnostics and classification. Firstly, projects from the Anglo-American countries and from WHO have to be mentioned. Their results confirmed — also in psychiatry — the scientific commonplace that diagnoses depend on methodology: the same methodology leads to the same results, a different methodology to different results. All those efforts were crowned with success in 1970 by the International Classification of Diseases of WHO (ICD-8 and -9) being introduced and accepted for psychiatric nosological classification in most countries of the world (WHO 1974, 1978; Mombour 1975).

At the level of symptoms and syndromes, the discovery of neuroleptics and antidepressants added to a worldwide standardization: their convincing effects on psychopathology and the change of psychopathology under treatment and during the longitudinal course could be operationalized and quantified by rating scales (see Mombour 1972; Möller and von Zerssen 1982, 1983). With these rating scales typical cross-sectional syndrome profiles were also found for specific diagnoses. This added to the typing and the standardization of nosological diagnoses (e.g. Mombour, 1974; Hiller et al. 1986).

The purpose was not to make psychiatric diagnoses more "right" — there is no right and wrong in psychiatric diagnostics as long as we have no provable etiology and etiopathogenesis for most psychiatric disorders — diagnoses should only be more standardized and correspond better with one another. This aim was certainly reached by world psychiatry in the years between 1970 and 1980 by using the ICD and some of the internationally known rating scales.

In spite of this undoubted success, there has been increasing criticism of ICD diagnostics, of which the "categorical" character was rejected. The criticism was made that ICD diagnoses were only general and vague descriptions and enumerations of symptoms and signs, of other variables, of behavior and course, etc. There were no clear definitions as to which and how many of the enumerated symptoms and signs had to be present in order to give a specific diagnosis to a single patient. In this form of so-called "typological" (or categorical-athetic) diagnosis a real patient is compared with an ideal patient out of a psychiatric textbook, who very often does not exist in reality; the real patient need not be totally identical to the ideal patient but only convincingly similar; nowhere is it defined how great the similarity has to be. Using these typological diagnoses of ICD-8/-9, one still comes across diagnostic discrepancies. To oppose these inconveniences criteria-based diagnoses were developed, first in 1972 in the United States with the so-called Feighner criteria (Feighner et al. 1972), then with the RDC (Research Diagnostic Criteria) (Spitzer et al. 1978) and finally with DSM-III (APA 1980), DSM-III-R (APA 1987), and ICD-10 (WHO 1990). The criteria are presented in two forms:

1. For each specific diagnosis a list of variables is presented, indicating which variables (e.g., symptoms, signs, time criteria, etc.) a real patient must have and must not have in order to receive this diagnosis.
2. There is a list of optional variables, of which a certain number are required for the diagnosis, without stating which ones.

The presently existing new diagnostic systems are a combination of both 1 and 2. These criteria define the diagnoses more exactly than previously, and single diagnostic groups are more homogeneous; many patients who in ICD-8/-9 have had a specific diagnosis fall into a remaining group.

The WHO has also joined the development toward criteria-based diagnostics; ICD-10 is copying DSM diagnostics in its formal structure and in headline terminology, but unfortunately there are many differences among the definitions of individual diagnoses.

Along with these developments, standardized and structured diagnostic interviews for each individual diagnostic system were created, e.g., SADS (Schedule for Affective Disorders and Schizophrenia) for RDC (Spitzer and Endicott 1985), SCID (Structured Clinical Interview for DSM-III-R (Spitzer et al. 1987), and in preparation SCAN (Schedules for Clinical Assessment in Neuropsychiatry) for ICD-10 (Wing et al. 1990). Standardized and structured interviews are supposed to reduce the variance in data collection compared with rating scales, which are mostly based on free interviews.

By introducing the criteria-based diagnostics of DSM-III in 1980 North American psychiatry left the rest of the World still committed to ICD. The worldwide coherence in diagnostic matters ended in 1980; French psychiatry always diagnosed patients by the national system of INSERM (1968), many research groups are diagnosing according to the Feighner criteria or RDC, and some countries are using ICD-8, and others ICD-9. At least eight different diagnostic systems are used in the world of psychiatry: ICD-8, -9 and in some projects -10; INSERM; Feighner; RDC; DSM-III; and DSM-III-R. For the mid-1990s the birth of DSM-IV is expected.

Most of these diagnostic systems of today — perhaps combined with their respective standardized interviews — are certainly better operationalized, quantified and standardized than the clinical diagnoses at the time of the classical schools of psychiatry which were dominant until the 1960s. Therefore it is not easy to dismiss the new systems as subjective isms.

Decades ago one was disconcerted by the noncomparability of psychiatric diagnoses and the ad libitum arbitrariness. One did everything to enhance their reliability. Methodologically one was very successful, even to the point that one created a great number of reliable diagnostic systems which did not agree with one other. The situation of today is the same as in the 1960s, only at a higher scientific level. It sometimes happens in the history of ideas that a principle, successfully and increasingly improved, becomes the very opposite. All endeavor to come to a better agreement by increasing reliability only has led to a worldwide dissent. Observing the operations with new diagnostic principles, one very often gets the impression that — by being obsessed with reliability — the notion of validity is lost.

Let me elaborate on this by discussing the diagnostics of schizophrenia and depression. French psychiatry (see Ey et al. 1967; Lemperière and Féline 1977) as well as "the old" Kraepelin (1909 -1915) diagnosed schizophrenia only if a chronic deterioration of personality could be observed. Schizophrenia-like psychoses without this personality change were given another diagnostic label. This is a strict concept. DSM-III took over this concept by defining "...with some signs of the illness at present."

In DSM-III-R this statement is again omitted; but the duration criterion of a 1/2 year is still preserved (the symptoms of an active phase and residual or prodromal symptoms can be added up, in order to result in a 1/2 year). Contrary to these 6 months of DSM-III-R, ICD-10 requires only 1 month. These different time criteria result in the very frequent forms of schizophrenia with a course between 1 and 6 months being counted as schizophrenia by ICD-10, but not by DSM-III-R. This will lead to great disparities in frequency distributions and in therapeutic results for schizophrenic patients, because ICD-10 includes cases with phases of short duration (and therefore better therapeutic results), which are excluded by DSM-III-R diagnostics. There are no empirically validated arguments either for the 1 or for the 6 months criterion; rather it is an arbitrary decision by the members of WHO or APA diagnostic committees. In a therapy group of schizophrenics, the proportion of phasic, short-lasting schizophrenics (usually responding well to therapy) to chronic cases will be dramatically changed depending on the use of ICD-10 or DSM-III-R criteria, because DSM-III-R eliminates short-lasting cases from the diagnosis of schizophrenia. So we can expect that in a group of treated schizophrenics we will get better results if their diagnosis is made according to ICD-10.

For the diagnosis of the depressions, terms like "endogenous depression" and "neurotic depression" have been eliminated, because they are etiologically controversial and for controversial points pure description is recommended. All forms of affective disorder — except for organic and reactive depressions, of which the etiology is not controversial — are collected in one single section called "affective (mood) disorders." Subdivisions are made first by the severity of the disorder (e.g., "major depression" in DSM-III-R and "severe depression" in ICD-10); secondly, by whether there is only one single episode or a recurrent course or chronicity. Appearance of a manic episode (by itself or together with depression) enforces the diagnosis of a bipolar disorder. Among the chronic forms we will also find the personality disorder "cyclothymia" (alternating episodes of hypomania and subdepression with a chronic course). The subdivision of depressions according to severity is emphasized even more in ICD-10 by terms such as "mild," "moderate,"and "severe," than in DSM-III-R, which distinguishes only between "major depression" and "nonmajor depression." In ICD-10 there are 18 diagnoses for depression, in DSM-III-R "only" 14. ICD-10 and DSM-III-R also give different time criteria for the free interval between the phases of depression or within the chronic states of depression. Today if the same patients are diagnosed by different systems there will be a considerable shift from one diagnosis to another (Fig. 1).

Classical psychiatry has made great efforts to improve differential diagnoses by concepts such as "endogenous," "neurotic," and "reactive," which have been supported by different features of symptomatology, in the course, by the reaction to treatment, and by other variables of the individual diagnostic groups. DSM-III-R and ICD-10 have reduced these concepts to differences in severity and course (= time criteria) only.

Nowhere else in medical science and practice is differential diagnosis considered in this way. The diagnosis of poliomyelitis is not changed to another diagnosis in patients with severe paralysis of muscles compared with patients with only a certain weakness of muscles. In multiple sclerosis recovery of the symptoms or their subsistence does not require another diagnosis to be made. Carcinoma of the

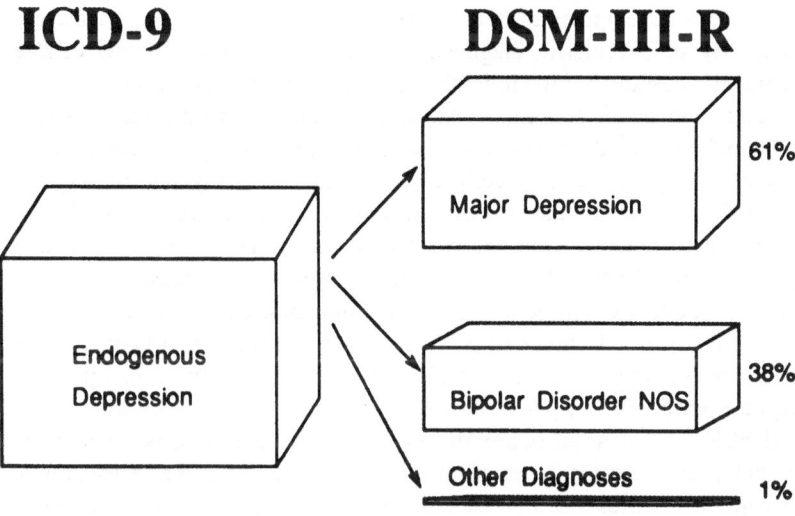

Fig. 1. The same patients, diagnosed by two different diagnostic systems (ICD-9 and DSM-III-R). (Hiller et al. 1988)

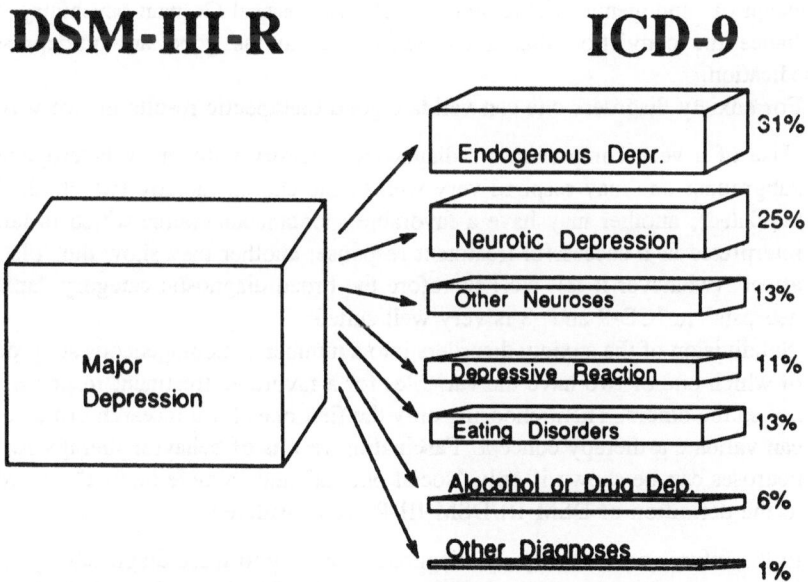

Fig. 2. The same patients, diagnosed by two different diagnostic systems (ICD-9 and DSM-III-R). (Hiller et al. 1988)

mamma with metastases, leading to an early death, does not lead to another diagnosis than the same carcinoma, operated upon successfully at the beginning and therefore resulting in no metastases.

All these developments in the recent years certainly have not increased the credibility of psychiatric diagnostics. Today there is worldwide difference in diagnostics despite the high reliability of methods and the substitution of etiological and etiopathogenetic concepts — however unsatisfactory they may be — by a kind of "cookbook" method with the idea that in the end by increasing reliability a psychiatric layman can also collect the elements for a psychiatric diagnosis.

The ability to manipulate research results by clever choice of statistical methods is supplemented today by an informed selection from the many existing diagnostic systems. There was a bestseller in the United States called *How to lie with statistics*. Soon we will be able to write a new bestseller *How to lie with psychiatric diagnostics*. A choice of possible arguments for such a book follows:

In order to support the hypothesis that schizophrenia has a bad prognosis and responds unsatisfactorily to treatment, one may diagnose schizophrenia according to INSERM whereas an ICD-9 diagnosis supports the opposite hypothesis (good prognosis and treatment response). To support the idea that a tranquilizer is a qualified antidepressant, one should diagnose depression using the term "major depression" (DSM-III-R and RDC) and improvement is demonstrated by a decrease in the Hamilton score (being very sensitive to changes in autonomic and other somatic symptomatology which — in all disorders — usually responds very well to tranquilizers; 24 points on the Hamilton scale out of a total of 63 points are based on somatic complaints). On the other hand diagnosing depression by the concept of "endogenous depression" (ICD and classical German psychiatry) will enhance the conviction that a tranquilizer is not as good an antidepressive medication.

For anxiety disorders one can validate good therapeutic results in two ways:

1. Use of a very comprehensive diagnostic category with many heterogeneous subgroups: one may respond very well to the chosen therapy (which shall be validated); another may have a favorable spontaneous course which is falsely interpreted as a successful treatment response; another may show the "placebo effect" (whatever it is), etc.; therefore the broad diagnostic category "anxiety neurosis" in ICD-9 and -8 is very well suited.
2. Subdivision of the anxiety disorders into a number of homogeneous subgroups, of which one or two have the variables for a favorable treatment response, but not so the others. Then, choosing only the first ones for a research project, one can validate a therapy concept. Fascinating results of behavior therapy for the neuroses can be shown if only "social phobia" and "simple phobia" according to the definition of DSM-III/DSM-III-R are considered.

In the future, one will have to diagnose according to these diagnostic systems. However, one should keep a critical mind and be able to see through the surface of all "make-beliefs," especially of scientific publications.

Many psychiatrists including the author have regarded concepts such as "endogenous, neurotic, and reactive" as not being satisfactory in the past, but many of the arbitrary descriptions offered today by the new diagnostic systems are even more unsatisfactory. Increasing reliability and better operationalisation are very important tools in the hands of experienced psychiatrists, but it is an illusion to think that by merely using these tools, an inexperienced beginner or layman will be able to make a valid psychiatric diagnosis.

Acknowledgements: Many coworkers of the Max Planck Institute of Psychiatry, Munich, took part in these new developments in diagnostics by writing and editing German translations, by evaluating rating scales, standardized and structured interviews, and new diagnostic systems, by preparing normative standards for German patients, by analyzing the diagnostic process, etc. We must mention especially: the Dept.of Adult Psychiatry under the guidance of Prof. von Zerssen, and in recent years the two groups of Psychiatric Evaluation Research under Prof. von Zerssen und Prof. Wittchen and the Psychiatric Outpatient Dept. under my guidance. Professor Ploog actively supported all these research projects by joining the very important and decision-making committees, sessions, meetings, etc., of the DGPN (German Society for Psychiatry and Neurology), of the association of German University professors, of the directors of German Mental Health Hospitals, and others.

References

American Psychiatric Association (APA) (1980) Diagnostic and Statistical Manual of Mental Disorders (Third Edition) DSM-III. APA, Washington DC

American Psychiatric Association (1987) Diagnostic and Statistical Manual of Mental Disorders (Third Edition Revised) DSM-III-R. APA, Washington DC

Ey H, Bernard P, Brisset Ch (1967) Manuel de Psychiatrie. Masson et Cie, Paris

Feighner JP, Robins E, Guze SB, Woodruff RA, Winokur G, Munoz R (1972) Diagnostic Criteria for Use in Psychiatric Research. Arch Gen Psychiat 26: 57-63

Hiller W, von Zerssen D, Mombour W, Wittchen HU (1986) Inpatient Multidimensional Psychiatric Scale (IMPS, deutsche Version). Manual und Testbögen. Beltz Test, Weinheim

Institut National de la Sante et la Recherche Medicale (INSERM); section psychiatrie (1968) Classification francaise des troubles mentaux. INSERM, Paris

Kraepelin E (1909-1915) Psychiatrie. 8. Aufl: Bd. I - IV. Barth, Leipzig

Lemperière Th, Féline A (1977) Psychiatrie de l'adulte. Masson, Paris New York Barcelone Milan

Möller HJ, von Zerssen D (1982) Psychopathometrische Verfahren: I. Allgemeiner Teil. Nervenarzt 53: 493-503

Möller HJ, von Zerssen D (1983) Psychopathometrische Verfahren: II. Standardisierte Beurteilungsverfahren. Nervenarzt 54: 1-16

Mombour W (1972) Verfahren zur Standardisierung des psychopathologischen Befundes. Teil 1: Psychiat Clin 5: 73-120; Teil 2: Psychiat Clin 5: 137-157

Mombour W (1974) Syndrome bei psychiatrischen Erkrankungen. Eine vergleichende Untersuchung mit Hilfe von zwei Schätzskalen für den psychopathologischen Befund (IMPS und AMP-Skala). Arch Psychiat Nervenkr 219: 331-350

Mombour W (1975) Klassifikation, Patientenstatistik, Register. In: Kisker KP, Meyer JE, Müller C, Strömgren E (Hrsg) Psychiatrie der Gegenwart, 2. Aufl: Bd. 3. Springer, Berlin Heidelberg New York.

Spitzer RL, Endicott J (1985) Schedule for Affective Disorders and Schizophrenia. Biometrics Research, New York State Psychiatric Institute. New York, USA

Spitzer RL, Endicott J, Robins E (1978) Research Diagnostic Criteria (RDC). Biometrics Research, New York State Psychiatric Institute. New York, USA

Spitzer RL, Williams JBW, Gibbon M (1987) Structured Clinical Interview for DSM-III-R. Biometrics Research, New York State Psychiatric Institute. New York, USA

Wing JK, Babor T, Brugha T, Burke J, Cooper JE, Giel R, Jablensky A, Regier D, Sartorius, N (1990) SCAN: Schedules for Clinical Assessment in Neuropsychiatry. Arch Gen Psychiat 47:589-593

World Health Organization (WHO) (1974) Glossary of Mental Disorders and Guide to their Classification. WHO, Geneva

World Health Organization (WHO) (1978) Mental Disorders: Glossary and Guide to their Classification in Accordance with the Ninth Revision of the International Classification of Diseases. WHO Geneva

World Health Organization (WHO) (1990) ICD-10. 1990 draft of Chapter V: Mental, Behavioural and Developmental Disorders. Revision 4. Clinical Descriptions and Guidelines. WHO Geneva [German translation: Dilling H, Mombour W, Schmidt MH (eds) (1991): Psychiatrische Klassifikation, klinisch-diagnostische Leitlinien. Huber, Bern]

17 Schizoaffective Psychosis: A Challenge to Kraepelin's Paradigm?

M. Zaudig

Introduction

The existence of schizoaffective psychosis has for many decades been a matter of much discussion and controversy. This diagnostic category has been the focus of two basic psychopathological hypotheses: Kraepelin's *"Zweiteilungsprinzip"* (two-disease entity) and Jaspers' *"Schichtenregel"* (Jaspers 1973).

Kraepelin (1913) himself felt obliged to follow the medical concept of disease entity and attempted early on to derive the course of the illness from the cross-sectional/psychopathological status. He, thereby, adopted Kahlbaum's concept, who had as early as 1874 insisted that the course of a psychiatric illness should be the basis of the diagnostic classification. Kraepelin (1896) defined dementia praecox (schizophrenia) as a chronic, progressively deteriorating illness, and considered manic-depressive insanity (bipolar affective disorder) to run a periodic course with complete remissions. However, in 1913 Kraepelin had to agree to certain exceptions (with regard to his chronic versus phasic dichotomy): he described a subgroup within dementia praecox, which was evidently periodic, and called this group "periodic type of dementia praecox": "Earlier, I had accounted these types to manic-depressive insanity, without a doubt this illness may produce exacerbations of similarly short duration. Nevertheless, the above mentioned states of agitation, which within a short period of time repeat themselfs, seem to be part of a otherwise clearly to dementia praecox belonging course... these experiences made me change my opinion" (Kraepelin 1913).

In this group Kraepelin ranked longitudinal characteristics below the psycho-pathological cross-sectional profile. The description in his textbook undoubtedly implies a catatonic syndrome. In 1909 Zendig reported a study on 468 patients which had been admitted between 1904 and 1906 to a Munich psychiatric hospital with the diagnosis of dementia praecox: 30% of these patients were living at home, some of them worked, were socially adapted, and showed no signs of psychopathology. Zendig reasoned that these patients must have been falsely diagnosed, "mainly due to misinterpretations of the so-called catatonic syndrome" and attributed most of these cases to the manic-depressive category, mainly because a chronic course was absent. In contrast to Kraepelin, Zendig valued the course above the psychopathological profile (Zendig 1909).

In 1915 Kraepelin concluded that 12.5% of all improved patients with a diagnosis of dementia praecox could be adequately described as completely remitted. This number increased to 13.3% when he included all patients "which were able to live without difficulties within the society and who were able to support themselves." According to Kraepelin many of these patients had a catatonic syndrome.

In 1920 Kraepelin critically reviewed his *Zweiteilungsprinzip*: "We will have to get used to the idea that the typical symptoms will not under all circumstances provide for a reliable distinction between the manic-depressive insanity and the schizophrenias" (Kraepelin 1920). Too many disorders could not be subsumed under the dichotomy concept, and too many schizophrenias (Bleuler 1972) showed a phasic course with remissions without a residuum. All these syndromes constantly showed a marked affective symptomatology which, among many authors, gave rise to a most varied terminology, e.g., mixed psychosis, cycloid psychosis, good prognosis schizophrenia, intermediate psychosis, borderline psychosis *"Legierungspsychose,"* atypical psychosis (Perris 1974; Pull et al. 1983; Leonhard 1980). Currently the term "schizoaffective psychosis" is commonplace, which goes back to Kasanin (1933), who in 1933 coined the term; in his original essay he described nine cases with the following characteristics:

- Patients were aged between 20 and 30 years.
- Premorbid personality, and social and occupational functioning were appropriate to age and showed no difference to those of the average population.
- There was evidence of a clearly defined and specific psychosocial factor which precipitated the psychotic episode.
- Patients showed a dramatic onset with emotional turmoil, delusions, and a destroyed perception of reality.
- Symptomatology was mixed with affective and schizophrenic symptoms.
- The psychosis lasted an average of some weeks to months.
- The psychosis finally terminated with complete remission.
- There was a pronounced tendency to relapse.
- The psychosis usually first manifested itself during late adolescence.

As one reason for his exact description, Kasanin (1933) cited his quest for homogeneous diagnostic groups without which further psychiatric research would not lead to reliable results.

Many psychiatrists nowadays believe that schizoaffective psychoses are a variant of affective psychoses (Procci 1976), although this concept has so far not been fully accepted within the new classification systems — a good example is the first draft of the ICD-10 system from 1987. Originally (ICD-10, 1987 draft) the schizoaffective psychoses were subsumed under affective disorders; 1 year later in 1988 and 1989, a revised version was presented which again included schizoaffective psychosis within the group of schizophrenias. According to the presently much used classification system ICD-9, schizoaffective psychoses belong to the schizophrenias; according to DSM-III and DSM-III-R they run under the heading "psychotic disorders not elsewhere classified." Principally, there are several ways of classifying schizoaffective psychoses:

- As a subgroup of affective psychosis
- As a subgroup of schizophrenic psychosis
- As a third entity by themselves
- As proof for the theory of the unity psychosis

In order to distinguish schizoaffective psychosis reliably from schizophrenia and affective disorders we need clear distinctions with regard to clinical profile, course and therefore prognosis, hereditary factors, therapeutic response, and finally etiology and pathogenesis.

Diagnosis of Schizoaffective Psychosis

Most studies on schizoaffective disorders (Berner and Lenz 1986; Angst 1986; Marneros et al.1986 a,b) use a cross-sectional, syndromal approach based on the existence of various symptoms of schizophrenia, concurrent with depressive or manic symptoms. Currently, a cross-sectional-based diagnosis distinguishes between schizomanic or bipolar schizoaffective psychosis and schizodepressive psychosis. Schizomanic patients generally show similar characteristics to patients with bipolar affective disorders with regard to course, therapeutic response, and family background. These results were confirmed mostly by Brockington et al. (1980a,b) and Kendell(1986), but also by Marneros et al.(1986a,b, 1989), Möller et al. (1988), and Zaudig and Vogl (1991).

The group of schizodepressive patients show strikingly more heterogeneous results, at least according to studies by Brockington et al. (1980a,b) and Kendell (1986).

Changes in symptomatology in the longitudinal course have been sparsely investigated. Two of the few studies were undertaken by Angst (1986) and Marneros et al. (1986 a,b; 1988 a,b), who were able to show that patients with schizoaffective psychosis showed a course which would begin with a manic depressive symptomatology and terminate with schizophrenic symptoms, or vice versa. How then do syndromes during the course change, e.g., do they remain stable or — using a term by Marneros et al.(1986 a,b) — do they remain "monomorphic" constituting the same syndrome longitudinally or do they change into a variety of psychopathological syndromes which Marneros would describe as a "polymorphic" course? The results of the Cologne longitudinal study (Marneros et al. (1986 a,b) as well as our own results (Munich Follow-up Study) (MFS) (Wittchen und von Zerssen 1988; Zaudig and Vogl 1991) indicate that more than half of all patients belong to the "polymorphic" category, e.g.,recurrent episodes may present as purely schizophrenic, then again as purely affective or schizoaffective, schizomanic, schizodepressive, etc. The longitudinal studies by Kendell (1986), Marneros (1989, Marneros et al. (1990), Möller et al. (1987), and Zaudig and Vogl (1991) gave ample evidence that schizomanic syndromes tend to run a "monomorphic" course, e.g., the probability of a repeated recurrence of similar syndromes is very high. At the same time, patients with a schizomanic syndrome show the highest frequency of episodes. Schizodepressive patients run a "polymorphic" course much more often.

With the exception of ICD-10 (1989), there are no distinct criteria in other classification systems for the diagnosis of schizoaffective disorders according to the longitudinal course. ICD-10 requires for the diagnosis of, e.g., a schizomanic state a preponderance of schizomanic episodes; the same holds true for schizo-depressive patients. The diagnoses of schizoaffective psychosis, therefore, should strictly differentiate between cross-sectional and longitudinal diagnosis, if this is at all possible.

Schizoaffective Psychosis as Subgroup of Schizophrenias

Based on Jaspers' *Schichtenregel* (Jaspers 1973), many authors would rather attribute patients with a mixture of affective and schizophrenic symptoms to schizophrenia, which is still an integral part of the currently used classification system, e.g., ICD-9. Consecutively, affective symptomatology plays a nosological-ly more unspecific role when compared with the schizophrenic symptomatology, e.g., schizophrenic symptoms would in the absence of organic factors preclude an affective disorder. According to Kraepelin and his successors the diagnosis of schizophrenia or dementia praecox would demand a long-term course. Only one follow-up study (Welner et al. 1977) substantiated a long-term course, for instance the development of residual symptoms in patients with schizoaffective psychosis.

However, most longitudinal studies agree that schizoaffective psychosis runs a phasic course with complete remission. This again is in concordance with the results of many investigators pointing to the prognostic relevance of affective symptoms. Pope and Lipinski (1978) concluded in a very detailed survey of the literature that a good prognosis could be forecast depending on the number of affective symptoms, while so-called schizophrenic symptoms per se were not prognostically relevant. Based on this and many other studies schizoaffective psychoses in DSM-III (1980) were more or less subsumed under affective disorders or remained a "melting pot or ragbag category" lacking further definition.

At this point it may be useful to remember that the development of DSM-III (operationalized diagnosis in psychiatry) can be traced back primarily to the "invisible college" of the neo-Kraepelinians (Klerman 1983). Their paradigm is evident from a very conservative concept of schizophrenia as a chronic illness and from the broader concept of affective disorders with a primarily phasic course.

Schizoaffective Psychosis as a Variant of Affective Disorders

What favors the hypothesis that schizoaffective psychosis belongs to the category of affective disorders?

Most longitudinal studies including the MFS (Wittchen and von Zerssen 1988) indicate that the course of schizoaffective psychosis is phasic with free intervals and complete remission. Moreover, the occupational and psychosocial integration remains even after many years at a premorbid level; there is a good therapeutic response to prophylaxis with lithium and a sex ratio of 2:1 (female/male) — all these results indicate the similarity to the group of affective psychosis. Pope and Lipinski in 1980 pointed out that schizophrenic symptoms should be regarded rather as unspecific manifestations of the syndrome whereas affective symptomatology should be more relevant with regard to nosology and prognosis. Based on these results, the concept of affective disorders in DSM-III was broadened to include mood incongruent (parathymic) psychotic symptoms in addition to mood congruent (synthymic) psychotic characteristics. Schizoaffective psychosis remained a "ragbag category," not classified elsewhere.

Schizoaffective Psychosis as a Third Entity

Much has been written about schizoaffective psychosis (SAP) especially under the term "cycloid psychosis". Brockington's (Brockington and Leff 1979), Kendell's (1986), and our results (Zaudig et al. 1988; Zaudig 1990) as well as the studies of Angst (1989) and Marneros (1989) indicate that cycloid psychosis according to Leonhard (1980) and Perris and Brockington (1981) must be differentiated from the modern concept of schizoaffective psychosis.

Schizoaffective psychosis with its mixture of depressive or manic and schizophrenic symptoms runs a course with a less favorable outcome compared with affective psychosis; however, the outcome of schizoaffective psychosis is definitely more favorable than that of schizophrenia. Several studies on hereditary factors have so far not provided conclusive results: some authors found a higher incidence of affective disorders among first-degree relatives, while others found a higher incidence of schizophrenia. Few studies have shown much schizoaffective psychosis among first-degree relatives. The polymorphic course (Marneros et al. 1986b) could also indicate that we are dealing with a diagnostic group in its own right.

How Can the Results of the MFS 5- to 8-Year Follow-up Clarify the Problem of Schizoaffective Psychosis?

Within the frame of our 5- to 8-year follow-up (Wittchen and von Zerssen 1988) on 103 former inpatients of the Psychiatric Dept. of the Max-Planck Institute for Psychiatry, we have tried to contribute empirical data to the question of nosology of schizoaffective psychosis. Our patients belonged to the schizophrenic, schizoaffective or purely affective categories and were evaluated mainly on the basis of their course. Of a total of 29 patients with schizoaffective psychosis within the period 1973 - 1976, 22 patients could be followed up, 5 (17%) died from suicidal actions, and 95% showed a phasic course with complete remissions and absence of residual symptoms and with full rehabilitation to their premorbid level of functioning. The sex ratio of men to women was 1:2, and the age of the first manifestation of the disorder was 24 years (average). Typically, in 82% of our cases there was an acute onset. On admission, psychopathological symptoms were clearly described as dramatic, turbulent, and with much emotional expression, affective and psychotic symptoms were both present at the same time, often maximum doses of psychopharmacenties were needed, and usually patients improved rapidly and lastingly. At the time of the follow-up evaluation these patients overall showed very favorable social integration. More than 90% of our patients lived with a partner or were married, and 95% were unimpared in their professional performance in the year before, e.g., they were able to function at their premorbid level.

For the whole group of schizoaffective psychosis the average frequency of psychotic episodes during catamnesis (5 - 8 years) was 3.7 phases. Psychopathometric tests were applied on admission, discharge, and catamnesis (5 -8 years later) on a self- and third-party rating basis. The tests employed were the Inpatient Multidimensional Psychiatric Scale (Lorr et al. 1969) (IMPS), self-rating scales such as the paranoid-depressive scale (PDS), and the adjective complaint list (BS) by von Zerssen (1976).

Almost all IMPS factors were much improved at the time of discharge when compared with the admission ratings.

Interestingly, the factor "psychomotor disturbances (catatonic syndrome)" was positive in 95% of all schizoaffective patients at the time of admission and for most patients resulted in strongly pathological ratings. It is this factor which indicates a favorable prognosis with regard to the course. Meanwhile this has been increasingly substantiated in the literature, e.g., Taylor and Abrahams (1975); Huber et al. (1979); Angst (1980, 1986). As already mentioned, Kraepelin 1913 also, recognized the catatonic syndromes as an indicator for a periodic course, as did Zendig (1909) and Lange in 1922. As early as 1907 Wilmanns commented that catatonic symptomatology could not only be observed in schizophrenias but also in manic-depressive insanity. When comparing the group of schizoaffective psychosis with other types of psychosis, the IMPS factors disorientation and incoherence/thought disorder ranked highest within the group of schizoaffective psychosis. As we were able to show, these factors also point to a favorable prognosis.

When analyzing the self-rating scales a marked tendency towards improvement of the three factors (scales) between admission and discharge, and also during follow-up, is striking. At follow-up psychopathological symptomatology showed almost no difference to the standard values from the average population. The comprehensive evaluation of psychopathological symptoms and disturbances of psychosocial adaptation at follow-up on the Global Assessment Scale (GAS) (Spitzer et al. 1978) showed that 80% of our patients had reached a GAS score of over 60, indicating that these patients had none or only moderately pronounced symptoms and impairment. The mean score for all our patients was 77.6 and, therefore, resembles the score of patients with affective psychosis and is definitely higher than the score of schizophrenic patients.

At follow-up the type and course of psychopathological disturbances was evaluated; the longitudinal course was determined by means of cluster analysis. For schizoaffective patients three types emerged: 64% of our patients followed a "mild course" with an average recurrence frequency of episodes of 1.9 during follow-up; 32% were of the "phasic type" with an average recurrence frequency of episodes of 5.57. Only one patient suffered from a chronic and severe course and phasic changes could not be found. In this case the investigator later diagnosed chronic schizophrenia.

In view of the multifactorial character of psychiatric disorders in addition to the cross-sectional psychopathological profile and the cluster analysis for the course, we employed three more criteria with reference to psychosocial adaptation: level of occupational functioning, ability to lead an independent life-style, and the GAS score, which were all summarized into an overall outcome score. Possible ratings were favorable, intermediate, and unfavorable. Under this aspect of a global outcome rating, 45.5% of our patients had a favorable outcome, 31.8% had an intermediate outcome, and 22.7% showed an unfavorable outcome. In comparison with both other diagnostic groups schizoaffective disorders ranked in between!

Of major importance for every follow-up study is the prognostic evaluation of relevant indices with regard to course and prognosis. A good prognosis refers to clinical course and social rehabilitation. Factors indicating a favorable prognosis were found to be: acute onset, stable relationship, female sex, and older age at first manifestation. Factors predicting an unfavorable course were: insufficient improvement at discharge, prolonged average duration of the index phase, divorce before index admission, and insidious onset of the disorder.

Among the psychopathological items at admission time some were of prognostic relevance: The IMPS factor "psychomotor disturbance" (catatonic disturbance) correlated highly significantly with a favorable course. Also favorable at admission were the following IMPS factors: irritability, incoherence/formal thought disorder. Which of the MFS results indicate that schizoaffective patients belong to the group of affective psychosis? A phasic course, repeated complete remission or lack of residual symptomatology, rehabilitation to the premorbid level of functioning, a certain sex ratio, a relatively high rate of suicide (17%), a high percentage of patients with a lasting (stable) relationship — all these factors indicate a close similarity of our patients to the group of affective psychosis.

Schizoaffective Psychosis as a Subgroup of Schizophrenia?

Similarities to schizophrenic psychosis are seen mainly in the clinical profile (Shenton et al.1987), whereby schizoaffective psychosis generally leads to a marked expression of psychotic symptoms, of psychomotor or catatonic symptoms, and of confusion, perplexity, and formal thought disorder. Moreover, the age at first manifestation of the illness, which averages 24 years, may indicate a similarity to schizophrenia.

Schizoaffective Psychosis as a Separate Diagnostic Entity?

The global outcome profile of our study indicated that schizoaffective psychosis occupies an intermediate status with more similarities to affective psychosis. The psychopathological profile was often a mixture between schizophrenic and affective symptoms and could also not clearly be attributed to schizophrenic or affective psychosis. It is this heterogeneity of the psychopathological profile and the polymorphic characteristics of the course (at times clearly schizophrenic, at other times schizodepressive, schizomanic, etc.) which seem typical for schizoaffective psychosis.

Conclusion

From all this we can conclude that the schizoaffective psychosis group should occupy an intermediate status between schizophrenic and affective psychosis with regard to symptomatology, course, and prognosis (Sauer 1990; Janzarik 1980). However, SAP seems to be closer to the group of affective psychosis and cannot be clearly attributed to one of the main groups. In agreement with the most important catamnestic studies of other authors, e.g., Angst (1986, 1989); Brockington et al.al (1980a,b); Kendell (1986); Marneros et al. (1986a, 1989), we have to assume that schizoaffective disorders occupy an intermediate status between affective disorders and schizophrenic psychosis, with regard to course, outcome, occupational level of functioning, and psychosocial rehabilitation. They should therefore — in spite of the nosological confusion — currently be treated as a separate group. Their nosological classification remains a challenge for future research.

References

American Psychiatric Association (1980) Diagnostic and statistical manual, DSM-III. Am Psychiatr Assoc, Washington

American Psychiatric Association (1987) Diagnostic and statistical manual, revised, DSM-III-R. Am Psychiatr Assoc, Washington

American Psychiatric Association (1989) Diagnostisches und Statistisches Manual psychischer Störungen — DSM-III-R, edited by Wittchen HU, Saß H, Zaudig M, Koehler K Beltz, Weinheim, p 500

Angst J (1980) Verlauf unipolar depressiver, bipolar manisch-depressiver und schizoaffektiver Erkrankungen und Psychosen. Fortschr Neurol Psychiatr 48: 3-30

Angst J (1986) The course of schizoaffective disorders. In: Marneros A, Tsuang NT (eds) Schizoaffective psychoses. Springer, Berlin Heidelberg New York Tokyo, pp 63-93

Angst J (1989) Der Verlauf schizoaffektiver Psychosen. In: Marneros A (ed) Schizoaffektive Psychosen. Springer, Berlin Heidelberg New York, pp 46-54

Berner P, Lenz G (1986) Definitions of schizoaffective psychoses. Mutual concordance and relationship to schizophrenia and affective disorder. In: Marneros A, Tsuang N T (eds) Schizoaffective psychoses. Springer, Berlin Heidelberg New York Tokyo, pp 31-49

Bleuler M (1972) Die schizophrenen Geistesstörungen im Lichte langjähriger Kranken- und Familiengeschichten. Thieme, Stuttgart

Brockington IF, Leff J P (1979) Schizoaffective psychosis: definitions and incidence. Psychol Med 9: 91-99

Brockington IF, Kendell RE, Wainwright S (1980a) Depressed patients with schizophrenic or paranoid symptoms. Psychol Med 10: 665-675

Brockington IF, Wainwright S, Kendell RE (1980b) Manic patients with schizophrenic or paranoid symptoms. Psychol Med 10: 73-83

Ciompi L, Müller C (1976) Lebensweg und Alter der Schizophrenen. Eine katamnestische Langzeitstudie bis ins Senium. (Monographien aus dem Gesamtgebiete der Psychiatrie, vol 12) Springer, Berlin Heidelberg New York

Feighner J P, Robins E, Guze S B, Woodruff R A, Winokur G, Munoz R (1972) Diagnostic criteria for use in psychiatric research. Arch Gen Psychiatr 26: 57-63

Huber, G., Gross G., Schüttler, R (1979) Schizophrenie. Springer, Berlin Heidelberg, New York

Janzarik B (1980) Der schizoaffektive Zwischenbereich und die Lehre von den primären und sekundären Seelenstörungen. Nervenarzt 51: 272-279

Jaspers K (1973) Allgemeine Psychopathologie, (9th edn). Springer, Berlin Heidelberg New York

Kahlbaum J (1874) Die Katatonie oder das Spannungsirresein. Eine klinische Form psychischer Krankheit, klinische Abhandlungen über psychische Krankheiten, vol 1. Hirschwald, Berlin

Kasanin J (1933) The acute schizoaffective psychosis. Am J Psychiatr 90: 97-126

Kendell RE (1986) The relationship of schizoaffective illness   to schizophrenic and affective disorders. In: Marneros A, Tsuang MT (eds) Schizoaffective psychoses. Springer, Berlin Heidelberg New York Tokyo

Klerman G L (1983) The significance of DSM-III in american psychiatry. In: Spitzer R, Williams E B W, Skodol A E (eds) International perspectives on DSM-III. American Psychiatric, Washington

Kraepelin E (1913) Psychiatrie: ein Lehrbuch für Studierende und Ärzte, 8th edn. Barth, Leipzig

Kraepelin E (1920) Die Erscheinungsformen des Irreseins. Z Gesamte Neurol Psychiatr 62: 1-29

Lorr M, Klett CJ (1967) Manual for the inpatient multidimensional psychiatric scale, Consulting Psychologists Press, Palo Alto

Lange, J (1972) Katatonische Erscheinungen im Rahmen manischer Erkrankungen. Springer, Berlin (Monographien aus dem Gesamtgebiet der Neurologie und Psychiatrie, Vol 31)

Langfeldt G (1937) The prognosis in schizophrenia and the factors influencing the course of the disease. Acta Psychiatr Scand Suppl 13: 1-128

Leonhard K (1980) Aufteilung der endogenen Psychosen. Akademieverlag, Berlin

Marneros A, Deister A, Rhode A (1986a) The Cologne study on schizoaffective disorders and schizophrenia suspecta. In: Marneros A, Tsuang N T (eds) Schizoaffective psychoses. Springer, Berlin Heidelberg New York Tokyo

Marneros A, Rohde A, Deister A, Risse A (1986b) Schizoaffective disorders. The prognostic value of the affective component. In: Marneros A, Tsuang N T (eds) Schizoaffective psychoses. Springer, Berlin Heidelberg New York Tokyo

Marneros A, Deister A, Rhode A, Jünemann H, Fimmers R (1988a) Longterm course of schizoaffective disorders. Definitions, methods, frequency of episodes and cycles. Eur Arch Psychiatry Neurol Sci 237: 264-275

Marneros A, Rhode A, Deister A, Jünemann H (1988b) Syndrome shift in longterm course of schizoaffective disorders. Eur Arch Psychiatry Neurol Sci 238: 97-104

Marneros A (1989)   Diagnose, Therapie und Prophylaxe. In: Marneros A (ed) Schizoaffektive Psychosen. Springer, Berlin Heidelberg New York London Paris Tokio Hong Kong

Marneros A, Rhode A, Deister A, Steinmeyer E N (1990) Behinderung und Residuum bei schizoaffektiven Psychosen Daten, methodische Probleme und Hinweise für zukünftige Forschung. Fortschr Neurol Psychiatr 58: 66-75

Möller H J, von Zerssen D (1986) Der Verlauf schizophrener Psychosen unter den gegenwärtigen Behandlungsbedingungen. Springer, Berlin Heidelberg New York Tokyo

Möller H J, Schmid-Bode W, Cording-Tömmel C, Wittchen H U, Zaudig M, von Zerssen D (1988) Psychopathological and social outcome in schizophrenia versus affective/schizoaffective psychoses and prediction of pure outcome in schizophrenia. Acta Psychiatr Scand 77: 379-389

Perris C (1974) Cycloid psychosis. Acta Psychiatr Scand Suppl 253: 7-77

Perris C, Brockington J F (1981) Cycloid disorders and their relation to the major psychoses. In: Perris C (ed) Biological psychiatry. Elsevier, Amsterdam, pp 447-450

Pope H G, Lipinski J F, Cohen B M, Axelrod D T (1980) Schizoaffective disorder: an invalid diagnosis? A comparison of schizoaffective disorder, schizophrenia and affective disorder. Am J Psychiatry 137: 921-927

Procci W R (1976) Schizoaffective psychosis: fact or fiction? Arch Gen Psychiatry 33: 1167-1178

Pull C B, Pull M C, Pichot P (1983) Nosological position of schizoaffective psychoses in France. Psychiatr Clin 16: 141-148

Sauer H (1990) Die nosologische Stellung schizoaffektiver Psychosen. Problematik und empirische Befunde. Nervenarzt 61: 3-15

Shenton M E, Sollovay M R, Holzman P (1987) Comparative studies of thought disorders. II. Schizoaffective disorder. Arch Gen Psychiatry 44: 21-30

Spitzer R, Endicott J, Robins E (1978) Research diagnostic criteria: rationale and reliability. Arch Gen Psychiatry 35: 773-782

Strömgren E (1986) Reactive (psychogenic) psychoses and variations to schizoaffective psychoses. In: Marneros A, Tsuang N T (eds) Schizoaffective psychoses. Springer, Berlin Heidelberg New York Tokyo

Taylor, MA, Abrams K (1975) Manic-depressive illness and good prognosis schizophrenia. Am J Psychiatr 132 : 741-742

Vogl G, Zaudig M (1985) Investigation of operationalized diagnostic criteria in the diagnosis of schizoaffective and cycloid psychoses. Compr Psychiatry 26: 1-10

Welner A, Croughan J L, Robins E (1974) The schizoaffective and related psychoses — critique, records follow-up and family studies. I. Persistent enigma. Arch Gen Psychiatry 31: 628-631

Wilmans K (1907) Zur Differentialdiagnostik der "funktionellen" Psychosen. Zentralbl Nervenheilk Psychiatr V F 18: 569-588

Wittchen H U, von Zerssen D (1988) Verläufe behandelter und unbehandelter Depressionen und Angststörungen. Springer, Berlin Heidelberg New York Paris Tokyo

World Health Organization (ICD 9) (1980) Mental disorders. Glossary and guide to their classification in accordance with the 9th revision of the international classification of diseases. In: Degkwitz R, Helmchen H, Kockott G, Mombour W (eds) Diagnosenschlüssel und Glossar psychiatrischer Krankheiten, (5th edn). Springer, Berlin Heidelberg New York

World Health Organization (ICD 10) (1989) Mental, behavioural and developmental disorders: clinical descriptions and diagnostic guidelines WHO, Geneva

Zaudig M (1990) Cycloid psychoses and schizoaffective psychoses — a comparison of different diagnostic classifications, systems and criteria. Psychopathology 23: 233-242

Zaudig M, Vogl G (1983) Zur Frage der operationalisierten Diagnostik schizoaffektiver und cycloider Psychosen. Arch Psychiatr Nervenkr 233: 385-396

Zaudig M, von Cranach M, Wittchen H U, Semler G, Steinböck H (1988) Schizoaffective psychosis: an examination of its historical and present status. An empirical study. In: Mezzich J, von Cranach M (eds) International classification in psychiatry: unity and diversity. Cambridge University Press, Cambridge, pp 122-134

Zaudig M, von Bose M, Weber M N, Bremer S, Ziegelgängsberger B (1989) Psychotoxic effects of ofloxacin. Pharmacopsychiatry 22:11-15

Zaudig M, Stieglitz R D, Gastpar M, Rösinger C (1990) Mood (affective) and schizoaffective disorders (section F3) results of the ICD-10 field trial. Pharmacopsychiatry [Suppl] 23:160-164

Zaudig M, Vogl G (1991) Schizoaffektive Psychosen. Hippokrates, Stuttgart

Zendig (1909) Beiträge zur Differentialdiagnose des manisch-depressiven Irreseins und der Dementia praecox. Allg Z Psychiatrie 66: 47-49

Zerbin-Rüdin E (1986) Schizoaffective and other atypical psychoses: the genetical aspect. In: Marneros A, Tsuang NT (eds) Schizoaffective psychoses. Springer, Berlin Heidelberg New York, pp 225-231

Zerssen von D, Keller D M (1976) Klinische Selbstbeurteilungsskalen KSB-S aus dem Münchner psychiatrischen Informationssystem (Psychis) Manual. Beltz, Weinheim

18 The Concept of Comorbidity in Psychiatry and Its Influence on Research of Risk Factors

T. Bronisch

Introduction

Comorbidity refers to the joint occurrence of two illnesses. Its use originated in general medicine and medical epidemiology (Feinstein 1970). Applied to mental disorders, the term refers to the joint occurrence of two or more mental disorders and/or with medical conditions. Comorbidity can take place during an episode of illness for the individual; within the lifetime of an individual; and among members of larger groups, such as patients, the general population, and families (Klerman 1990).

Two recent developments in the classification of psychiatric disorders and in the assessment of psychopathology promoted the application of the concept of comorbidity to psychiatry:

The first development refers to the introduction of semi-standardized interviews (Present State Examination, PSE, Wing et al. 1974; Structured Clinical Interview for DSM-III diagnoses, SCID, Spitzer et al. 1986) and standardized interviews (Schedule of Affective Disorders and Schizophrenia, SADS, Endicott and Spitzer 1978; Diagnostic Interview Schedule, DIS, Robins et al. 1981) for the assessment of symptoms. With the help of computerized algorithms symptoms can be combined into syndromes and psychiatric diagnoses.

The second development refers to the omission of the hierarchical classification of psychiatric diagnoses originally proposed by K. Jaspers (1913), the so-called *Jaspers'sche Schichtenregel*, and still clinically used in ICD-8 (WHO 1965) and in ICD-9 (WHO 1979). This omission took place in North America with the introduction of DSM-III (APA 1980) and DSM-III-R (APA 1987), which have in the meantime also been widely used in Europe for research. In DSM-III, and more pronouncedly in DSM-III-R, the hierarchy of psychiatric diagnoses is replaced by the possibility of making more than one diagnosis without a certain rank order.

Two epidemiological studies, one with a semistandardized interview for the assessment of psychiatric syndromes according to ICD-9 (Sturt 1981) and one with a standardized interview for the assessment of psychiatric disorders according to DSM-III (Boyd et al. 1984), found a general tendency toward co-occurrence with regard to syndromes (Sturt 1981) and to diagnoses (Boyd et al. 1984): the presence of any syndrome/disorder increased the odds of having almost any other syndrome/disorder. The authors concluded that empirical studies are needed to study the assumptions underlying the use of a hierarchy of syndromes as well as of diagnoses.

In this article, I refer to an empirical investigation of risk factors which could be responsible for the development of comorbidity of mainly anxiety disorders in patients with a major depression.

Subjects

The patients were selected from a sample of inpatients who had been admitted consecutively for treatment to the Crisis Intervention Ward of the Max-Planck Institute of Psychiatry (MPIP) during 1983 and 1984 ($N=670$). Of this sample, 165 patients met the ICD-9 diagnosis of a brief or prolonged depressive reaction lasting no longer than 3 months. Only patients older than 20 years with German as their first language and with a stay of at least 5 days for a rigorous assessment were included in the study. A total of 76 patients were examined.

These 76 patients had been assessed by a standardized diagnostic interview (DIS, Robins et al. 1981) for assessment of DSM-III diagnoses.
According to DIS/DSM-III, four groups emerged:

1. Major depressions with comorbidity ($N=25$)
2. Major depressions without comorbidity ($N=22$)
3. Adjustment disorders with depressed mood ($N=22$), i.e., the depressed mood did not last long enough, and/or the number of depressive symptoms was not sufficient to meet the criteria for the diagnosis of a major depression
4. Other diagnoses

Results are related to the 25 patients with major depression with comorbidity (MDC) and 22 patients without an additional co-existing DSM-III diagnosis (pure major depression, PMD).

Patients with MDC were given the following cross-sectional DSM-III diagnoses besides a major depression. Of the 25 patients, 3 reported a panic disorder, 12 agoraphobia, 9 a simple phobia, 4 an obsessive compulsive disorder, and 5 also a somatization disorder as lifetime diagnoses. Twelve (48%) had more than one additional diagnosis. Both groups are comparable regarding age of onset (PMD: $x=29.0$, SD$=9.3$; MDC: $x=25.7$, SD$=8.5$), duration of the longest depressive episode (PMD: $x=26.1$ weeks, SD$=38.0$; MDC: $x=41.0$, SD$=60.1$), and the frequency of depressive episodes before the index manifestation (PMD: $x=3.0$, SD$=2.7$; MDC: $x=3.6$, SD$=3.9$). Additionally, the course of depressive symptoms during index treatment, assessed by self and observers' rating scales, was not significantly different between PMD and MDC. Twelve patients reported that the anxiety disorder had begun before the depressive disorder, six patients reported that the depressive disorder preceded the anxiety disorder, and two patients reported that the beginning of the depressive disorder and panic disorder had coincided.

Control Group

Because the availability of specific social roles depends on sex and life stage, the patients were compared with (mentally healthy) matched control subjects with regard to sex and age in analyses of the social variables. The data of the control groups were taken from a representative general population sample (the Munich Follow-up Study, MFS; see Wittchen and von Zerssen 1988), which had been examined with the same instruments (DIS, SIS).

Study Instruments

Psychiatric Diagnoses

DSM-III diagnoses were assessed on the 3rd day (or 4th day in the case of a weekend) after admission with the Diagnostic Interview Schedule (DIS, Version II, Robins et al. 1981; German version, Wittchen and Rupp 1982). The test-retest and the interrater reliabilities of the DIS can be regarded as being sufficiently high (Semler and Wittchen 1983).

Social Functioning and Social Support

In order to evaluate the kind and degree of social impairment, the German version of the Social Interview Schedule (SIS; Clare and Cairns 1978; Hecht et al. 1987; Hecht and Wittchen 1988) was applied. The SIS assesses the subject's social situation and covers 13 social role areas (e.g., work, children) in three "dimensions," namely, objective social conditions (O), management of social difficulties (M), and satisfaction with social roles (S). In contrast to the first two dimensions, the third dimension (S) is rated by the patient him- or herself. The ratings for each category are evaluated according to a 4-point scale on which (1) is equivalent to no restrictions/no difficulties/very satisfied and (4) to severe restrictions/severe difficulties/very dissatisfied. On the basis of empirically derived results, cutoff scores are defined for objective social restrictions, social dysfunction, and dissatisfaction (for each role area). Additional items allow the construction of two social support indices which are comparable to the indices defined by Surtees (1980). "Close social support" comprises the quality and number of close ties (confiding relationship other than partner, contact with close relatives, living group), and "diffuse social support" the quality and amount of superficial contacts (contact with colleagues, contact with neighbors, contact through attendance at clubs/associations/church). High global scores indicate a lack of social support. The SIS is a cross-sectional instrument assessing the level of social functioning and social support during the previous 4 weeks. The interrater reliability of the SIS can be judged to be sufficiently high (Faltermaier et al. 1985).

Personality Features

Personality features were assessed with the Munich Personality Test (MPT, von Zerssen et al. 1988). This self-rating test consists of 51 items, representing 6 dimensions that are based upon several factor analytical studies. The scales are labeled: Extraversion, Neuroticism, Frustration Tolerance, Rigidity, Isolation Tendency, and Esoteric Tendencies. In addition, an orientation toward social norms in a subject's attitude to self-evaluation and/or possibly also to real life is measured with a six-item "lie" scale and the motivation for adequate performance in a three-item test. The corresponding scales of the MPT self-rating and relative rating versions are significantly correlated with each other ($r=0.30$-0.50). Most of the scale values are not markedly affected by the depressive state: the scores of patients with a major depression at the index admission but without a major depression at follow-up, 4-6 years later, are highly correlated (Extraversion, 0.83; Rigidity, 0.67; Frustration Tolerance, 0.61; Esoteric Tendencies, 0.60; Isolation Tendency, 0.55). Only the coefficient for the Neuroticism scale is lower (0.37) (Bronisch and Hecht 1989, 1990).

Statistical Procedures

For statistical analysis, the chi-square, Fischer's exact test, and the Mann-Whitney U-test with a correction for ties (if necessary) were used.

Results

Sociodemographic Characteristics

Table 1 shows the sociodemographic characteristics of patients with PMD and MDC. There are significant differences between PMD and MDC mainly with regard to sex distribution. The MDC group consists nearly exclusively of females, but in the PMD group females are also overrepresented. Furthermore, 52% of the MDC group were never married, whereas only 23% of the PMD group married, but this difference is not statistically significant.

Table 1. Sociodemographic characteristics of patients with pure major depression (PMD) and major depression with comorbidity (MDC)

	PMD (N=22)		MDC (N=25)	
Age x SD (years)	36.7	10.8	32.4	7.5
Sex Male	7	32%	2	8%
Female	15	68%	23	92%
Marital status				
Never married	5	23%	13	52%
Married	12	55%	8	32%
Divorced	1	5%	3	12%
Separated	4	18%	1	4%
Occuptional status				
Employed (full time\ half time)	15	68%	19	76%
Prematurely retired	1	5%	-	-
In training	1	5%	2	8%
Housewife	3	14%	4	16%
Unemployed	2	9%	-	-
Other status	-	-	-	-
Social class[a]				
Upper class	4	18%	5	20%
Middle class	9	41%	11	44%
Lower class	9	41%	9	36%

[a] According to Moore and Kleining (1960)

Social Functioning and Social Support

Table 2 compares the PMD and MDC groups as well as both patient groups with the age- and sex-matched control groups. With regard to "objective social conditions," there were no differences between PMD and MDC groups or between the patient groups and the control groups. With "social dysfunctions" and "satisfaction," there were no differences between patient groups, but both patient groups had significantly more social dysfunction and were more dissatisfied than their control groups. The direct comparison of "close" and "diffuse social support" between the PMD and MDC groups reveals less "close social support" in terms of less confidants for MDC. However, neither patient group differed from the respective control group.

Table 2. Objective social conditions, social dysfunctions, satisfaction, and social support prior to index admission (medians)

	MDC	Controls	PMD	Controls
Objective conditions	1.45	1.45	1.57	1.44
Social dysfunctions	2.11	1.44	2.12	1.38
Satisfaction	2.64	1.89	2.42	1.90
Close social support	5.00	4.00	2.50	4.00 *
Diffuse social support	1.00	1.00	1.00	2.00

* MDC vs. PMD: $p < 0.05$

Premorbid Personality Features

Figure 1 shows the personality features of the MPT of both patient groups, demonstrated by boxplots. Patients with MDC reported more frequently the personality features Neuroticism and Isolation Tendency than patients with PMD. There was a tendency toward more Extraversion in PMD patients than with MDC patients, but this was not statistically significant.

Discussion

The introduction of the concept of comorbidity in psychiatry facilitates the investigation of risk factors predisposing to multiple psychiatric disorders such as depressive and anxiety disorders. Summarizing the differences between patients with PMD and MDC in sociodemographic characteristics, social functioning, social support, and premorbid personality features, MDC patients are more conspicuous in terms of the personality features of Neuroticism and Isolation Tendency, and are less extroverted than PMD patients. MDC patients are more often never married and have less close social support in terms of fewer confidants than PMD patients which both point to the isolation tendency of MDC patients. Therefore, MDC patients display personality traits such as Neuroticism, Introversion, and Isolation Tendency, which point to a "neurotic personality" of MDC patients in comparison with PMD patients.

There are two hypotheses for the more pronounced "neurotic personality traits" in patients with a concurrence of multiple psychiatric disorders such as Major Depression and anxiety disorders when compared with a pure Major Depression:

1. Since the onset of anxiety disorders was mostly prior to the onset of depressive disorders in our sample (see also Robins et al. 1984; Wittchen et al. 1988), anxiety could alter the personality and/or alter the perception of the patient's

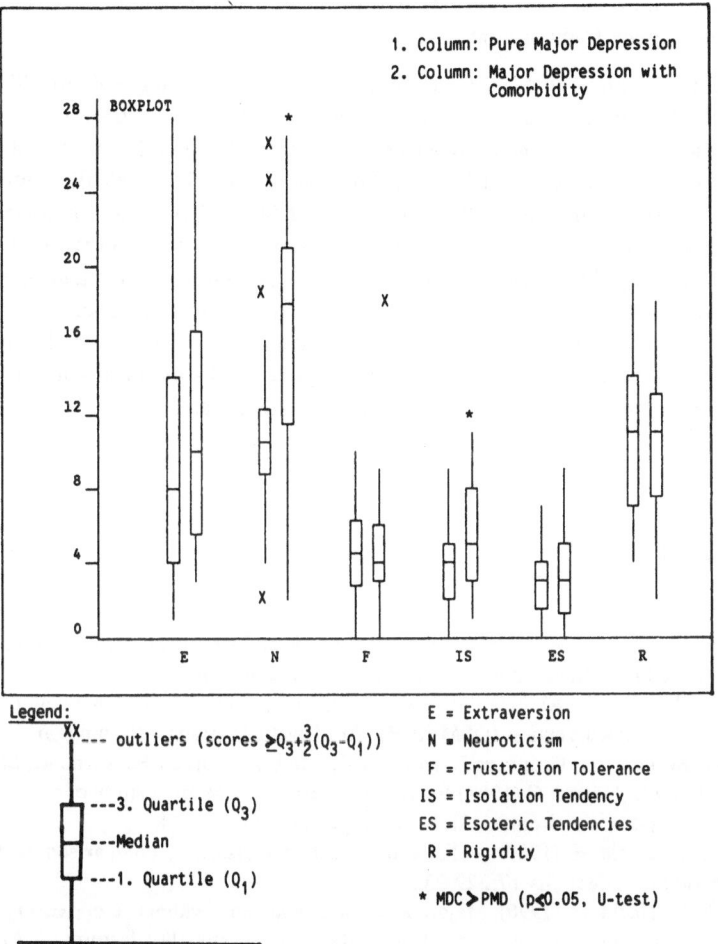

Fig. 1. Personality features of both patient groups, measured by the Munich Personality Test (MPT)

own personality. However, there is only some empirical evidence that a depressive disorder alters the perception of the personality (Hirschfeld et al. 1983), but so far no empirical evidence has existed for such an effect of anxiety disorders. Additionally, the MPT is not a state-dependent instrument, and the course before the assessment of the personality as well as the severity of the depression during the assessment of the personality were comparable between PMD and MDC.

2. Multiple psychiatric disorders such as anxiety and depressive disorders are consequences of a vulnerable personality in terms of a personality with neurotic traits. This hypothesis was initially introduced to genetic research by Slater and Slater (1944), and later backed by Eysenck (1947). However, the authors had

different opinions about the putative gene-environment interactions as well as modes of gene transmission.

Personality features such as Neuroticism, Introversion, and Isolation Tendency could also be closely connected with personality features and personality disorders within the families of patients suffering from depressive disorders with and without comorbidity of anxiety disorders. Leckman et al. (1983), VanValkenburg et al. (1984), and Coryell et al. (1988) investigated familial patterns of anxiety and depression in first-degree relatives of major depressives with and without comorbidity of anxiety disorders, but did not assess personality features and personality disorders in the patient groups as well as in their families. Therefore, further family and genetic studies looking at the transmission of anxiety and depression in families of patients with anxiety and/or depressive disorders should include the assessment of personality traits and personality disorders.

References

American Psychiatric Association (1980) Diagnostic and statistical manual. Mental disorders, 3rd edn. DSM-III. Am Psychiatr Assoc, Washington
American Psychiatric Association (1987) Diagnostic and statistical manual of mental disorders. Revised version (DSM-III-R). Am Psychiatr Assoc, Washington
Boyd JH, Burke jr JD, Grünberg E, Holzer CE, Rae DS, George LK, Karno M, Stoltzman R, McEvoy L, Nestadt G (1984) Exclusion criteria of DSM-III: a study of co-occurrence of hierarchy-free syndromes. Arch Gen Psychiatry 41:983-988
Bronisch T, Hecht H (1989) Validity of adjustment disorder, comparison with major depression. J Affect Dis 17:229-236
Bronisch T, Hecht H (1990) Major depression with and without a coexisting anxiety disorder: social dysfunction, social integration, and personality features. J Affect Dis 20:151-157
Clare A, Cairns V (1978) Design, development and use of a standardized interview to assess social maladjustment and dysfunction in community studies. Psychol Med 8:589--604
Coryell W, Endicott J, Andreasen NC, Keller MB, Clayton PJ, Hirschfeld RMA, Scheftner WA, Winokur G (1988) Depression and panic attacks: the significance of overlap as reflected in follow-up and family study data. Am J Psychiatry 145:293-300
Endicott J, Spitzer RL (1978) A diagnostic interview. The schedule for affective disorders and schizophrenia. Arch Gen Psychiatry 35:837-844
Eysenck HJ (1947) Dimensions of personality. Routledge & Kegan Paul, London
Faltermaier T, Wittchen H-U, Ellmann R, Lässle R (1985) The social interview schedule (SIS) — content, structure and reliability. Soc Psychiatry 20:115-124
Feinstein AR (1970) The pre-therapeutic classification of comorbidity in chronic disease. J Chron Dis 21:455-468
Hecht H, Faltermaier T, Wittchen H-U (1987) Social interview schedule (SIS). Ein Verfahren zur Beschreibung sozialer und sozialpsychologischer Faktoren der Lebenssituation. Roderer, Regensburg

Hecht H, Wittchen H-U (1988) The frequency of social dysfunction in a general population sample and in patients with mental disorders: a comparison using the social interview schedule (SIS). Soc Psychiatry Psychiatr Epidemiol 23:17-29

Hirschfeld RMA, Klermann GL, Clayton PJ, Keller MB, McDonald-Scott P, Larkin BH (1983) Assessing personality: effects of the depressive state on trait measurement. Am J Psychiatry 140:695-699

Klerman GL (1990) Approaches to the phenomena of co-morbidity. In: Mases JD, Cloninger CR (eds) Co-morbidity of mood and anxiety disorders. American Psychiatric, Washington, DC, pp 13-37

Leckman JF, Weissman MM, Merikangas KR, Pauls DL, Prusoff BA (1983) Panic disorder and major depression. Increased risk of depression, alcoholism, panic, and phobic disorders in families of depressed probands with panic disorder. Arch Gen Psychiatry 40:1055-1060

Moore H, Kleining G (1960) Das soziale Selbstbild der Gesellschaftsschichten in Deutschland. Kölner Z Soziol Sozialpsychol 12:86-119

Robins LN, Helzer JE, Croughan J, Ratcliff KS (1981) National Institute of Mental Health, Diagnostic Interview Schedule: its history, characteristics and validity. Arch Gen Psychiatry 38:381-389

Robins LN, Helzer JE, Weissman MM, Orvaschel H, Gruenberg E, Burke JD, Regier DA (1984) Lifetime prevalence of specific psychiatric disorders in three sites. Arch Gen Psychiatry 41:949-958

Semler G, Wittchen H-U (1983) Das Diagnostik-Interview-Schedule. Erste Ergebnisse zur Reliabilität und differentiellen Validität der deutschen Fassung. In: Kommer D, Röhrle B (eds) Gemeindepsychologische Perspektiven 3. GwG, Cologne. DGVT, Tübingen, pp 109-117

Slater E, Slater P (1944) A heuristic theory of neurosis. J Neurol Psychiatry 7:49-55

Spitzer RL, Williams JB, Gibbon M (1986) Structured Clinical Interview for DSM-III-R patient version (SCID-P, 8/1/86). Biometric Research Department, New York State Psychiatric Institute, New York

Sturt E (1981) Hierarchical patterns in the distribution of psychiatric symptoms. Psychol Med 11:783-794

Surtees PG (1980) Social support, residual adversity and depressive outcome. Soc Psychiatry 15:71-80

VanValkenburg C, Akiskal HS, Puzantian V, Rosenthal T (1984) Anxious depressions: clinical family history, and naturalistic outcome-comparisons with panic and major depressive disorders. J Affective Disorders 6:67-82

Von Zerssen D, Pfister H, Köller D-M (1988) The Munich Personality Test (MPT): a short questionnaire for self-rating and relatives' rating of personality traits: formal properties and clinical potential. Eur Arch Psychiatr Neurol Sci 238:73-93

Wing JK, Cooper JE, Sartorius N (1974) Measurement and classification of psychiatric symptoms. Cambridge University Press, Cambridge

Wittchen H-U, Hecht H, Zaudig M, Vogl G, Semler G, Pfister H (1988) Häufigkeit und Schwere psychischer Störungen in der Bevölkerung Eine epidemiologische Feldstudie. In: Wittchen H-U, von Zerssen D (eds) Verläufe behandelter und unbehandelter Depressionen und Angststörungen. Springer, Berlin, Heidelberg, New York, pp 232-251

Wittchen H-U, Rupp H-U (1982) Diagnostic interview schedule. Dt.Version II. Max-Planck Institut für Psychiatrie (unpublished data)

Wittchen H-U, von Zerssen D (1988) Verläufe behandelter und unbehandelter Depressionen und Angststörungen. Springer, Berlin, Heidelberg, New York

World Health Organization (WHO) (1965) Manual of the international statistical classification of diseases, injuries and causes of death. Sect 5, 8th rev. World Health Organization, Geneva

World Health Organization (WHO) (1979) Manual of the international statistical classification of diseases, injuries and causes of death. Sect 5, 9th rev. World Health Organization, Geneva

19 Results of Inpatient Treatment of Alcoholics: Follow-ups After 18 and 48 Months [Munich Evaluation of Alcoholism Treatment, MEAT]*

W. Feuerlein, H. Küfner

Central Aims

The central aims of the study were to find out:

1. What are the overall results of treatment for alcoholism?
2. What patient variables does outcome depend on?
3. What treatment variables are favorable for the outcome?

Description

The study can be characterized as:

- A multicenter study
- A prospective panel study
- A field, not an experimental study
- Outcome research, rather than process research
- A study taking an empirical, pragmatic approach, without
  any closed theory behind it

This multicenter study involved 1410 consecutively admitted alcoholics (73% of them men) with an average age of 39 years (range 17-66, SD 8.5 years) in 21 treatment units which can be considered to be representative of the residential treatment in the Federal Republic of Germany (including West Berlin). The representativeness of the sample of centers selected out of the roughly 220 then existing can be described as "typical." The following aspects were considered: length of treatment (short term, 6-8 weeks; medium term, 4-5 months; long term, 6 months), selection of patients, type of treatment program, size of center, regional distribution, sponsor organization.

In this study, started in 1980, patient data were collected at five different times: at the patient's admission for treatment, at discharge, and 6, 18, and 48 months

* The project was carried out in cooperation with and funded by the Federation of German Pension Insurance Institutions, Frankfurt/M.

after discharge. At the follow-ups, the intention was to assess every patient by means of personal interview and mailed questionnaire or vice versa. Patients who did not answer the mailed follow-up questionnaire or refused to fill them out were visited by an interviewer for a "substitute interview." The interviews were carried out by specially trained persons not members of the treatment staff. All interviewers were recruited and worked locally. There were also some cases in which the patient gave written forms each time.

The refusal rate was 18% (range, 0%-50%). A comparison carried out (in the center having the extreme refusal rate) between an anonymous, unselected sample and the original sample showed no significant differences in the prognosis index.

The outcome was assessed with reference to alcohol and drug consumption, social integration, physical health, and personality using the *Freiburger Persönlich-keits-Inventar* (Freiburg Personality Inventory) (FPI) (Fahrenberg et al. 1973) and the *Unsicherheits-Fragebogen* (U-Fb) (Self-Assertiveness Questionnaire) (Ullrich-de Muynck and Ullrich 1977). Life events were estimated by self-ratings (cf. Holmes and Rahe 1967), the global psychophysical condition by the *Beschwerden-Liste* (Complaints List) (von Zerssen 1967).

For characterization of the alcohol consumption drinking was divided into three rough categories:

1. Totally abstinent
2. Improved [less than 60/30 g alcohol/day (male/female), no signs of physical or psychic consequences of alcohol abuse or of any pathological element in their drinking patterns (that is to say "controlled drinking")]
3. Unimproved: all other cases

For the 48-month follow-up we set up four different classifications of drinking behavior. Classifications 1-3 covered the total follow-up period and classification 4 covered only the last 6 months prior to 48-month follow-up:

Classification 1: abstinent versus relapsed (in the whole follow-up period)
Classification 2: abstinent, improved, unimproved according to the strict criteria of 6 and 18 months follow-up
Classification 3: abstinent, improved, unimproved, but with the category improved defined in less strict terms: either: abstinent after a relapse period of at most 1 month and no inpatient treatment due to alcohol or: "social drinking": no signs of pathological drinking and no inpatient treatment due to alcohol abuse
Classification 4: abstinent, improved, unimproved in the sense of classification 2 (but only covering the previous 6 months)

In addition, data were collected from health insurance and pension insurance institutions concerning periods of sick leave taken, days of inpatient treatment, and granting of pensions.

The data concerning the variables of the treatment units were acquired by means of semistructured interviews. The main variables were length of treatment (short-term, 6-8 weeks; medium-term, 4-5 months; long-term, 6 months), size, staffing, methods of treatment (e.g., individual therapy, group therapy, therapeutic community, involvement of the partners, etc.), general orientation (e.g., behavior therapy versus psychodynamic orientation), admission criteria, and source of referral, altogether about 150 variables. There was a broad consensus as to the goal of the treatment: in none of the units was controlled drinking regarded as a goal.

Assessment of the Validity and Reliability of the Data

We tried to assess reliability and validity of the data by using various approaches:

1. A comparison between the patients' data given at the three follow-ups. In cases of discrepant data the unfavorable data were employed for further analysis.
2. A comparison of patients' data relating to particular issues with other sources of information (e.g., inpatient treatment during follow-up, comparison with the data from the pension insurance institutions).
3. A comparison of data provided by the patient with the personal impression of the interviewer during the interviews (recorded in nearly all interviews and for some of the patients with partial data).
4. A comparison of the reports given by family members and/or significant others (i.e., relatives) with the patients' data (available in 41 cases).
5. A comparison of the outcome data from the health insurance and pension insurance companies regarding days sick leave and days in inpatient treatment.
6. A comparison of the original data at the 48-month follow-up with an additional control interview. Ninety-three patients from the 48-month follow-up were involved in this. This subgroup proved to be comparable with the original sample as to sex distribution and prognosis index (see below). The following hypotheses could be confirmed:
   - Global data are more consistent than more detailed data.
   - Data concerning a particular time window are more reliable the closer their time window to the follow-up time.
   - There are no major discrepancies between written versus interview follow-ups or phone versus personal interviews.

Findings at the 18-Month Follow-up

The response (including 2.5% patients with partial data) was 84% out of the original 1410 patients. During the 18 months 37 (3%) died. (The data from those who died were excluded from this and the other follow-up evaluations.)

There were no appreciable changes in marital status in comparison to the time of admission. Seventeen percent are unemployed now, whereas at admission this figure was 23%. There was a trend toward social stabilization with respect to home life, partners, and work.

After exclusion of discrepant data, 53% (55% of the males, 47% of the females) remain as the rate of total abstinence over the whole 18-month period; this is 17% less than at the 6-month follow-up. Improvement was seen in 8.5% (9% of the males, 8% of the females), whereas 38% (39% of the males and 44.5% of the females) had not improved. Taking account of only the previous 6 months, 63% of the patients were abstinent, nearly as many as the 67% at the 6-month follow-up. For patients with at least one previous period of treatment in an addiction treatment center,the rate of abstinence was noticeably lower: 39% at the 18-month follow-up.

Of the alcohol-abstinent patients, 3% had been taking sleeping pills, painkillers, tranquillizers, or stimulants regularly for several months. According to the information from the patients, consumption of illegal drugs was extraordinarily low, the most frequently used being hashish (1.5% occasionally or regularly).

Patients with a secondary ICD diagnosis of abuse of medicaments did not have a lower rate of abstinence than those with no secondary did not have a lower rate of abstinence than those with no secondary abuse. By contrast, those with a secondary diagnosis of medicament or drug dependence had a lower rate of abstinence (45% alcohol abstinent, 27 % abstinent from alcohol and medicaments/drugs).

The FPI indicated that the trend toward normalization, first noticeable at the discharge interview, was continuing. The only raised value of the U-Fb was on the scale "being able to make demands." The mean score on the Complaints List was lower than at the 6-month follow-up: 15.7.

Findings at the 48-Month Follow-up

Complete or partial follow-up data could be obtained from 1068 patients (81% of the original sample minus 92 dead). An overview on the drinking behavior of the two follow-ups is given in Table 1.

During the whole follow-up period the overall abstinence rate was 46% (48.5% of the men, 41% of the women). Twelve percent had improved (11% of the men, 13% of the women) and 42% had not improved (40% of the men, 46% of the women), according to the less strict terms of classification 3.

Looking only at the previous 6 months prior to the data collection, we found 66% (males 65%, females 70%) abstinent, 4% (4% males and 2% females) improved, and 30% (31% males and 28% females) unimproved (according to the strict terms of classification 2). Of the patients who dropped out during the index treatment, only 23% were abstinent during the whole follow-up period (vs 46% of the whole sample). It should in addition be remembered that only 62% of these patients could be traced in the 48-month follow-up (vs. 81% of the whole sample).

Table 1. Drinking behavior in the three follow-up periods

		18 months n = 1118	48 months n = 1057
Abstinent		53.2%	46.4%
Improved	(class 2)	8.5%	2.6%
	(class 3)		11.9%
Unimproved	(class 2)	38.3%	51.0%
	(class 3)		41.7%

Patients who had to repeat the inpatient treatment during the whole follow-up period had a significantly worse outcome than patients without such treatment: the abstinence rate (previous 6 months) was only 35% (vs 73% of the patients without repeated treatment).

Forty-three percent of the patients abstained from all kinds of addictive substances (alcohol, misuse of medicaments, illegal drugs) for the whole follow-up period. Thirty-three (7%) of the alcohol abstinent patients regularly consumed addictive substances of various kinds, i.e., 3% of the whole sample.

In comparison to the situation at admission the proportion of patients who were single, married, and living alone decreased slightly: the number of divorcees rose from 17.5% to 24%. The number of patients living together with their parents decreased from 11% to 6%.

The *working situation* continued to improve (on average). During the whole follow-up period the number of unemployed persons decreased by 8% (contrasting with the increasing unemployment rates in the country in general). Now 15% of the patients are unemployed. However, about 25% of the unemployed had been continuously out of work for 4 years.

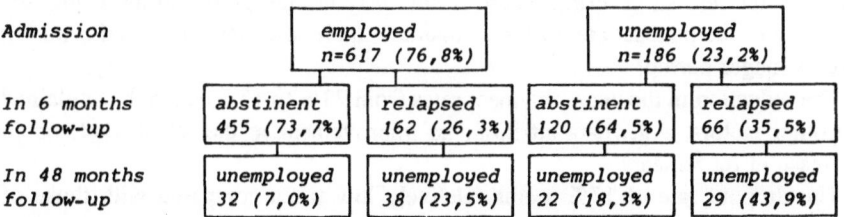

Fig. 1 Relationship between work situation and abstinence: 6-month and 48-month follow-up

A clear influence of the abstinence on the rate of unemployment could be shown. Only 7% of the patients employed at admission and abstinent at the 6-month follow-up were unemployed at the 48-month follow-up, whereas 23.5% of the employed (at admission) and relapsed (at the 6-month follow-up) patients were unemployed at the 48-month follow-up.

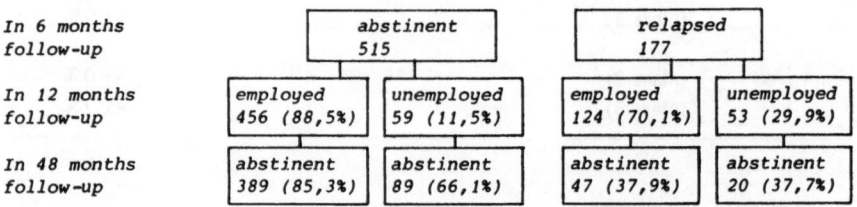

Fig.2 Relationship between abstinence and work situation: 6-month and 48-month follow-up

Unemployment became a risk factor mainly in abstinent patients: in abstinent patients (6-month follow-up) the abstinence rate after 48 months was 85% in employed patients, but only 66% in unemployed patients. In relapsed patients no influence of unemployment could be demonstrated.

In comparison to the 18-month follow-up the proportion of (selected) complaints showed only small changes, i.e., the positive development after the index treatment proved to be stable. The data of the personality tests (FPI, U-Fb) indicate a similar situation.

The abstinence rates of 53% at the 18-month and 46% at the 48-month follow-up are high in comparison to those in the international literature (e.g., Emrick 1974, 34% abstinent; Polich 1980, 7% abstinent; for overview see Hoellen and Hoellen 1985). In comparison to other German-speaking studies (e.g., Keup 1985; Klein 1981; Koester et al. 1981; Krampen 1986; Scheller and Klein 1982, Watzl 1986), the abstinence rates of this study are about average. The number of "improved" patients is relatively small: 8.5% at the 18-month follow-up. At the 48-month follow-up the rate was 3% (according to the strict term) and 12% (according to the less strict term). These results may be interpreted to mean that the majority of the patients are unable to maintain their so-called controlled drinking over a longer period.

The reduction in the unemployment rates from 23% to 15% cannot be explained by other factors, e.g., data attrition, an improvement in the job market, or an increase in retirements.

The dropout rate of 17% seems relatively low when compared with those of other studies (e.g., Keup: 24%). The differences between dropout rates in the various centers of this study are great (range, 4.5% - 32%). Dropping out of treatment is generally regarded as a treatment failure: the abstinence rate of dropouts was 30%, in comparison to the 57% of patients who completed their treatment (18-month follow-up).

Data from Health Insurance and Pension Insurance Institutions

In the 18-month follow-up the insurance institutions were asked for information on a random sample ($n= 297$) of the patients, stratified according to the length of treatment. We obtained data on 65% of these cases.

The average overall number of days sick leave went down from 118 days in the 18-month period prior to the index treatment to 43 days in the 18-month period after discharge. This reduction of 64% can mainly be attributed to the drastic fall in absences caused probably or possibly by alcohol-related conditions. Similarly, the proportion of days in inpatient treatment decreased from 34.7 days prior to index treatment to 14.6 days after discharge. Patients who abstained from alcohol and those who relapsed differ significantly on number of days sick leave (34 vs. 47 days).

In the 48-month follow-up we tried to include all the patients in a survey of their days on sick leave and in inpatient treatment. Sixty-three percent of the patients concerned agreed to let us ask the insurance institutions for information. Thus data on 651 patients were obtained. The data cover the periods 2 years prior to and after the index treatment as well as the period 2 years prior to the collection of the data of the 48-month follow-up.

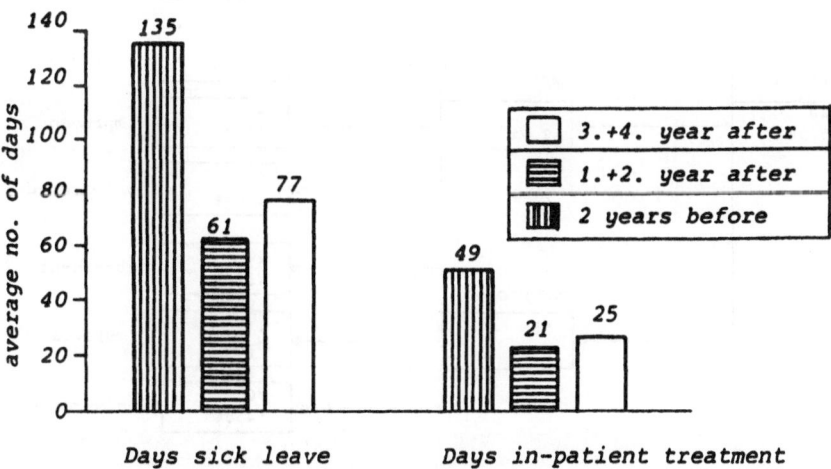

Fig.3 Average days sick leave and inpatient treatment (2 years before treatment, during the 1st and 2nd year and 3rd and 4th year after treatment)

Altogether the number of patients without sick leave time increased considerably during the periods after treatment. As a consequence, there was a marked reduction in the mean values of sick leave taken: by 55% (from 135 to 61) during the first 2-year period and by 43% (from 135 to 77) during the second 2-year period (each compared with the period prior to index treatment). This reduction prevails in patients probably or possibly suffering from alcohol-related conditions. There was a similar decrease in the number of days in inpatient treatment (from 49 to 21 or 25). The reduction of the mean values was 58% during the first 2-year period and 48% during the second 2-year period, the greatest effect being seen in connection with probably or possibly alcohol-related conditions. The reduction in number of days on sick leave and on inpatient treatment depends on the drinking behavior after index treatment. Although there was also a slight reduction among relapsed patients (e.g., sick leave probably alcohol- related conditions: 71.7 vs 51.5 days), this reduction was much greater in abstinent patients (73 vs 7.5 days).

Data were provided on 60 patients receiving pensions, of whom 55% were 50 years of age or less. For 19 patients alcoholism was indicated as the reason for the pension being given; in three other cases carcinoma of the upper digestive tract was specified which can probably be attributed to the alcohol abuse.

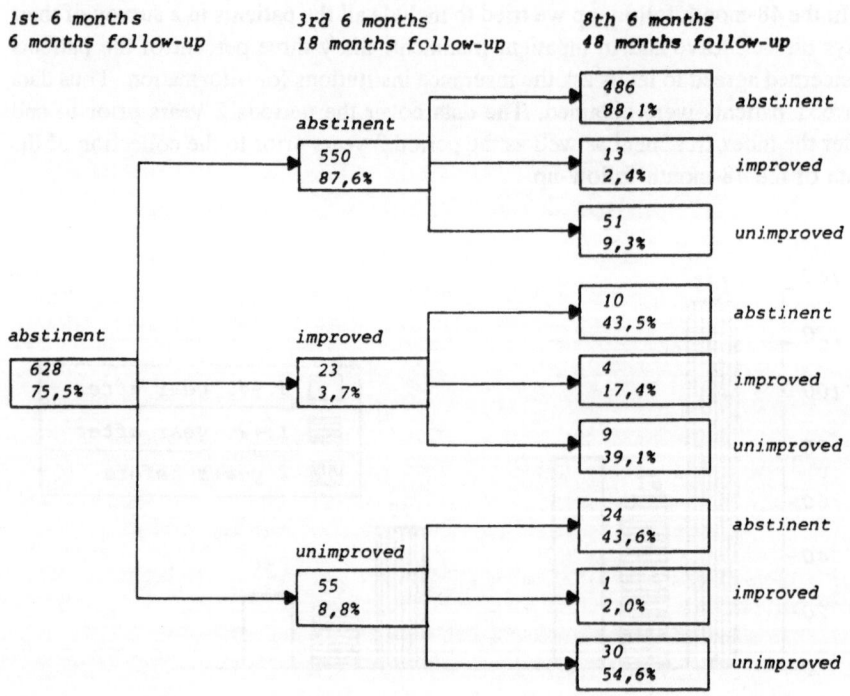

Fig.4 Course over time of drinking behavior: abstinent patients in 6-month follow-up (n=832)

Changes in Drinking Behavior over the Course of the Study

Of the patients who were abstinent ($n = 628$) in the first 6 months, 77% continued to be so to the end of the 18-month and 48-month period. Fourteen percent were classified as "unimproved" and 3% as "improved" in the 48-month follow-up (previous 6 months).

Of the 130 patients who were classified as "unimproved" in the 6-month follow-up, 52% continued to be so during the whole follow-up period. At the time of the 48-month follow-up (previous 6 months), 31.5% were classified as abstinent and 2% as improved.

The group of "improved" patients ($n = 74$) seemed to be the least stable. Only two (3%) continued to be "improved" during the whole follow-up period. At the 48-month follow-up (previous 6 months) 7% could be identified as "improved," whereas 38% were found to be "abstinent" and 55% "unimproved," It may thus be concluded that only a rather small percentage of patients are able to maintain their "controlled drinking" over a long time.

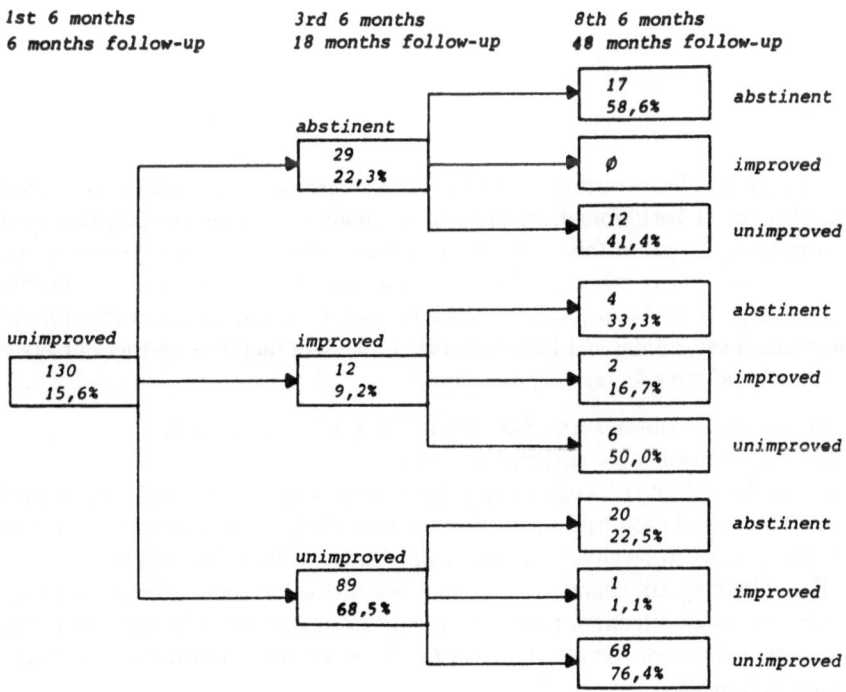

Fig.5 Course over time of drinking behavior: unimproved patients in 6-month follow-up ($n=832$)

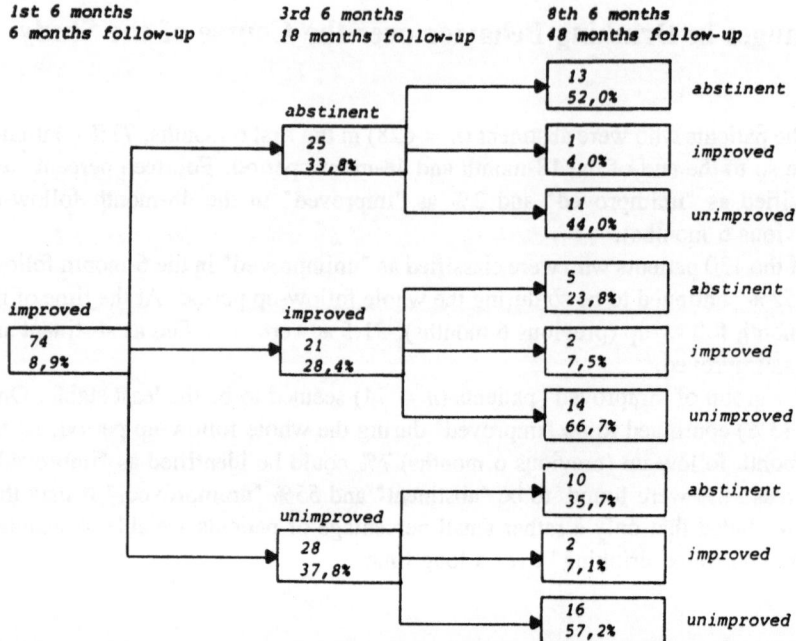

Fig.6 Course over time of drinking behavior: improved patient in 6 month follow-up (n=832)

Prognosis

The prognosis of the treatment may depend upon patient characteristics (e.g., age and sex, social background, severity of alcoholism) as well as upon treatment factors (e.g., length of treatment, details of treatment). Assessment of the prognosis involves many other problems we have tried to take into account, mainly methodological problems, which cannot be discussed here in detail (for further information see Küfner and Feuerlein 1989). We will therefore restrict ourselves to some basic remarks on the procedure:

- All patient variables were taken as possible prognostic variables.
- Men and women were analyzed separately.
- To test the stability of a relationship the study population was randomly divided into halves and each half analyzed separately. Only if the relationship in both halves proved to be significant was a prognostic relationship assumed.
- The following six characteristics were selected as outcome criteria: drinking behavior, work situation, partner relationship, satisfaction with work and with partner, subjective complaints. Data on these criteria were available from the three follow-ups.

Patient Variables as Prognostic Factors

For setting up the prognosis factors we used only the abstinence rate as the outcome criterion. The prognostic relationships could only be examined under the conditions of the inpatient treatment studied here. It is possible that different prognostic factors may arise from different treatment forms. Our central problem was to develop a search strategy for prognostic factors or combinations of such factors. A simple method is summarizing the selected predictors (prognosis index). Its correlation with abstinence can nevertheless be regarded as more than moderate: $r = .29$ for men, $r = .28$ for women (on the basis of the 18-month follow-up). When factors from the discharge interview are included and with optimum weighting in a multiple regression analysis, the correlation was: $r = .4$.

The following variables indicated a more favorable prognosis:

In men:
- Living with spouse
- Home town population smaller than 100 000
- Only one place of work in the previous 2 years
- Not unemployed
- Home owner
- Not living in a hostel or homeless
- Never lost a job because of alcohol
- No history of suicide attempts
- No previous treatment in an addiction unit

In women:
- Less than two suicide attempts
- No previous treatment in an addiction unit
- Less than 625 g pure alcohol drunk per week
- Low score on U-Fb scale: "being able to make demands"
- High score on U-Fb scale: "social decency"

The prognostic factors were combined in to prognostic indices by summation (divided into three levels). The scores of the prognosis index for men have a range from 0 - 9 points (Cronbach's α, 0.61), and the scores of the prognosis index for women have a range of 0 - 5 points (Cronbach's α, 0.31).

In men the relationships between the prognosis index (divided into three levels) and abstinence rates are different. In men with the poorest prognosis (score 0-3) the abstinence rate is 31 %; in those with the best prognosis (score 7-9) it is 69 %, i.e., a difference of 38 %. The difference between the men with the poorest prognosis and the men with a moderate prognosis (score 4-6) is 15 %, and that between the latter and those with a good prognosis 23 %. In women with the poor prognosis (score 0-1) the abstinence rate is very low (17 %); in women with the best prognosis (score 3-5) it is 60 %, the difference being 43 %. The difference between the poor and the moderate (score 2) prognosis group is 26%, and between the latter and the best prognosis group 17%.

The correlation coefficients for selected predictors with the other five outcome criteria ranged between .36 (satisfaction with partner relationship) and .64 (subjective complaints) for the men and between .13 (work situation) and .62 (subjective complaints) for the women.

Some new, prognostically unfavorable factors appeared at discharge:

Men:
- Dropping out
- Alcohol relapse during treatment
- Poor or doubtful clinical prognosis (assessed by the therapists)
- Low involvement (i.e., few hours) of significant persons

Women:
- Dropping out
- Low complaints list score (moderate score favorable!)

Using the outcome data from the 48-month follow-up, these prognostic factors and indices were reestablished. In men, all were confirmed. In women, only three of the five prognostic factors could be confirmed, in the remaining two a trend in the expected direction was found.

In addition to the abstinence several other outcome criteria were assessed: working situation, partner, satisfaction with the working situation and with the partner respectively, and complaint list. The highest correlations (at the 48-month follow-up) were found between the complaint list score and the patient variables (in men .62, in women .69). In other criteria there were substantial differences between male and female patients: working situation: .48 vs .18 and satisfaction with the partner: .33 vs. .12.

Showing good agreement with the literature (for reviews see Gibbs and Flanagan 1977; Küfner 1984), some markers of social stability proved to be favorable prognostic factors, but only for men. Occupational status and age were not relevant in our study. The latter did show a weak positive correlation with abstinence in the overall group, but did not meet the selection criteria for a prognostic factor. There were similar differences in the prognosis index: the older the patients, the higher the index. The conclusion which must be drawn from this is that the effect of age is probably due to the effect of the different prognostic factors.

Treatment Variables and Outcome

The effects of treatment variables are difficult to analyze, mainly because they are mixed up with the effects of patient variables.

Remarks on the Procedure. The units of analysis are now represented by the treatment centers. For controlling patient selection in the various treatment centers patients were divided into two subgroups (on the basis of the prognosis index): a negative prognosis group (scores men, 0-6; women, 0-2) and a positive prognosis group (scores men, 7-9; women, 3-5). For evaluation two strategies were carried out:

- Correlations between a center's treatment variables and its abstinence rate (strategy 1)
- Comparison of variables of the most successful and the least successful centers (strategy 2)

1. By means of the prognosis index homogeneous subgroups were established and abstinence rates in these subgroups of every treatment center were calculated. The relationship between treatment variables and abstinence rates was analyzed. Separate analysis for patients with positive and negative prognosis (in both strategies as mentioned above) showed that very different treatment variables were having a demonstrable effect in each group.
2. At the level of treatment centers the effect of treatment variables independent of patient variables was assessed by means of multiple regression analysis using the abstinence rates of the centers as dependent variables, and the prognosis index and selected treatment variables as independent variables. The results indicated the following: the prognosis index explains 37% of the variance of the abstinence rates. The selected treatment variables explain 63% of the abstinence rates of the centers. These two packages of variables taken together explain 73.2% of the variance of the abstinence rates of the centers. That means that 36% of the abstinence can be explained solely by the treatment variables.

The relationship between treatment variables and outcome is variously regarded in the literature. We may conclude that the inconsistency of results as to the effects of treatment variables is due to the heterogeneity of patient samples. In most studies, however, this interaction is not taken into account.

Results. The following variables were positively connected with the abstinence rate:

Treatment Variables (Positive Prognosis Group)
- Higher minimum age limit for admission (21 years)
- Regular individual therapy
- Broad spectrum of therapeutic techniques
- Therapeutic response to unpunctuality
- Flexible control for drugs sent in by post
- Intensive involvement of relatives

Treatment Variables (Negative Prognosis Group)
- Segregation of men and women
- Information and discussion groups for life planning
- Extended waiting list for admission

Treatment Variables (Whole Patient Group)
- Referral from counseling centers
- Extended waiting list
- No referrals from social welfare
- No part-time staff
- Segregation of men and women
- Physical therapy
- Relapse a ground for discharge

The effect sizes of these treatment variables are characterized by differences in the abstinence rates ranging between 7.7% and 15.9% (analyzed at the patient level).

Because of lack of sufficient variance there were some problems with several variables. If variables were very rare (e.g., acupuncture, offered only in one center) or very common (e.g., group therapy, sport), they could not be used to assess the relationship to outcome.

In the 48-month follow-up the treatment variables mentioned above were reconsidered on the basis of abstinence as an outcome criterion. The abstinence rates of the 21 treatment centers did not assimilate to each other after the 4-year period. On the contrary, the differences between the centers increased slightly (maximal difference 35.3% vs. 32.9% in the 18-month follow-up). As to the various treatment variables, in the negative prognosis group only one item (life planning groups) could be confirmed. In the positive prognosis group four out of five treatment items were confirmed: higher minimum age limit, regular individual therapy, flexible management regarding drugs sent in, intensive involvement of relatives. Three additional significant treatment variables (different for each of the prognostic subgroups) were identified. The item life planning was the only one that proved to be relevant for the two subgroups.

Length of treatment means lengths of scheduled (not actual) treatment. The effect of the length of the treatment (short-term, medium-term, long-term) as a variable of great practical significance was an object of particular interest. Neglecting differences in patient groups long-term treatment produced the highest abstinence rate, 60%, while medium-term treatment achieved 45% and short-term 54%. However, comparing the patients from the three lengths of treatment we found significant differences in the mean values of the prognosis index. The medium-term treatment had the highest percentage of patients with the poor prognosis. In males, 59% of the patients with the poor prognosis were allotted to medium-term treatment, but only 33% of the patients with the moderate prognosis and 18% of the patients with the best prognosis. In females, the situation was similar: 37% vs 22% vs 12% in the medium-term treatment. Therefore the abstinence rates of the three treatment lengths should not be compared unless the differences in the prognosis indices are controlled.

Regardless of the fact that the three different lengths of treatment have significantly different abstinence rates, the question of the comparability of their patient groups must be raised. Comparisons of prognosis indices and of numerous individual items show up clear variations in the patient selections of these three treatment lengths: the patients in medium-term centers are consistently those with the worst prognosis. In order to control the influence of this patient selection (which is likely, but is not to be specified) in the three treatment lengths we carried out several analyses. We could not show relationships between length of treatment and abstinence rate at every level. Only at the top (good prognosis) level was a positive effect of long-term treatment empirically verifiable.

Out of 27 studies in the literature regarding length of treatment (see Küfner 1984), 16 found positive effects of longer treatment, 9 found no difference, and 2 found negative effects. The often-cited finding of Orford and Edwards (1977), that a single individual counseling session is at least as effective as quite lengthy outpatient treatment (average 9.6 contacts), cannot be extended to inpatient treatment.

Summary

1. The percentage of alcoholics who were abstinent over 18 months and 48 months is relatively high: 53% and 46%, respectively.
2. The abstinence rate of the 6-month time windows prior to each follow-up (6 months, 18 months, 48 months) is almost invariable: about 66%.
3. The days of sick leave and inpatient treatment decreased considerably after the index treatment.
4. There is a relatively high percentage of patients who could be classified as abstinents in the last 6 months of the 48-month follow-up although they had to be classified as unimproved at the 18-month follow-up (22.5%).
5. Only 3% of all patients succeeded in controlled drinking over the period of 48 months.
6. The group of patients abstinent at the 6-month follow-up remained stable during the whole follow-up period: 88% at the 18-month and also 88% at the 48-month follow-up.
7. The effects of treatment can be demonstrated in different areas: besides the drinking behavior in the areas of occupation, partnership, and psychophysical condition.
8. Patients who had to repeat the inpatient treatment during the 48-month follow-up period had a significantly worse prognosis. However, even 35% of them succeeded in being abstinent at the last 6-month follow-up.

9. Patients who dropped out during treatment had a significantly worse prognosis (30% abstinent in dropouts vs.57% in completers).
10. There are significant interactions between unemployment and drinking behavior (in both directions).
11. There are considerable differences between the various treatment centers as to their abstinence rates (range 30% 65.5% at the 48-month follow-up).
12. There are remarkable differences between both sexes as to outcome (drinking behavior), prognosis, and indication factors.
13. The effects of treatment lengths depend on the patients' characeristics. There are remarkably large subgroups of patients who did better in short-term or medium-term treatment than in long-term treatment. However, the long-term treatment programs should not be given up totally since a considerable percentage of patients did best in this treatment.

Acknowledgements. It is impossible to list here all the persons who helped us carry out this study. Only some of these are mentioned. We thank:
- The Federation of German Pension Insurance Institutions (Verband Deutscher Rentenversicherungsträger) Frankfurt/Main for sponsorship and advice; particularly Dr. R. Buschmann-Steinhage, Dr. F. Kaufmann, PD Dr. M. Schuntermann, and Prof. Dr. H. Weber-Falkensammer.
- Dr.phil.habil. K. Antons, Büsingen, Dipl.-Psych. T. Flohrschütz, Gräfelfing, and M. Huber, Munich, for their substantial and effective help in planning, carrying out, and evaluating the study.
- Dr. E. Hansert and Dr. A. Yassouridis, Munich, and Prof. Dr. H. Wottawa, Bochum, for their advice on statistical problems.

References

Emrick CD (1974) A review of psychologically oriented treatment of alcoholism. I. The use and interrelationship of outcome criteria and drinking behavior following treatment. J Stud Alcohol 35:523-549
Emrick CD (1975) A review of psychologically oriented treatment of alcoholism. II. The relative effectiveness of different treatment approaches and the effectiveness of treatment versus no treatment. J Stud Alcohol 36:88-108
Fahrenberg I, Selg H, Hampel R (1973) Das Freiburger Persönlichkeitsinventar (FPI), 2.edn. Hogrefe, Göttingen
Gibbs L, Flanagan I (1977) Prognostic indicators of alcoholism treatment outcome. Int J Addict 12:1097-1141
Hoellen BM, Hoellen B (1985) Neue Ergebnisse der Alkoholismustherapie: Ein Überblick. Suchtgefahren 31:402-413
Holmes TH, Rahe RH (1967) The social adjustment rating scale. J Psychosom Res 11:213-218

Keup W (1985) Jahresstatistik 1983 der Fachkrankenhäuser für Suchtkranke (DOSY 83): Katamnesen. In: Ziegler H (ed) Jahrbuch 85 zur Frage der Suchtgefahren. Neuland, Hamburg

Klein KH (1981) Probleme bei Katamnesen von Alkoholiker- Therapie. Katamnestische Untersuchung in einer Fachklinik für Alkoholabhängige. Thesis. University of Freiburg

Koester W, Schneider R, Hachmann E, Mai N (1981) Dokumentation und Evaluation der stationären Behandlung von Alkohol- und Medikamentenabhängigen nach einem verhaltenstherapeutischen Programm. Beschreibung des Dokumentationssystems und Ergebnisse. Suchtgefahren 27:193-206

Krampen G (1986) Zum indikativen Wert handlungstheoretischer Persönlichkeitsvariablen für die Alkoholismusbehandlung. In: Ladewig D (ed) Drogen — Alkohol. Der aktuelle Stand in Behandlung Drogen- und Alkoholabhängiger. ISPA, Lausanne

Küfner H, Feuerlein W (1989) In-patient treatment for alcoholism. Springer, Berlin, Heidelberg, New York

Küfner H, Feuerlein W, Flohrschütz T (1986) Die stationäre Behandlung von Alkoholabhängigen: Merkmale von Patienten und Behandlungseinrichtungen, katamnestische Ergebnisse. Suchtgefahren 32:1-86

Küfner H, Feuerlein W, Huber M (1988) Die stationäre Behandlung von Alkoholabhängigen: Ergebnisse der 4-Jahreskatamnesen, mögliche Konsequenzen für Indikationsstellung und Behandlung. Suchtgefahren 34:157- 271

Orford J, Edwards G (1977) Alcoholism. Oxford University Press, Oxford

Polich JM, Armor DJ, Braiker HB (1980a) The course of alcoholism: four years after treatment. Rand, Santa Monica

Polich JM, Armor DJ, Braiker HB (1980b) Patterns of alcoholism over four years. J Stud Alcohol 41:397-416

Scheller R, Klein M (1982) Persönlichkeitspsychologische Determinanten des Therapieerfolgs bei Alkoholabhängigen. Z Differentielle Diagn Psychol 3:47-54

Ullrich-de Muynck R, Ullrich R (1977) Der Unsicherheitsfragebogen, Testmanual. Pfeiffer, München

Watzl H (1986) Die Vorhersage des Behandlungserfolgs bei alkoholkranken Frauen — eine empirische Untersuchung. Röttger, München

von Zerssen D (1976) Beschwerden-Liste, Manual. Beltz, Weinheim

20 Psychophysical Differentiation of Pain by Threshold Methods

F. Strian

Aims of Pain Measurement

Pain represents an unpleasant, distressing, and agonizing sensation. It cannot be described in terms of perception only, but refers to a complex experience with concomitant psychophysical components. Acute pain serves warning and protection functions, whereas chronic pain is also characterized by emotional reactions such as anxiety and depression, generalization, potentiation, and perpetuation. Thus, pain is always a complex phenomenon with at least three levels of reactions: the level of subjective and psychological experience, the level of behavioral responses, and the level of neurophysiological and biochemical findings. Because in clinical pain syndromes these levels are involved in different ways and with different interrelationships, it is important that pain measurement should refer to at least some components of these levels (Fig. 1; Birbaumer 1984; Handwerker 1984). For example, pain questionnaires refer solely to the subjective pain experience.

One entry to pain measurement including both peripheral sensory and central psychological pain components is the evaluation of pain thresholds. They connect subjective and neurophysiological pain mechanisms and enable peripheral and CNS factors of pain to be differentiated. The philosophy of this experimental pain measurement is to prove pain reactions at various levels of pain processing provoked by defined pain stimuli, e.g., by heat pain stimuli. In comparison to other pain stimuli (e.g., electrical stimuli) the examination of heat pain thresholds has the advantage that thermal pain refers to a physiological system. Because the peripheral sensory thresholds not only represent peripheral sensory function (e.g., A-delta and C-fiber function), but are controlled via spinal and descending CNS influences (Iggo 1982; Kenshalo 1984; Darian-Smith 1984; Dyck et al. 1984, 1987; Lynn and Baranowski 1987), heat pain thresholds represent a type of "interface" between peripheral and CNS influences.

Therefore by means of heat pain thresholds it should also be possible to discriminate between peripheral and CNS components of pain reactions. This type of measurement, however, needs a modification of the simple psychophysical threshold method. According to the various pain components, suitable modifications of threshold methods need to be developed.

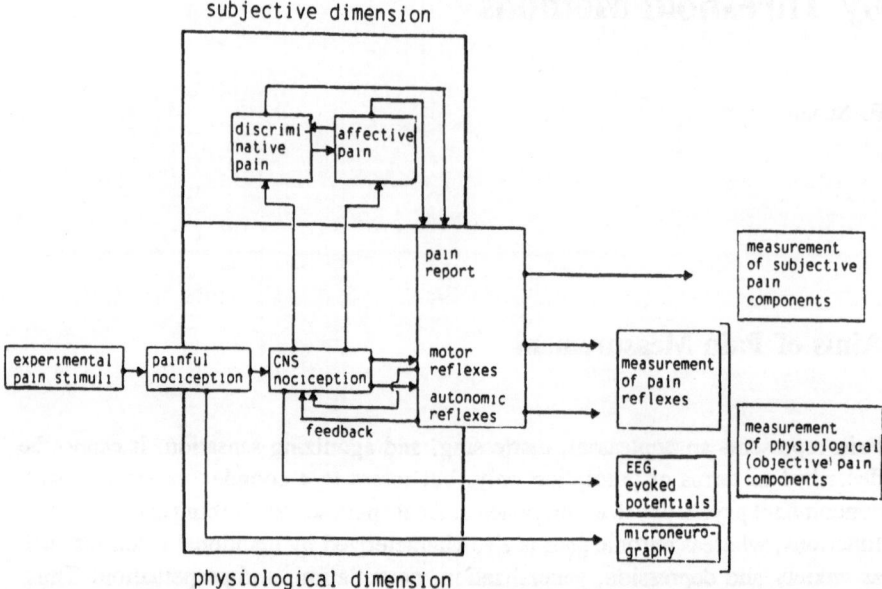

Fig.1. Somatic and psychological processes in pain and nociception (pain measurement techniques *on the right*). (from Handwerker 1984)

Measuring Methods for Heat Pain Threshold

Heat pain thresholds can be determined by radiation or contact heating. Each method has its advantages and shortcomings, e.g., radiation heat warms up the skin more intensively, whereas contact heating also includes tactile stimulation. Therefore, in contact heating it is necessary to keep the thermode at a constant pressure.

The contact heating Peltier elements, which are integrated in a thermode (Marstock thermode, according to Fruhstorfer et al. 1974, 1976), are the most widely used. These elements produce cold or warmth in relation to the direction of the applied current. The intensity of the cold or heat stimuli can be varied by modification of the intensity of the current. We have developed various thermodes suited for applications on different locations of the body surface (e.g., hands, feet, face) or for special pain measurement methods. Stimulus criteria as well as pain measurement programs are computer controlled (Fig.2). Patients have to press a lever if they perceive cold, warmth, or heat pain. For pain measurement the following measures were used, each referring to a particular aspect of pain.

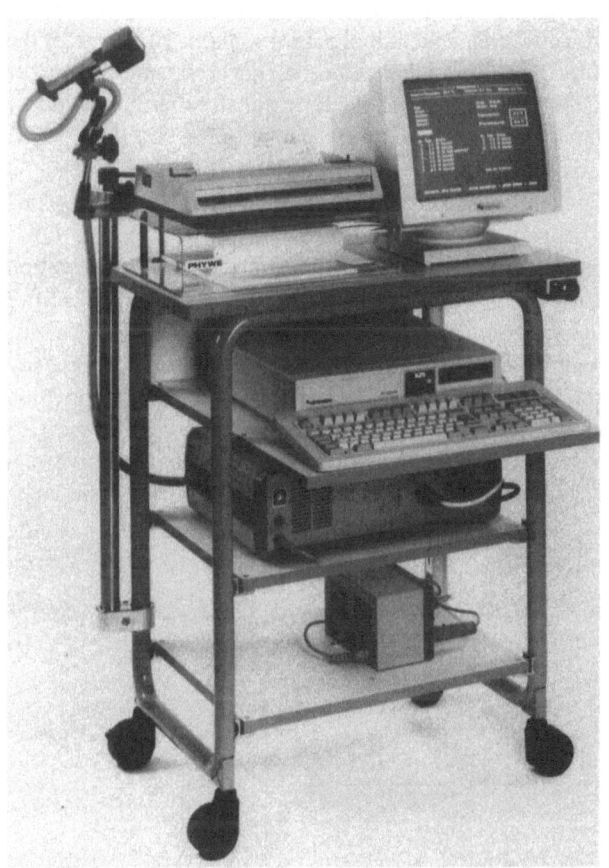

Fig.2. PATH Tester
MPI 100. (Photo
courtesy of Phywe AG,
Göttingen)

Measurement of Simple Pain Threshold ("Method of Limits")

The most elementary procedure of measuring heat pain threshold is to determine the borderline of heat pain sensation. The patient has to press a lever as soon as the heat sensation changes into a heat pain sensation. The method therefore examines the pain experience within the range of minimal pain and does not expose the patient to severe stress or pain. Some variables have to be controlled, however, e.g., thermode size, skin and room temperature, stimulus type (Ebaugh and Thauer 1950; Gray et al. 1982; Petrovaara and Kojo 1985; Kojo and Petrovaara 1987).

Sensitization Procedure

A specific phenomenon which characterizes chronic pain syndromes is pain sensitization, i.e., pain becomes more and more painful with time. It is well known from psychophysiological studies that long-lasting "tonic" heat pain stimuli are perceived as much more painful than the initial pain sensation. However, if the initial perception is not painful, the opposite phenomenon occurs, namely a weaker sensation, i.e., adaptation. Thus the pain threshold discriminates thermoception by adaptation and nociception by sensitization (Perl et al. 1976; LaMotte 1979; Kenshalo et al. 1979; Campbell and Meyer 1983; LaMotte et al. 1984).

This polar phenomenon can be used to differentiate "pain" and "non pain" perception, but also to prove pain sensitization itself.

Sensitization in clinical pain syndromes can be demonstrated by the sensitization method as follows (Severin et al. 1985; Lehmann and Strian 1986): 30 s after application of a tonic heat stimulus the patient is asked to reduce the stimulus intensity if the stimulus is painful (sensitization) and increase the stimulus intensity if it is not painful (adaptation). The difference (delta T) between initial perception and up- and downregulation is a criterion of the intensity of sensitization or adaptation (Fig.3). Pilot studies using the sensitization method have shown differences between analgesic and placebo conditions in clinical pain syndromes (see "Application in Clinical Pain Syndromes" below).

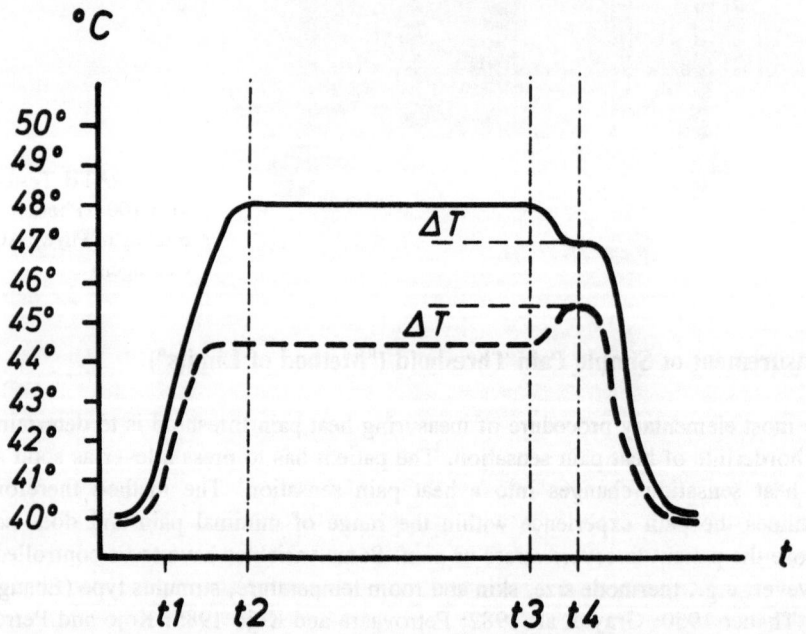

Fig. 3. Pain sensitization: increase in sensitivity to pain under painful stimulation ("downward adjustment": *upper curve*); decrease in sensitivity to pain under nonpainful stimulation ("upward adjustment": *lower curve*). (From Severin et al. 1985)

Signal Detection Procedure

The signal detection (SD) theory has been regarded as a very suitable model for differentiation of discriminative and evaluative pain factors, i.e., discrimination of sensory and emotional pain in the broadest sense. In recent years, however, there have been various objections against SD in pain measurement — most are true for pain as well as for other sensory modalities (Rollman 1977; Gracely 1980; Chapman et al. 1985). A strong argument has been that the reference point in regard to the series of stimuli is not determined physically (as in auditory or visual SD), but represents a solely subjective estimation. To eliminate this objection, we adjusted the pain threshold (the reference point) prior to SD using the sensitization method (Lautenbacher et al 1989a). The corrected sensitization threshold was used as the reference point for SD. This adjustment eliminates some of the problems in pain SD, resulting from lack of physical determination. Studies in normal subjects support this strategy (Lautenbacher et al. 1989a).

Tracking Procedures

A pain measurement which may give information about longterm adaptation or long term sensitization mechanisms is the tracking procedure. In this procedure the patient him- or herself adjusts the pain threshold (Lautenbacher et al. 1989b). Similar to the modified SD-method, the patient first adjusts the pain threshold (reference point) by the sensitization method and thereafter learns to discriminate between a just noticeable painful and a just noticeable nonpainful heat stimulus. During the subsequent tracking procedure every "hit" (i.e., adequate discrimination between painful and nonpainful stimulus) will be reinforced by an approximation of the next stimulus to the pain threshold and every "false alarm" (i.e., wrong discrimination) will be punished by more distancy of the next stimulus being further from the pain threshold. Thus, the patient exhibits a more cautious or more "heroic" strategy in response to pain stimuli. These behavioral tendencies may also be interpreted as an indicator of pain behavior and pain expression.

Stevens' Function (Relation of Stimulus Intensity and Probability of Pain Perception)

The above-mentioned procedures are time-consuming and expensive. Various aspects of pain experience and pain behavior can only be appreciated using various procedures. One of the most long-standing procedures in sensory physiology is "Stevens' function," i.e., the correlation between intensity of stimulus and probability of subjective pain sensation. The advantage of this method is that almost all the criteria relating to pain measurement can be evaluated in only one examination procedure. It was necessary to modify the original method as follows by reducing the number of stimuli to obtain a practicable procedure (Fig.4).

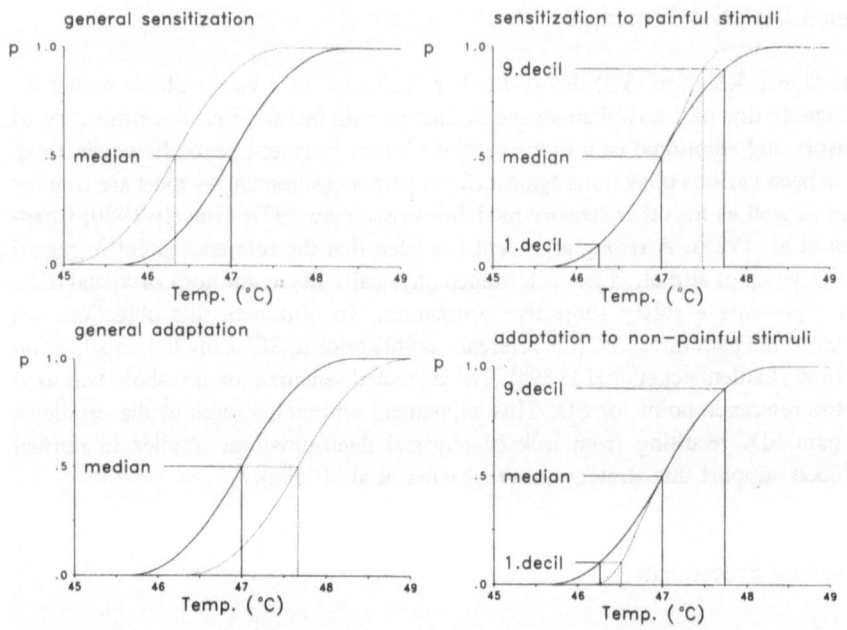

Fig. 4. Pain measurement according to the Stevens procedure. p, subjective intensity of pain

Using an adaptive procedure the poicilitic function is estimated, from which everything else can be computed. The procedure is as follows: firstly, the heat stimuli are adjusted to increase roughly in steps of 0.5°C. The upper and lower deciles are taken as cutoff points. Then only stimuli within the remaining range are applied. The temperature intervals of the second series of stimuli are 0.1°C. These are applied repeatedly to obtain a reliable estimation of the poicilitic function. Both the steepness and the midpoint of this function can be used as indices of discrimination for bias, adaptation, and sensitization.

Autonomic Pain Responses - A Nonverbal Indicator of Pain?

The subjective estimation also plays an important role in the measurement of pain thresholds. A possible method of objective measurement of pain sensations is recording the autonomic components of pain response, e.g., heart rate response. We also recorded various autonomic functions including heart rate (Möltner et al. 1990). Results show that autonomic pain responses can be discriminated into peripheral sensory and CNS-components: We found a strong correlation between the initial heart rate response, which had a weak phasic reaction, and stimulus intensity, and between the late part of the heart rate response, which showed a tonic heart rate elevation, and the subjective estimation of pain intensity. Thus the autonomic pain response seems to represent an initial phasic and nocifensive component and a late tonic and cognitive component, which we can suppose to represent spinal versus cortical and/or limbic processing of pain.

Applications in Clinical Pain Syndromes

With the above-described pain measurement methods, using heat stimuli to induce experimental pain it is possible to examine various aspects of pain perception and pain responses, e.g., the discrimination of peripheral (neuropathic) and CNS ("psychological") factors in clinical pain syndromes, adaptive or sensitizing mechanisms, long-term course of pain development, and finally analgesic mechanisms. The following studies give some examples of clinical applications.

Time Course of Pain Perception: Circadian Variations

Pain measurement within the lower range of pain sensitivity (i.e., pain thresholds) does not burden subjects with severe stress or pain. Therefore it is possible to study pain reactions within short intervals, e.g., to examine the circadian course of pain thresholds. This was performed in a study in 11 healthy subjects for cold, warmth, and heat pain stimuli at intervals of 3 h and during a period of 2 days (Strian et al. 1989). It could be shown that pain thresholds exhibit a slight circadian varation with the lowest pain thresholds (i.e., highest pain sensitivity)

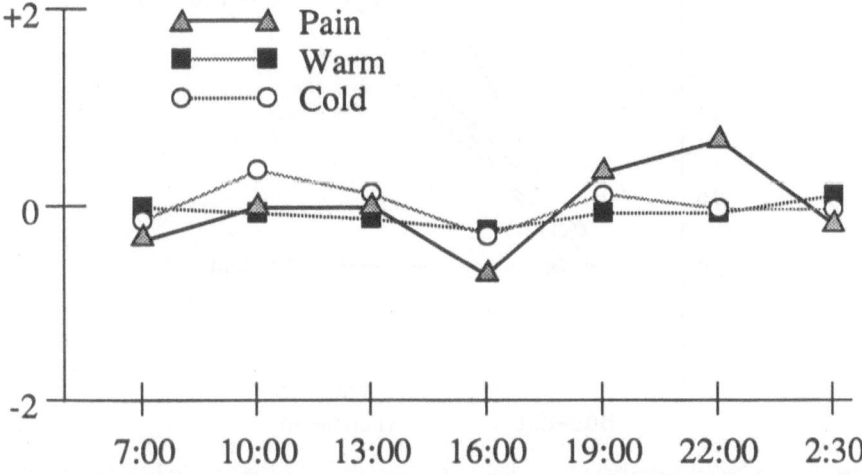

Fig. 5. Circadian changes in thermal and nociceptive thresholds (From Strian et al. 1989)

during the late afternoon. This agrees well with the clinical observation that patients have the highest demand for analgesic drugs in the late afternoon and moreover with studies about circadian variations of electrical pain sensitivity. No circadian rhythms of cold and warm thresholds could be found, indicating that the peak of pain sensitivity is not due to peripheral sensory mechanisms but is more likely due to psychological influences (Fig.5). A study to clarify these central or peripheral factors has not been performed so far.

Pain Sensitization

The evaluation of sensitization mechanisms in patients with chronic pain would also be a helpful marker for diagnostic and therapeutic decisions. Therefore a study was performed to evaluate the sensitization mechanisms in experimental pain conditions and their interference with an analgesic intervention, namely transcutaneous electrical stimulation (TENS; Lehmann and Strian 1986). Partcipants in the study were 114 healthy volunteers. Subjects received heat pain stimuli to the

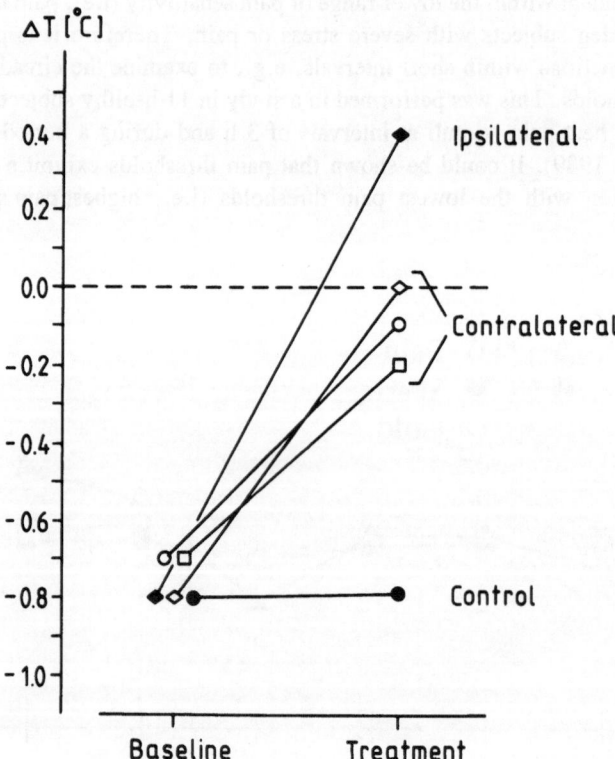

Fig. 6. Ipsilateral sensitization and improved contralateral adaptation to heat pain during TENS (From Lehmann and Strian 1986)

thenar of both hands with a Marstock thermode as described above. In the "ipsilateral" group (n=25) TENS was applied to the arm stimulated with the heat pain stimulus. In the "contralateral" group (n=48) TENS was delivered with three different intensities to the same trigger points on the arm not stimulated with the conditioned heat pain stimulus. The control group performed without applications of TENS electrodes. It could be shown that in the ipsilateral group the pain-relieving effect of TENS was visible in an inversion from sensitization to adaptation. This could also be shown for three intensities of TENS. In the contralateral group a significant analgesic effect was also found with a smaller grade of sensitization (Fig.6) that did not change from sensitization to adaptation. Thus the study demonstrates that the pain-relieving effects of TENS also involve spinal mechanisms.

Another clinical pain study was performed in patients with pain sensitization of the lumber disk syndrome and radiculopathy (Strian 1990). In these patients there is often a discrepancy between only mild or even absent clinical and radiological findings on the one hand and severe complaints of pain on the other hand. Neuro-physiological examinations often do not contribute very much to the elucidation of this problem. Therefore 20 patients with chronic low back pain were bilaterally examined by cold, warmth, and pain thresholds at the level of the discopathia and at neighboring levels. In patients with chronic low back pain the pain thresholds were lowered at the neighboring levels of the discopathia. At the level of disco-

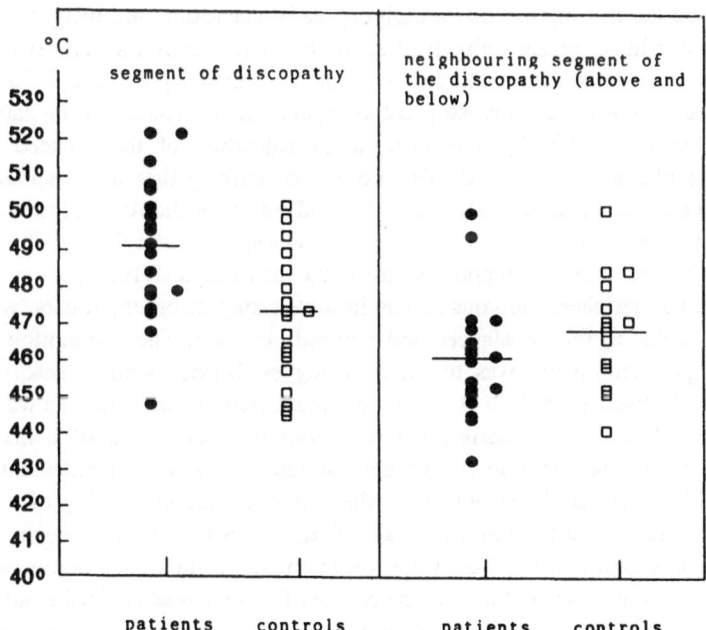

Fig. 7. Pain threshold to heat pain stimuli applied to segment diskopathy and neighboring segments (From Strian 1990)

pathia itself heightened cold, warmth, and pain thresholds were found. Thus the local findings seem to indicate a peripheral damage of A-delta- and C-fibers. The findings at the neighboring levels seem to indicate a pain sensitization at the spinal level (Fig.7). A similar finding was reported in experimentally induced gonarthritis. To summarize, these findings confirm that the described methods of pain measurement are helpful in the elucidation of the neurophysiological mechanisms of pain sensitization in both somatic and psychosomatic pain syndromes.

Pain Sensitivity in Psychiatric Patients

In a series of studies we observed a reduced sensitivity for heat pain in both anorexia and bulimia nervosa (Lautenbacher et al. 1991a; Fig.8). Most of the patients had had their eating disorder for a prolonged period and had been newly admitted for an inpatient behavioral treatment program. They showed the typical endocrine, metabolic, and physical signs of restrictive eating, but there were no major medical findings. The result in the anorectic patients of a negative correlation between pain threshold and peripheral skin temperature suggests an association of thermoregulatory and pain sensitivity disturbances. The positive correlation between body weight and pain threshold in the patients with bulimia nervosa made the assumption that a high degree of starvation and weight loss is a necessary condition appear unlikely. Reports of alterations in the activity of the endogenous opioids in these patients — found both in the plasma and CSF — prompted us to conduct a naloxone-placebo experiment with some of the patients (Lautenbacher et al. 1991b). However, a normalization of the reduced pain sensitivity could not be achieved. Therefore it is unlikely that we observed an acute, opioid mediated stress analgesia of the kind Abraham and Joseph (1987) had found in one patient with bulimia nervosa as a consequence of episodes of vomiting. We derived another hypothesis from the neurological findings on dysfunctions of the peripheral nervous system in some eating disorder patients, which seemed to be due to the unbalanced and reduced nutrition. The assumption of a subclinical polyneuropathy was tested by using established somatosensory indicators of this disease (Pauls et al. 1991), but the deficit pattern observed was not pathognostic. The findings correspond well with the assumption of a marked disturbance in the pain system and of mild deficits of perceptual processing in general, which had also been observed when studying the processing of visual stimuli in anorexia and bulimia nervosa. Relating to a few measurements after clinical improvement it seems that, whatever the pain system affects in our eating disorder patients, it is reversible over the course of several weeks. Further studies will be conducted to investigate the relationship of the pain sensitivity disturbance of eating disorder patients to that of depressive patients and to additional neuroendocrine dysfunctions in anorexia and bulimia nervosa.

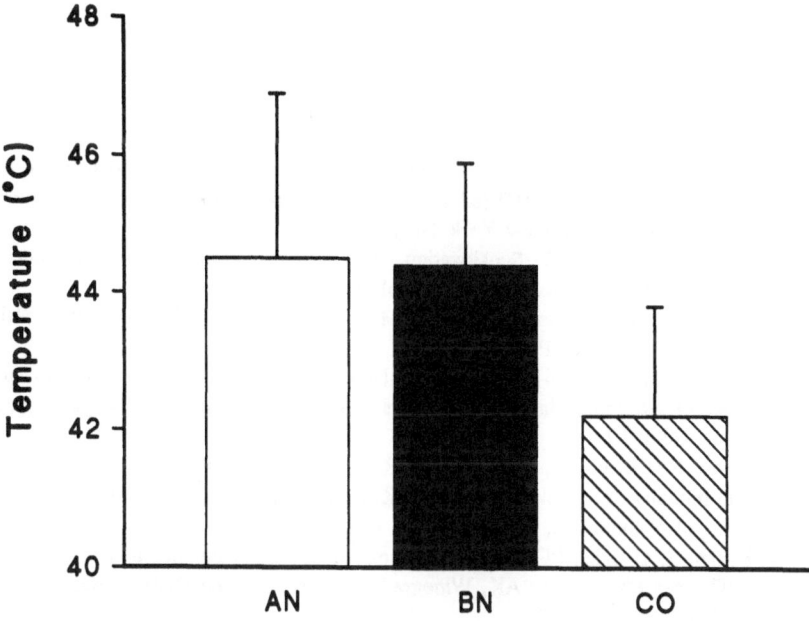

Fig. 8. Pain thresholds of 19 patients with anorexia nervosa (AN), 20 patients with bulimia nervosa (BN) and 21 healthy control subjects (CO)

Outlook

The measurement of pain thresholds — as demonstrated by means of the measurement of heat pain perception and their modifications of type of stimulation — seems to be a helpful approach to clinical pain problems. One line of interest is peripheral influences as shown by painful sensations in neuropathies, radiculopathies, entrapment syndromes, etc., and the related spinal pain mechanisms. Another line of interest is evaluations of CNS factors including evaluative, emotional, and cognitive components as evidenced by long-term pain, pain symptoms in psychosomatic diseases, and severe pain syndromes in affective disorders (e.g., major depression or eating disorders). There is still much work to be done in validating the methods described above as well in studying the different pain mechanisms in somatic and psychological disorders with pain syndromes.

References

Abraham HD, Joseph AB (1987) Bulimic vomiting alters pain tolerance and mood. Int J Psychiatry Med 16:311-316

Birbaumer N (1984) Psychologische Analyse und Behandlung von Schmerzzuständen. In: Zimmermann M, Handwerker HO (eds) Schmerz — Konzepte und ärztliches Handeln. Springer, Berlin Heidelberg New York Tokyo, p 124

Campell JN, Meyer RA (1983) Sensitization of unmyelinated nociceptive afferents in monkey varies with skin type. J Neurophysiol 49:98-110

Chapman CR, Casey KL, Dubner R, Foley KM, Gracely RH, Reading AE (1985) Pain measurement: an overview. Pain 22:1-31

Darian-Smith I (1984) Thermal sensibility. In: Brookhart JM, Mountcastle VB, Darian-Smith I, Geiger SR (eds) Handbook of physiology, vol III. American Physiological Society, Bethesda p 87

Dyck PJ, Karnes J, O'Brien PC, Zimmermann IR (1984) Detection thresholds of cutaneous sensation in humans. In: Dyck PJ, Thomas PK, Lambert EH, Bunge R (eds) Peripheral neuropathy, vol 1. Saunders, Philadelphia, p 1103

Dyck PJ, Karnes J, O'Brien PC (1987) Detection thresholds of cutaneous sensation. In: Dyck PJ, Thomas PK, Asbury AK, Winegrad AI, Porte D (eds) Diabetic neuropathy. Saunders, Philadelphia, p 107

Ebaugh F, Thauer R (1950) Influence of various environmental temperatures on the cold and warmth thresholds. J Appl Physiol 3:173-182

Fruhstorfer H, Zenz M, Nolte H, Hensel H (1974) Dissociated loss of cold and warm sensibility during regional anaesthesia. Pflügers Arch 349:73-82

Fruhstorfer H, Goldberg JM, Lindblom U, Schmidt WG (1976) Temperature sensitivity and pain thresholds in patients with peripheral neuropathy. In: Zotterman Y (ed) Sensory functions of the skin in primates. Pergamon, Oxford, p 507

Gracely RH (1980) Pain measurement in man. In: Ng LKY, Bonica JJ (eds) Pain, discomfort and humanitarian care. Elsevier, New York, p 111

Gray L, Stevens JC, Marks LE (1982) Thermal stimulus thresholds: sources of varibility. Physiol Behav 29:335-360

Handwerker HO (1984) Experimentelle Schmerzanalyse beim Menschen. In: Zimmermann M, Handwerker HO (eds) Schmerz — Konzepte und ärztliches Handeln. Springer, Berlin Heidelberg New York Tokyo, p 87

Iggo A (1982) Cutaneous sensory mechanisms. In: Barlow HB, Mollon JD (eds) The senses. Cambridge University Press, Cambridge, p 369

Kenshalo DR, Leonard RB, Chung JM, Willis WD (1979) Responses of primate spinothalamic neurons to graded and to repeated noxious heat stimuli. J Neurophysiol 42:1370-1389

Kenshalo DR (1984) Cutaneous temperature sensitivity. In: Dawson WW, Enoch JM (eds) Foundations of sensory science. Springer, Berlin Heidelberg New York Tokyo, p 419

Kojo I, Pertovaara A (1987) The effects of stimulus area and adaptation temperature on warm and heat pain thresholds in man. Int J Neurosci 32:875-880

LaMotte RH (1979) Intensive and temporal determinants of thermal pain. In: Kenshalo DR (ed) Sensory functions of the skin of humans. Plenum, New York, pp 327-361

LaMotte RH, Torebjörk HE, Robinson CJ, Thalhammer JG (1984) Time-intensity profiles of cutaneous pain in normal and hyperalgesic skin: a comparison with c-fiber nociceptor activities in monkey and human. J Neurophysiol 51:1434-1451

Lautenbacher S, Möltner A, Lehmann WP, Galfe G, Hölzl R, Strian F (1989a) SDT analysis of experimental thermal pain, with "signal" and "no-signal" being determined psychophysically. Percept Mot Skills 68:1019-1030

Lautenbacher S, Galfe G, Hölzl R, Strian F (1989b) Threshold tracking for assessment of long-term adaptation. Percept Mot Skills 69:579-589

Lautenbacher S, Pauls AM, Strian F, Pirke KM, Krieg JC (1990a) Pain sensitivity in anorexia nervosa and bulimia nervosa. Biol Psychiatry, in press

Lautenbacher S, Pauls AM, Strian F, Pirke KM, Krieg JC (1990b) Pain perception in patients with eating disorders. Psychosom Med 52:673-682

Lehmann WP, Strian F (1986) Comparative effects of ipsilateral and contralateral TENS on subjective sensitization to tonic heat. Clin J Pain 1:211-216

Lynn B, Baranowski R (1987) A comparison of the relative numbers and properities of cutaneous nociceptive afferents in different mammalian species. In: Schmidt RF, Schaible HG, Vahle-Hinz C (eds) Fine afferent nerve fibres and pain. VCH Weinheim, p 87

Möltner A, Hölzl R, Strian F (1990) Heart rate changes as an autonomic component of the pain response. Pain (to be published)

Pauls AM, Lautenbacher S, Strian F, Pirke KM, Krieg JC (1990) Somatosensory indicators of polyneuropathy in patients with eating disorders. Eur Arch Psychiatry Clin Neurosci, (to be published)

Perl, ER, Kumazawa T, Lynn B, Kenins P (1976) Sensitization of high threshold receptors with unmyelinated (C) afferent fibers. In: Iggo A, Ilyinsky OB (eds) Somatosensory and visceral receptor mechanisms. Prog Brain Res, vol 43. Elsevier, Amsterdam, p 263

Pertovaara A, Kojo I (1985) Influence of the rate of temperature change on thermal thresholds in man. Exp Neurol 87:439-445 Rollman GB (1977) Signal detection theory measurement of pain: a review and critique. Pain 3:187-211

Severin F, Lehmann WP, Strian F (1985) Subjective sensitization to tonic heat as an indicator of thermal pain. Pain 21:369-378

Strian F, Lautenbacher S, Galfe G, Hölzl R (1989) Diurnal variations in pain perception and thermal sensitivity. Pain 36:125-131

Strian F (1990) Diagnostische und klinische Aspekte der Neuropathie der kleinen Nervenfasern. Fortschr Neurol Psychiatr 58:51-65

21 Problems with the Precise Treatment of Imprecise "Givens"

E. Hansert

What Are the Attributes of a Science?

What makes a science a science? Theories of science provide criteria that are either very abstract and difficult to apply or are as trivial as, say, "Science consists of what scientists write in journals that are accepted by scientists as being scientific journals" or "Acting as a scientist means not disregarding any of the rules of the scientific game" (Seiffert and Radnitzky 1989). If these definitions are accepted at face value, it follows that a "science" can be described by:

- its rules, i.e., the body of methods used
- the kind of propositions it yields

Certain things should be emphasized in this connection:

1. "Empirical" sciences, e.g., psychiatry or physics, are based on "observations"(or "measurements").
2. It is through the rules for observation and measurement that the results become a possible basis for scientific procedures.

But results of observation and measurement and conclusions drawn from them are of little value if the rules applied are not reported or are not stated clearly.

When conclusions are drawn from empirical findings the rigor of the argumentation can vary widely. If in the publications in a given field, e.g., psychiatry, the argumentation is characterized by expressions such as "indicates," "suggests", or "is evidence for" [for a recent example see Holsboer (1988)], one can conclude that the field deals essentially with statistical phenomena and therefore is dependent upon scientific rules of statistical reasoning. In such fields, therefore, it is equally important to state the rules by which one draws conclusions from the observations and measurements as it is to state the rules of observation and measurement themselves. These rules, too, are rules of the scientific game.

Precise Treatment of Givens

Two sciences are regarded as preeminent, mathematics and physics, the latter being the model for all of the other "natural sciences." Mathematics plays an especially important role in the sciences; Hilbert (1918), for example, once said:

"Ich glaube: alles, was Gegenstand wissenschaftlichen Denkens überhaupt sein kann, verfällt, sobald es zur Bildung einer Theorie reif ist, der axiomatischen Methode und damit mittelbar der Mathematik." I believe: If a topic is at all accessible to scientific thought, then, when thinking about this topic has matured to the stage of theory building, one will always fall back upon the axiomatic method and hence indirectly upon mathematics. And it is physics that is thought to have attained the highest possible degree of mathematization. It is therefore considered to be *the* exact natural science, and serves as a model for all other empirical sciences (Seiffert and Radnitzky 1989).

But what makes physics an "exact" science? Is this just a consequence of its using so many mathematical models, and almost nothing but mathematical models?

And is mathematics itself an "exact" science?

As an aid to understanding the topic under discussion I shall distinguish between "precise" and "exact" as follows (it may be that such a distinction will not find general agreement):

- The following expression for the circumference of a circle

$$C = 2 r \pi \qquad (1)$$

shall be called "exact."

- The following expression, defined for a physical field of force whose component parallel to the x-axis of a given coordinate system is constant over time,

$$\ddot{x} = c, \text{ where } c \text{ is constant,} \qquad (2)$$

shall also be called "exact."

- The following numerical expression for the number π,

$$\pi = 3.14, \qquad (3a)$$

shall be called "imprecise"; the numerical expression for the result of a radius measurement

$$r = 1.2 \pm 0.02 \text{ m}$$

shall be called a description of an "imprecise (and quantitative) given." This expression is short for

$$1.18 \text{ m} < r < 1.22 \text{ m.} \qquad (3b)$$

- The following numerical expression for the acceleration of a falling body near the ground

$$g = 10 \text{ m/s}^{-2} \qquad (3c)$$

is "imprecise." Under certain conditions such an expression corresponds to the specification of the value of c in (2).

Even if a mathematical expression is known to be exact, imprecise givens and imprecise values for parameters will lead to imprecise givens as results.

But the kind of imprecision of the givens deduced can itself be deduced from the underlying givens, parameter values, and exact formulae. For example, in the case of expressions 1 and 3b, the conclusion can be drawn that:

$$7.41 \text{ m} < C < 7.67 \text{ m}.$$

These inequalities are the logical consequence of Eq 1 and 3b and the properties of π. They are the result of a precise treatment of the "information" just referred to.

For the case of Eq 2 and 3c, a precise treatment is quite complicated and is therefore not outlined here.

I propose the term "precise treatment of givens" for any procedure by which conclusions are drawn from givens in a completely logical manner. With such procedures, mathematicians deduce exact formulae from exact formulae, and empirical scientists arrive at unambiguous conclusions from observations.

What Types of Imprecision Can Givens in Psychiatry Have?

According to the view formulated here, the exactitude of any proposition, for instance of a mathematical formula, lies in the fact that the proposition or formula is the only possible way (equivalent expressions not being regarded as different ways) to express what is intended to be expressed. And the impreciseness of any given of a quantitative nature (a quantitative given) lies in the fact that it is described by not one but a whole set (e.g., an interval) of numbers each of which is a possible representation of the given concerned.

In psychiatry, however, the usual observational results are not of a quantitative nature. Typical examples are the bodies of individual results obtained with questionnaires requiring "yes/no" responses or a response from a given sequence such as "never — sometimes — frequently — always" or from some other similarly ordered sequence. Any representation of such sequences by numbers is completely arbitrary, as has been well known in measurement theory from the start (see e.g., Suppes and Zinnes 1963). And experts on measurement theory have strongly emphasized the fact that the exactitude (in the sense formulated earlier) of any representation of such sequences by numbers lies in an exact representation of the order only, not in the character of the numbers chosen for representation.

But what are the typical procedures met with in the analysis of such data?

With the intention of creating a "natural science," psychologists and psychiatrists began assigning precise numbers to givens such as those just described (something not done even with physical measurements!) and basing their scientific argumentation on these numbers — it is my impression that some kind of inferiority complex must have been at work here. A possible explanation for this behavior may be found in a "paradigm" that seems to have played a role for the past several decades. The argument goes like this:

- "Measurement" is a characteristic of the "natural sciences."
- "Measurement" yields quantitative givens that can function as a basis for further research.

- Because there are quantitative givens, the natural sciences can apply mathematics.
- The use of mathematics makes the natural sciences more "exact" than other sciences.
- Because any natural science is more exact than other sciences [e.g. the humanities (*Geisteswissenschaften*)], it is a superior kind of science.

This paradigm can be found in the basic ideas of the measurement theories of the 1960s and 1970s: According to these theories, "to measure" means to assign numbers (but there are exceptions, see Hansert 1966; M.Hengst 1986: Merkmal und Messen, unpublished paper). It is strange that although measurement theorists have demonstrated in detail the relevance of relations between assigned numbers and the irrelevance of these numbers as measured values for the scales typically used in psychology and psychiatry, the fiction that ordinal scales, and even nominal scales, are precise quantitative scales has continued to be maintained by researchers in these fields.

When Galois introduced the concept of "groups," and especially when G. Cantor developed a theory of sets, it became clear that numbers and related concepts are no more than a special kind of mathematical object. So the idea that measurement lies in assigning numbers to observed givens may be as transitory as the view that mathematics consists in considering numbers and related concepts only. It is easy to see that a more general concept of measurement is inherent even in existing theories of measurement: As already pointed out, ordinal scales are to be represented, if at all, by any set of numbers fulfilling given conditions, and not by numbers chosen in a fixed way. For example, any single number attributed to a given ordinal scale is meaningless — only its relations to other assigned numbers are meaningful.

A typical given in psychiatry consists of someone's ratings of a person on nominal and/or ordinal scales. The question of interest here is: How can a "degree of imprecision" be defined for such givens? The important point is not the mathematical aspect of this problem. It is enough if we consider one common practice, namely, establishment of a "degree of certainty" for each rating by asking the raters to specify how sure they are about their ratings, e.g., 70%, 90%, or 100% sure.

In the end, except when a rater is 100% sure, it is implicit in such a response that another rating may in fact be more appropriate. Consequently, this situation is analogous to those with quantitative givens: In both situations it is *sets* of elements on a scale that are considered to be the results of the measurement or rating procedure. Although in the natural sciences (where measurement procedures in the strict sense are usually available) there is usually an awareness of the fact just described, in the "natural science of psychiatry" such an awareness seems not to have developed as yet. In the latter field, there appear to be only a few approaches so far to analyzing the imprecision of qualitative givens (e.g. scores obtained on questionnaires), and the available approaches have not been applied systematically. Hence psychiatry has become a "natural science" on the outside only.

Fictitious Givens — Useful Scientific Tools?

There are no fundamental problems in formulating exact probabilistic models for random variables whose possible values form a qualitative scale. The general mathematical structure of such models is known from the start — contrary to the case where the possible values form a quantitative scale of the continuous type. Probabilistic models for qualitative scales are defined by what might be termed "intrinsic probabilities." By taking these probabilities into consideration, a precise treatment of qualitative scales is possible, though for mathematical reasons not always easy, as will become evident later (see "Exact and Precise Values of Probabilities", below).

In contrast, quantitative scales allow the application of mathematical concepts that cannot even be formulated for qualitative scales (e.g., the concepts of "expected value" and "standard deviation"). Furthermore, in the case of quantitative scales of the continuous type the mathematical concept of a "normal distribution" may be applicable, which allows the precise treatment of many statistical problems. But by treating scales of a qualitative nature in this way, the "degree of fictitiousness," so to speak, becomes still greater: Random variables with scales that are sets of only a few numbers whose fictitiousness consists in their being regarded as both exact and precise are additionally treated as having a continuous scale and as being normally distributed. Now what can the scientific value of such fourfold complexes of fictions possibly be? Doubtless, such complexes allow one to produce large quantities of computer printouts, but it is no easy task to determine which of the results shown are fictional and which are not.

My personal view can be stated as follows (see also "Concluding Remarks"): On the one hand, it must be conceded that there are cases where a precise treatment of qualitative scales results in the same, or almost the same, propositions as when treatment is based on fictitious assumptions of the kind just described. On the other, the nearly ubiquitous use of fictitious probabilistic models has hindered the process of realizing that the purpose of scientific statistics and scientific data evaluation is not to produce great quantities of calculations but rather to develop logical and mathematical, i.e. good scientific argumentation. And I am sure that the stereotyped use of fictitious models leads quite often either to fictional results or to a loss of important information.

Precise Treatment of Scientific Problems

In any science the precise treatment of givens is only one part of the precise treatment of scientific problems, and it gains its importance from the more general task. Whatever the "rules of the game" of a science, they must always allow the deduction of scientific results from observations that are accepted as being scientific. As outlined earlier, statistical/biometric/mathematical methods of data evaluation are a key part of these rules of deduction. The question now posed is: Under what conditions can such methods yield scientifically acceptable results?

The formal acceptability of statistical results depends on the precise application of exact mathematical propositions. The material acceptability of deduced results, however, depends on the material acceptability of the premises.

Since a prerequisite for the application of mathematical concepts to scientific problems is that the problems have been "translated" into the language of mathematics, it follows that the acceptability of statistical results depends mainly on:

- As careful a translation as possible of a given scientific question into a mathematical-statistical question
- An analysis of the logical connections between the facts associated with the question and the facts characterizing the mathematical representation

For only an accurate model of the real world permits us to deduce propositions concerning the real world.

The goal of any precise treatment of scientific problems must therefore be to develop a method of data evaluation that is a logical consequence of the facts, the givens and the problem posed.

Exact and Precise Values of Probabilities

In a somewhat simplified form it can be said that the reason for applying mathematical concepts in statistical methodology is to enable probabilities to be calculated, especially probabilities for certain classes of phenomena, and probability distributions of statistical parameters. The most important probabilities concern the statistical significance of differences, for instance between different values for a particular parameter. The validity of a statement of significance depends on the mathematical demonstration that under certain precisely defined conditions the probability of a certain phenomenon or of a certain set of parameter values is below a given limit. Here it is not sufficient to apply a computational model or computer program and then attach one, two or three asterisks to the numerical result, as is currently in vogue. Rather, a careful analysis is required to demonstrate that the prerequisites for use of the proposed method of evaluation follow logically from the question addressed and the given situation. If this is not possible in all respects — and nature sees to it that we rarely have ideal situations — the mathematical problems that arise from the actual situation need to be investigated. In some cases, the probabilities of interest may be calculated on a hypothetical basis, i.e., on a basis that seems plausible but is not demonstrable at the moment.

An important consequence of all this should be realized: There are several very different types of calculated probabilities, as summarized in Fig.1.

What is meant by these different types of probabilities should generally be clear from the discussion so far; exceptions are the terms "asymptotically exact," "approximate", and "calculated approximately," which are illustrated in the

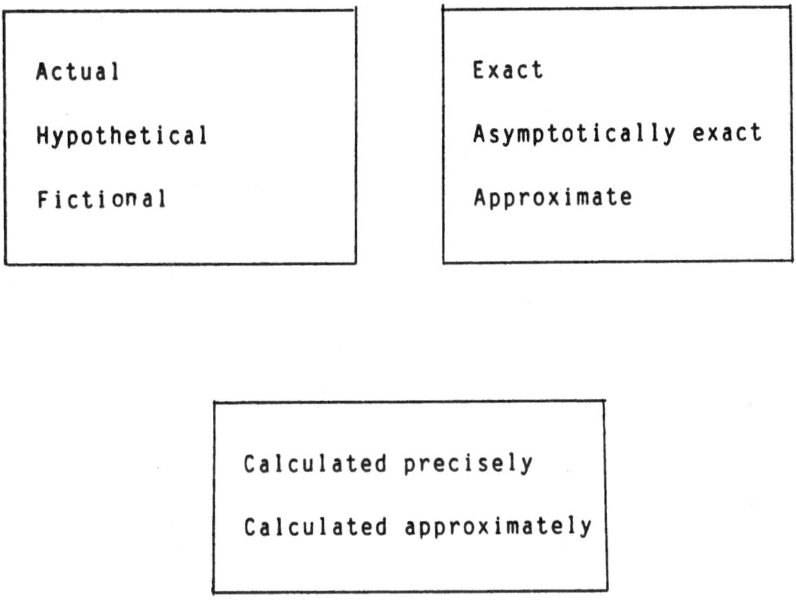

```
┌─────────────────────────────┐    ┌─────────────────────────────┐
│                             │    │                             │
│   Actual                    │    │   Exact                     │
│                             │    │                             │
│   Hypothetical              │    │   Asymptotically exact      │
│                             │    │                             │
│   Fictional                 │    │   Approximate               │
│                             │    │                             │
└─────────────────────────────┘    └─────────────────────────────┘


          ┌─────────────────────────────┐
          │                             │
          │   Calculated precisely      │
          │                             │
          │   Calculated approximately  │
          │                             │
          └─────────────────────────────┘
```

Fig. 1. Types of probability according to logical nature, accuracy, and properties of calculation

following example: Imagine a situation where the stochastic dependence of two variables has been described by an $r * s$ contingency table. As is well known, the classical criterion for analyzing the stochastic dependence of two such variables is the chi-square criterion X^2. Its exact distribution under the "null hypothesis of stochastic independence" must be the basis for calculating the critical region for a given level of significance. However, the exact distribution under the null hypothesis depends on the "intrinsic probabilities" of the contingency table deduced from the two marginal distributions. This kind of dependence decreases as the sample size increases. The asymptotic distribution of X^2 under certain very general assumptions is independent of the intrinsic probabilities of the contingency table, and is a chi-square distribution with $(r-1)(s-1)$ degrees of freedom. If this asymptotic distribution is used to calculate the critical region of the statistical test, the probabilities calculated on this basis are "asymptotically exact" (see Fig.2).

All this is textbook knowledge, and people often believe that common knowledge as expressed in textbooks is a sufficient basis for analyzing real situations. But the foregoing example has been chosen to demonstrate typical gaps in such knowledge: There exists no explicit and generally applicable mathematical criterion for answering the question of how to decide that the asymptotically exact probabilities are so little different from the true probabilities that they can be considered "approximate probabilities." And what is more, it is not uncommon that the facts

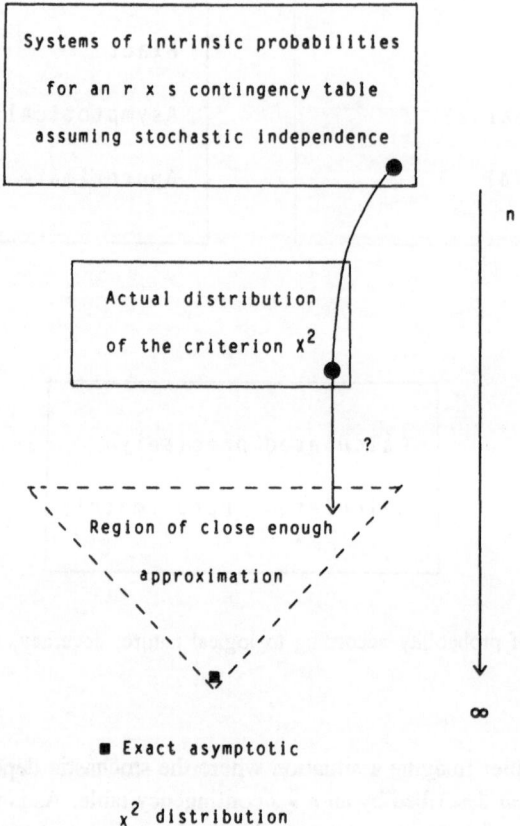

Fig. 2. Relationship between intrinsic distribution and asymptotic distribution for a situation where the chi-square criterion X^2 has been applied

give the impression that the probands or patients in the sample do not all have the same intrinsic probabilities associated with them (or in mathematical language, that the random variables considered are not identically distributed), and textbooks usually do not even discuss the possible existence of such situations. Figure 3 illustrates such a more complex situation, where the underlying intrinsic probabilities are, for example, a mixture of two or more sets of intrinsic probabilities, and thus lead to a broader class of exact probability distributions of the X^2 statistic as well as to a broader class of possible asymptotic distributions.

Finally, it should be mentioned that for many problems "nonparametric" or "distribution-free" methods offer a solution to the dilemma just described, i.e., that the exact probability distribution of a statistical criterion depends in a complex way on the unknown values of the distribution parameters. It is typical for nonparametric methods that they involve statistical criteria for whose probability distributions exact formulae are known (given a general null hypothesis and a sample of observations). However, a precise numerical evaluation of such formulae for samples that are not small usually presupposes the development of complex algorithms and the availability of adequate computer facilities and processing time. A new field of mathematical-statistical research, "computational statistics," has developed in recent years. It deals with such numerical problems and may lead to "approximately calculated" probabilities. The point made at the beginning of this paragraph should be repeated here: In most applications of probabilistic methods the essential task is to demonstrate by precise treatment of exact mathematical formulae that the probability (probabilities) sought is (are), with mathematical certainty, below a given limit. The application of parametric correlation theory to, for example, a contingency table, disregards all mathematical and logical facts, and any result calculated in this way must be considered "fictitious."

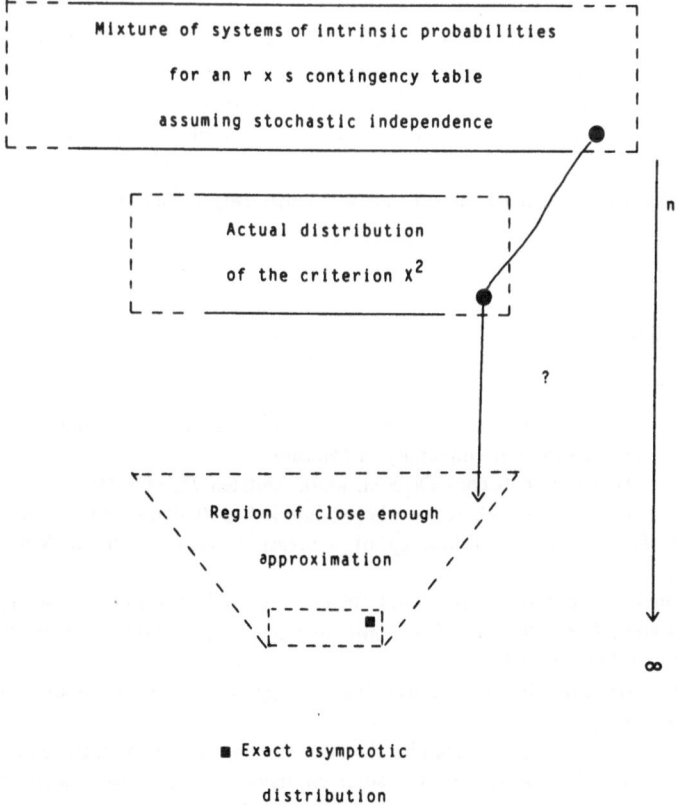

Fig. 3. Relationship between intrinsic distribution and asymptotic distribution for a situation where the chi-square criterion X^2 has been applied but the data cannot be assumed to be homogeneous

Concluding Remarks

1. One might get the impression that all of the foregoing arguments are nothing more than a collection of personal views. So I am glad to have found the following statements in the preface of a modern textbook (Krauth 1988) about which I first learned after I had presented an earlier version of this paper at the Ringberg Symposium:

- Even today most researchers in the behavioral and neurosciences use so-called parametric significance tests for evaluating their data.

- Examination of real data reveals that the assumption of a normal distribution is not justified in the majority of cases.

- Another assumption of parametric procedures that is often not taken into consideration is the assumption that the data are at least on an interval-scale level.

2. Since the Symposium, at least one of the issues addressed here has been given attention on an international level. I cite from the foreword of the *International Vocabulary of Basic and General Terms in Metrology* (1989): "Every measurement is tainted by imperfectly known errors, so that the significance which one can give to the measurement must take account of this uncertainty. We must therefore express with precision that self-same impreciseness."

References

Hansert E (1966) Begriff und Grundlegung einer phänomenologischen Wahrscheinlichkeitstheorie. Dissertation University of Münster

Hilbert D (1918) Axiomatisches Denken. Math Annalen 78: 405-415

Holsboer F (1988) Implications of altered limbic-hypothalamic-pituitary-adrenocortical (LHPA)-function for neurobiology of depression. Acta Psychiatr Scand Supp 77 (341):72-111

International Vocabulary of Basic and General Terms in Metrology, ISO/TAG4/WG1, August 1989. Available from ISO Central Secretariat, 1 Rue de Varembe, BP 56, 1211 Geneva 20, Switzerland

Krauth J (1988) Distribution-free statistics: an application-oriented approach. Elsevier, Amsterdam

Seiffert H , Radnitzky G (1989) Handlexikon zur Wissenschaftstheorie. Ehrenwirth, Munich

Suppes P, Zinnes IL (1963) Basic measurement theory. In: Luce RD, Bush RR, Galanter E (eds) Handbook of mathematical psychology. Wiley, New York

Subject index